CARBS, FAT, &
CALORIE COUNTER

SWEET
WATER
PRESS

Copyright ©2005 Sweetwater Press
Produced by Cliff Road Books

ISBN 1-58173-310-0

Printed in China

Source of Information: Nutritional content was taken from the U.S. Department of Agriculture, food labels, and information provided by certain national restaurants. All units are rounded to the nearest whole number. Because numbers on manufacturers' labels have also been rounded, figures in this book may vary slightly from the label.

Abbreviations:
carb = carbohydrate(s)
chol = cholesterol
fl = fluid
g = gram(s)
lb = pound(s)
mg = milligram(s)
oz = ounce(s)
prot = protein
sod = sodium
tbsp = tablespoon(s)
tsp = teaspoon(s)
"NA" indicates that the information was not available. Net carbs were derived by subtracting fiber grams from carbohydrate grams.

Feedback: Any corrections to or suggestions for entries in this book should be sent to fatcal@cliffroadbooks.com. Please note that due to the amount of correspondence received, we are unable to reply, but thank you for your input.

Order additional copies at www.booksamillion.com.

Table of Contents

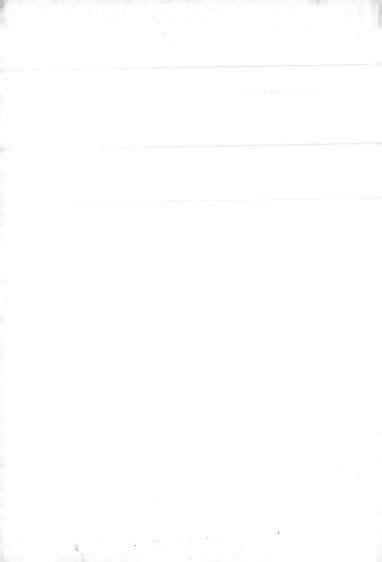

Description	Serving Size	Cal	Prot (g)	Fat (g)	Carbs (g)	Net Carb(g)	Fiber (g)	Sod (mg)	Chol (mg)
Brisket									
FLAT HALF									
Lean and fat, trimmed to 1/4" fat, all grades, braised	3 oz	309	21	21	0	0	0	48	81
Lean and fat, trimmed to 1/4" fat, all grades, raw	1 oz	82	5	6	0	0	0	18	20
Lean and fat, trimmed to 1/8" fat, all grades, braised	3 oz	263	23	15	0	0	0	50	81
Lean and fat, trimmed to 1/8" fat, all grades, raw	1 oz	67	5	4	0	0	0	19	19
Lean only, trimmed to 0" fat, all grades, braised	3 oz	183	26	7	0	0	0	53	81
Lean only, trimmed to 0" fat, all grades, raw	3 oz	162	27	4	0	0	0	54	81
Lean only, trimmed to 1/4" fat, all grades, braised	3 oz	189	27	7	0	0	0	54	81
Lean only, trimmed to 1/4" fat, all grades, raw	1 oz	42	6	1	0	0	0	21	17
POINT HALF									
Lean and fat, trimmed to 0" fat, all grades, braised	3 oz	304	20	21	0	0	0	58	78
Lean and fat, trimmed to 1/4" fat, all grades, braised	3 oz	343	19	25	0	0	0	55	78
Lean and fat, trimmed to 1/4" fat, all grades, raw	1 oz	94	5	7	0	0	0	18	22
Lean and fat, trimmed to 1/8" fat, all grades, braised	3 oz	297	21	20	0	0	0	59	78
Lean and fat, trimmed to 1/8" fat, all grades, raw	1 oz	75	5	5	0	0	0	20	20
Lean only, trimmed to 0" fat, all grades, braised	3 oz	207	24	10	0	0	0	65	77
Lean only, trimmed to 1/4" fat, all grades, braised	3 oz	222	24	12	0	0	0	65	77
Lean only, trimmed to 1/4" fat, all grades, raw	1 oz	46	6	2	0	0	0	24	18
WHOLE									
Lean and fat, trimmed to 0" fat, all grades, braised	3 oz	247	23	14	0	0	0	55	79
Lean and fat, trimmed to 1/4" fat, all grades, braised	3 oz	327	20	23	0	0	0	52	80
Lean and fat, trimmed to 1/4" fat, all grades, raw	1 oz	88	5	7	0	0	0	18	21

Description	Serving Size	Cal	Prot (g)	Fat (g)	Carbs (g)	Net Carb(g)	Fiber (g)	Sod (mg)	Chol (mg)
BRISKET (continued)									
Lean and fat, trimmed to 1/8" fat, all grades, braised	3 oz	281	22	18	0	0	0	54	79
Lean and fat, trimmed to 1/8" fat, all grades, raw	1 oz	71	5	5	0	0	0	20	19
Lean only, all grades, raw	1 oz	44	6	2	0	0	0	22	18
Lean only, trimmed to 0" fat, all grades, braised	3 oz	185	25	7	0	0	0	60	79
Lean only, trimmed to 1/4" fat, all grades, braised	3 oz	206	25	9	0	0	0	60	79

Chuck

ARM POT ROAST

Description	Serving Size	Cal	Prot (g)	Fat (g)	Carbs (g)	Net Carb(g)	Fiber (g)	Sod (mg)	Chol (mg)
Lean and fat, trimmed to 0" fat, all grades, braised	3 oz	238	25	12	0	0	0	53	85
Lean and fat, trimmed to 0" fat, choice, braised	3 oz	249	25	13	0	0	0	53	85
Lean and fat, trimmed to 0" fat, select, braised	3 oz	221	26	11	0	0	0	54	85
Lean and fat, trimmed to 1/2" fat, prime, braised	3 oz	332	22	24	0	0	0	49	84
Lean and fat, trimmed to 1/2" fat, prime, raw	1 oz	83	5	6	0	0	0	16	20
Lean and fat, trimmed to 1/4" fat, all grades, braised	3 oz	282	23	17	0	0	0	51	84
Lean and fat, trimmed to 1/4" fat, all grades, raw	1 oz	69	5	5	0	0	0	17	19
Lean and fat, trimmed to 1/4" fat, choice, braised	3 oz	296	23	19	0	0	0	50	84
Lean and fat, trimmed to 1/4" fat, choice, raw	1 oz	72	5	5	0	0	0	17	20
Lean and fat, trimmed to 1/4" fat, select, braised	3 oz	268	24	16	0	0	0	51	85
Lean and fat, trimmed to 1/4" fat, select, raw	1 oz	66	5	4	0	0	0	17	19
Lean and fat, trimmed to 1/8" fat, all grades, braised	3 oz	263	24	15	0	0	0	52	85
Lean and fat, trimmed to 1/8" fat, all grades, raw	1 oz	66	5	4	0	0	0	17	19
Lean and fat, trimmed to 1/8" fat, choice, braised	3 oz	275	24	16	0	0	0	52	85
Lean and fat, trimmed to 1/8" fat, choice, raw	1 oz	69	5	4	0	0	0	17	19

Description	Serving Size	Cal	Prot (g)	Fat (g)	Carbs (g)	Net Carb(g)	Fiber (g)	Sod (mg)	Chol (mg)
Lean and fat, trimmed to 1/8" fat, select, braised	3 oz	247	25	14	0	0	0	52	85
Lean and fat, trimmed to 1/8" fat, select, raw	1 oz	62	5	4	0	0	0	17	19
Lean only, trimmed to 0" fat, all grades, braised	3 oz	179	28	5	0	0	0	56	86
Lean only, trimmed to 0" fat, choice, braised	3 oz	186	28	6	0	0	0	56	86
Lean only, trimmed to 0" fat, select, braised	3 oz	168	28	4	0	0	0	56	86
Lean only, trimmed to 1/2" fat, prime, braised	3 oz	222	28	10	0	0	0	56	86
Lean only, trimmed to 1/2" fat, prime, raw	1 oz	44	6	2	0	0	0	19	17
Lean only, trimmed to 1/4" fat, all grades, braised	3 oz	184	28	6	0	0	0	56	86
Lean only, trimmed to 1/4" fat, all grades, raw	1 oz	37	6	1	0	0	0	19	17
Lean only, trimmed to 1/4" fat, choice braised	3 oz	191	28	6	0	0	0	56	86
Lean only, trimmed to 1/4" fat, choice, raw	1 oz	39	6	1	0	0	0	19	17
Lean only, trimmed to 1/4" fat, select, braised	3 oz	175	28	5	0	0	0	56	86
Lean only, trimmed to 1/4" fat, select, raw	1 oz	35	6	1	0	0	0	19	17
BLADE ROAST									
Lean and fat, trimmed to 0" fat, all grades, braised	3 oz	284	23	18	0	0	0	55	88
Lean and fat, trimmed to 0" fat, choice, braised	3 oz	296	23	19	0	0	0	55	88
Lean and fat, trimmed to 0" fat, select, braised	3 oz	266	23	16	0	0	0	56	88
Lean and fat, trimmed to 1/2" fat, prime, braised	3 oz	354	22	26	0	0	0	54	88
Lean and fat, trimmed to 1/2" fat, prime, raw	1 oz	93	5	7	0	0	0	18	21
Lean and fat, trimmed to 1/4" fat, all grades, braised	3 oz	293	23	19	0	0	0	54	88
Lean and fat, trimmed to 1/4" fat, all grades, raw	1 oz	72	5	5	0	0	0	19	20
Lean and fat, trimmed to 1/4" fat, choice, braised	3 oz	309	22	20	0	0	0	54	88

Description	Serving Size	Cal	Prot (g)	Fat (g)	Carbs (g)	Net Carb(g)	Fiber (g)	Sod (mg)	Chol (mg)
CHUCK (continued)									
Lean and fat, trimmed to 1/4" fat, choice, raw	1 oz	77	5	6	0	0	0	19	20
Lean and fat, trimmed to 1/4" fat, select, braised	3 oz	277	23	17	0	0	0	55	88
Lean and fat, trimmed to 1/4" fat, select, raw	1 oz	67	5	4	0	0	0	19	20
Lean and fat, trimmed to 1/8" fat, all grades, braised	3 oz	290	23	18	0	0	0	55	88
Lean and fat, trimmed to 1/8" fat, all grades, raw	1 oz	70	5	5	0	0	0	19	20
Lean and fat, trimmed to 1/8" fat, choice, braised	3 oz	305	22	20	0	0	0	54	88
Lean and fat, trimmed to 1/8" fat, choice, raw	1 oz	75	5	5	0	0	0	19	20
Lean and fat, trimmed to 1/8" fat, select, braised	3 oz	270	23	16	0	0	0	56	88
Lean and fat, trimmed to 1/8" fat, select, raw	1 oz	65	5	4	0	0	0	20	20
Lean only, trimmed to 0" fat, all grades, braised	3 oz	215	26	10	0	0	0	60	90
Lean only, trimmed to 0" fat, choice, braised	3 oz	225	26	11	0	0	0	60	90
Lean only, trimmed to 0" fat, select, braised	3 oz	202	26	8	0	0	0	60	90
Lean only, trimmed to 1/2" fat, prime, braised	3 oz	270	26	16	0	0	0	60	90
Lean only, trimmed to 1/2" fat, prime, raw	1 oz	58	5	3	0	0	0	22	18
Lean only, trimmed to 1/4" fat, all grades, braised	3 oz	213	26	9	0	0	0	60	90
Lean only, trimmed to 1/4" fat, all grades, raw	1 oz	42	5	2	0	0	0	22	18
Lean only, trimmed to 1/4" fat, choice, braised	3 oz	224	26	10	0	0	0	60	90
Lean only, trimmed to 1/4" fat, choice, raw	1 oz	45	5	2	0	0	0	22	18
Lean only, trimmed to 1/4" fat, select, braised	3 oz	201	26	8	0	0	0	60	90
Lean only, trimmed to 1/4" fat, select, raw	1 oz	39	5	2	0	0	0	22	18

Description	Serving Size	Cal	Prot (g)	Fat (g)	Carbs (g)	Net Carb(g)	Fiber (g)	Sod (mg)	Chol (mg)
Cured									
Breakfast strips, cooked	3 slices	153	11	11	0	0	0	766	40
Breakfast strips, raw or unheated	3 slices	276	9	25	0	0	0	649	56
Corned beef, brisket, cooked	3 oz	213	15	14	0	0	0	964	83
Corned beef, brisket, raw	1 oz	56	4	4	0	0	0	35	15
Corned beef, canned	1 oz	71	8	4	0	0	0	285	24
Corned beef, canned	1 slice	53	6	3	0	0	0	211	18
Dried	1 oz	47	8	1	0	0	0	984	12
Dried	5 slices	35	6	1	0	0	0	729	9
Dried	1 oz	50	8	1	2	2	0	408	12
Dried	5 slices	37	6	1	1	1	0	302	9
Luncheon meat, jellied	1 slice	31	5	1	0	0	0	375	10
Pastrami	1 slice	99	5	7	1	1	0	348	26
Sausage, smoked	1 oz	88	4	7	1	1	0	321	19
Sausage, smoked	1 sausage	134	6	11	1	1	0	486	29
Smoked, chopped beef	1 slice	38	6	1	1	1	0	357	13
Flank									
Lean and fat, trimmed to 0" fat, choice, braised	3 oz	224	23	12	0	0	0	60	61
Lean and fat, trimmed to 0" fat, choice, broiled	3 oz	192	22	9	0	0	0	69	58
Lean and fat, trimmed to 0" fat, choice, raw	1 oz	51	6	3	0	0	0	20	15
Lean only, trimmed to 0" fat, choice, braised	3 oz	201	24	10	0	0	0	61	60
Lean only, trimmed to 0" fat, choice, broiled	3 oz	176	23	8	0	0	0	71	57
Lean only, trimmed to 0" fat, choice, raw	1 oz	44	6	2	0	0	0	21	14
Ground									
Extra lean, (approx 17% fat), raw	1 oz	66	5	4	0	0	0	19	20
Extra lean, baked, medium	3 oz	213	21	12	0	0	0	42	70
Extra lean, baked, well done	3 oz	233	26	12	0	0	0	54	91
Extra lean, broiled, medium	3 oz	218	22	12	0	0	0	60	71
Extra lean, broiled, well done	3 oz	225	24	12	0	0	0	70	84
Extra lean, pan-fried, medium	3 oz	217	21	12	0	0	0	60	69
Extra lean, pan-fried, well done	3 oz	224	24	12	0	0	0	69	79
Lean, (approx 21% fat), raw	1 oz	75	5	5	0	0	0	20	21

Description	Serving Size	Cal	Prot (g)	Fat (g)	Carbs (g)	Net Carb(g)	Fiber (g)	Sod (mg)	Chol (mg)
GROUND (continued)									
Lean, baked, medium	3 oz	228	20	14	0	0	0	48	66
Lean, baked, well done	3 oz	248	25	14	0	0	0	60	84
Lean, broiled, medium	3 oz	231	21	14	0	0	0	65	74
Lean, broiled, well done	3 oz	238	24	13	0	0	0	76	86
Lean, pan-fried, medium	3 oz	234	21	14	0	0	0	65	71
Lean, pan-fried, well done	3 oz	235	23	13	0	0	0	74	81
Patties, frozen, (approximately 23% fat), raw	3 oz	240	15	17	0	0	0	58	67
Patties, frozen, broiled, medium	3 oz	240	21	14	0	0	0	65	80
Regular, (approx 27% fat), raw	1 oz	88	5	7	0	0	0	19	24
Regular, baked, medium	3 oz	244	20	15	0	0	0	51	74
Regular, baked, well done	3 oz	269	24	16	0	0	0	64	92
Regular, broiled, medium	3 oz	246	20	15	0	0	0	71	77
Regular, broiled, well done	3 oz	248	23	14	0	0	0	79	86
Regular, pan-fried, medium	3 oz	260	20	17	0	0	0	71	76
Regular, pan-fried, well done	3 oz	243	23	14	0	0	0	79	83
USDA Commodity, beef patties (100%), frozen, cooked	1 patty	159	15	10	1	1	0	42	55
USDA Commodity, beef patties w/VPP, frozen, cooked	1 patty	168	11	10	5	4	1	45	26

Ribs

Description	Serving Size	Cal	Prot (g)	Fat (g)	Carbs (g)	Net Carb(g)	Fiber (g)	Sod (mg)	Chol (mg)
Large end (ribs 6-9), lean and fat, trimmed to 0" fat, all grades, roasted	3 oz	300	20	21	0	0	0	55	72
Large end (ribs 6-9), lean and fat, trimmed to 0" fat, choice, roasted	3 oz	316	19	22	0	0	0	54	72
Large end (ribs 6-9), lean and fat, trimmed to 0" fat, select, roasted	3 oz	281	20	19	0	0	0	55	71
Large end (ribs 6-9), lean and fat, trimmed to 1/2" fat, prime, broiled	3 oz	361	17	29	0	0	0	51	74
Large end (ribs 6-9), lean and fat, trimmed to 1/2" fat, prime, raw	1 oz	109	4	9	0	0	0	15	21
Large end (ribs 6-9), lean and fat, trimmed to 1/2" fat, prime, roasted	3 oz	346	19	27	0	0	0	54	72
Large end (ribs 6-9), lean and fat, trimmed to 1/4" fat, all grades, broiled	3 oz	295	18	21	0	0	0	54	69
Large end (ribs 6-9), lean and fat, trimmed to 1/4" fat, all grades, raw	1 oz	92	5	7	0	0	0	16	20
Large end (ribs 6-9), lean and fat, trimmed to 1/4" fat, all grades, roasted	3 oz	310	19	22	0	0	0	54	72

Description	Serving Size	Cal	Prot (g)	Fat (g)	Carbs (g)	Net Carb(g)	Fiber (g)	Sod (mg)	Chol (mg)
Large end (ribs 6-9), lean and fat, trimmed to 1/4" fat, choice, broiled	3 oz	312	18	23	0	0	0	54	69
Large end (ribs 6-9), lean and fat, trimmed to 1/4" fat, choice, raw	1 oz	98	4	8	0	0	0	15	21
Large end (ribs 6-9), lean and fat, trimmed to 1/4" fat, choice, roasted	3 oz	326	19	24	0	0	0	54	72
Large end (ribs 6-9), lean and fat, trimmed to 1/4" fat, prime, broiled	3 oz	351	17	27	0	0	0	52	73
Large end (ribs 6-9), lean and fat, trimmed to 1/4" fat, prime, raw	1 oz	107	4	9	0	0	0	15	21
Large end (ribs 6-9), lean and fat, trimmed to 1/4" fat, prime, roasted	3 oz	342	19	26	0	0	0	54	72
Large end (ribs 6-9), lean and fat, trimmed to 1/4" fat, select, broiled	3 oz	275	18	19	0	0	0	54	68
Large end (ribs 6-9), lean and fat, trimmed to 1/4" fat, select, raw	1 oz	86	5	6	0	0	0	16	20
Large end (ribs 6-9), lean and fat, trimmed to 1/4" fat, select, roasted	3 oz	289	20	20	0	0	0	55	72
Large end (ribs 6-9), lean and fat, trimmed to 1/8" fat, all grades, broiled	3 oz	287	18	20	0	0	0	54	68
Large end (ribs 6-9), lean and fat, trimmed to 1/8" fat, all grades, raw	1 oz	90	5	7	0	0	0	16	20
Large end (ribs 6-9), lean and fat, trimmed to 1/8" fat, all grades, roasted	3 oz	302	20	21	0	0	0	54	72
Large end (ribs 6-9), lean and fat, trimmed to 1/8" fat, choice, broiled	3 oz	315	18	23	0	0	0	54	69
Large end (ribs 6-9), lean and fat, trimmed to 1/8" fat, choice, raw	1 oz	94	5	7	0	0	0	15	20
Large end (ribs 6-9), lean and fat, trimmed to 1/8" fat, choice, roasted	3 oz	321	19	23	0	0	0	54	72
Large end (ribs 6-9), lean and fat, trimmed to 1/8" fat, prime, broiled	3 oz	343	18	26	0	0	0	53	73
Large end (ribs 6-9), lean and fat, trimmed to 1/8" fat, prime, raw	1 oz	104	4	8	0	0	0	15	21
Large end (ribs 6-9), lean and fat, trimmed to 1/8" fat, prime, roasted	3 oz	334	19	25	0	0	0	54	72
Large end (ribs 6-9), lean and fat, trimmed to 1/8" fat, select, broiled	3 oz	275	18	19	0	0	0	54	68
Large end (ribs 6-9), lean and fat, trimmed to 1/8" fat, select, raw	1 oz	84	5	6	0	0	0	16	20
Large end (ribs 6-9), lean and fat, trimmed to 1/8" fat, select, roasted	3 oz	283	20	19	0	0	0	55	71
Large end (ribs 6-9), lean only, trimmed to 0" fat, all grades, roasted	3 oz	202	23	10	0	0	0	62	69

Description	Serving Size	Cal	Prot (g)	Fat (g)	Carbs (g)	Net Carb(g)	Fiber (g)	Sod (mg)	Chol (mg)
RIBS (continued)									
Large end (ribs 6-9), lean only, trimmed to 0" fat, choice, roasted	3 oz	215	23	11	0	0	0	62	69
Large end (ribs 6-9), lean only, trimmed to 0" fat, select, roasted	3 oz	187	23	8	0	0	0	62	69
Large end (ribs 6-9), lean only, trimmed to 1/2" fat, prime, broiled	3 oz	250	21	16	0	0	0	60	70
Large end (ribs 6-9), lean only, trimmed to 1/2" fat, prime, roasted	3 oz	241	23	14	0	0	0	62	69
Large end (ribs 6-9), lean only, trimmed to 1/4" fat, all grades, broiled	3 oz	190	21	9	0	0	0	61	65
Large end (ribs 6-9), lean only, trimmed to 1/4" fat, all grades, raw	1 oz	47	6	2	0	0	0	19	17
Large end (ribs 6-9), lean only, trimmed to 1/4" fat, all grades, roasted	3 oz	201	23	9	0	0	0	62	69
Large end (ribs 6-9), lean only, trimmed to 1/4" fat, choice, broiled	3 oz	204	21	11	0	0	0	61	65
Large end (ribs 6-9), lean only, trimmed to 1/4" fat, choice, raw	1 oz	50	6	2	0	0	0	19	17
Large end (ribs 6-9), lean only, trimmed to 1/4" fat, choice, roasted	3 oz	213	23	11	0	0	0	62	69
Large end (ribs 6-9), lean only, trimmed to 1/4" fat, prime, broiled	3 oz	250	21	16	0	0	0	60	70
Large end (ribs 6-9), lean only, trimmed to 1/4" fat, prime, raw	1 oz	60	6	4	0	0	0	19	17
Large end (ribs 6-9), lean only, trimmed to 1/4" fat, prime, roasted	3 oz	241	23	14	0	0	0	62	69
Large end (ribs 6-9), lean only, trimmed to 1/4" fat, select, broiled	3 oz	175	21	8	0	0	0	61	65
Large end (ribs 6-9), lean only, trimmed to 1/4" fat, select, raw	1 oz	43	6	2	0	0	0	19	17
Large end (ribs 6-9), lean only, trimmed to 1/4" fat, select, roasted	3 oz	187	23	8	0	0	0	62	69
Shortribs, lean and fat, choice, braised	3 oz	400	18	32	0	0	0	43	80
Shortribs, lean and fat, choice, raw	1 oz	110	4	9	0	0	0	14	22
Shortribs, lean only, choice, braised	3 oz	251	26	14	0	0	0	49	79
Shortribs, lean only, choice, raw	1 oz	49	5	3	0	0	0	18	17
Small end (ribs 10-12), lean and fat, trimmed to 0" fat, all grades, broiled	3 oz	252	21	16	0	0	0	54	71
Small end (ribs 10-12), lean and fat, trimmed to 0" fat, choice, broiled	3 oz	265	21	17	0	0	0	54	71
Small end (ribs 10-12), lean and fat, trimmed to 0" fat, choice, broiled	3 oz	261	21	16	0	0	0	54	71

Description	Serving Size	Cal	Prot (g)	Fat (g)	Carbs (g)	Net Carb(g)	Fiber (g)	Sod (mg)	Chol (mg)
Small end (ribs 10-12), lean and fat, trimmed to 0" fat, choice, raw	1 oz	78	5	5	0	0	0	16	19
Small end (ribs 10-12), lean and fat, trimmed to 0" fat, select, broiled	3 oz	242	21	15	0	0	0	54	71
Small end (ribs 10-12), lean and fat, trimmed to 1/2" fat, prime, broiled	3 oz	309	20	22	0	0	0	53	71
Small end (ribs 10-12), lean and fat, trimmed to 1/2" fat, prime, raw	1 oz	99	5	8	0	0	0	15	20
Small end (ribs 10-12), lean and fat, trimmed to 1/2" fat, prime, roasted	3 oz	357	19	28	0	0	0	54	72
Small end (ribs 10-12), lean and fat, trimmed to 1/4" fat, all grades, roasted	3 oz	295	19	21	0	0	0	54	71
Small end (ribs 10-12), lean and fat, trimmed to 1/4" fat, choice, roasted	3 oz	312	19	22	0	0	0	53	71
Small end (ribs 10-12), lean and fat, trimmed to 1/4" fat, prime, broiled	3 oz	307	20	22	0	0	0	53	71
Small end (ribs 10-12), lean and fat, trimmed to 1/4" fat, prime, raw	1 oz	97	5	8	0	0	0	15	20
Small end (ribs 10-12), lean and fat, trimmed to 1/4" fat, prime, roasted	3 oz	354	19	27	0	0	0	55	71
Small end (ribs 10-12), lean and fat, trimmed to 1/4" fat, select, roasted	3 oz	281	19	19	0	0	0	54	71
Small end (ribs 10-12), lean and fat, trimmed to 1/8" fat, all grades, broiled	3 oz	281	20	19	0	0	0	53	71
Small end (ribs 10-12), lean and fat, trimmed to 1/8" fat, all grades, raw	1 oz	82	5	6	0	0	0	15	20
Small end (ribs 10-12), lean and fat, trimmed to 1/8" fat, all grades, roasted	3 oz	290	19	20	0	0	0	54	71
Small end (ribs 10-12), lean and fat, trimmed to 1/8" fat, choice, broiled	3 oz	292	20	20	0	0	0	53	71
Small end (ribs 10-12), lean and fat, trimmed to 1/8" fat, choice, raw	1 oz	86	5	6	0	0	0	15	20
Small end (ribs 10-12), lean and fat, trimmed to 1/8" fat, choice, roasted	3 oz	305	19	22	0	0	0	54	71
Small end (ribs 10-12), lean and fat, trimmed to 1/8" fat, prime, broiled	3 oz	301	21	21	0	0	0	54	71
Small end (ribs 10-12), lean and fat, trimmed to 1/8" fat, prime, raw	1 oz	95	5	7	0	0	0	15	20
Small end (ribs 10-12), lean and fat, trimmed to 1/8" fat, prime, roasted	3 oz	349	19	26	0	0	0	55	71
Small end (ribs 10-12), lean and fat, trimmed to 1/8" fat, select, broiled	3 oz	268	20	17	0	0	0	54	71

Description	Serving Size	Cal	Prot (g)	Fat (g)	Carbs (g)	Net Carb(g)	Fiber (g)	Sod (mg)	Chol (mg)
RIBS (continued)									
Small end (ribs 10-12), lean and fat, trimmed to 1/8" fat, select, raw	1 oz	78	5	6	0	0	0	15	20
Small end (ribs 10-12), lean and fat, trimmed to 1/8" fat, select, roasted	3 oz	275	19	19	0	0	0	54	71
Small end (ribs 10-12), lean only, trimmed to 0" fat, all grades, broiled	3 oz	181	24	7	0	0	0	59	68
Small end (ribs 10-12), lean only, trimmed to 0" fat, choice, broiled	3 oz	191	24	9	0	0	0	59	68
Small end (ribs 10-12), lean only, trimmed to 0" fat, choice, broiled	3 oz	191	24	9	0	0	0	59	68
Small end (ribs 10-12), lean only, trimmed to 0" fat, choice, raw	1 oz	46	6	2	0	0	0	18	17
Small end (ribs 10-12), lean only, trimmed to 0" fat, select, broiled	3 oz	168	24	6	0	0	0	59	68
Small end (ribs 10-12), lean only, trimmed to 1/2" fat, prime, broiled	3 oz	221	24	12	0	0	0	59	68
Small end (ribs 10-12), lean only, trimmed to 1/2" fat, prime, roasted	3 oz	258	23	16	0	0	0	64	68
Small end (ribs 10-12), lean only, trimmed to 1/4" fat, all grades, raw	1 oz	43	6	2	0	0	0	18	17
Small end (ribs 10-12), lean only, trimmed to 1/4" fat, all grades, roasted	3 oz	185	23	8	0	0	0	60	67
Small end (ribs 10-12), lean only, trimmed to 1/4" fat, choice, broiled	3 oz	198	24	9	0	0	0	59	68
Small end (ribs 10-12), lean only, trimmed to 1/4" fat, choice, raw	1 oz	46	6	2	0	0	0	18	17
Small end (ribs 10-12), lean only, trimmed to 1/4" fat, choice, roasted	3 oz	197	23	10	0	0	0	60	67
Small end (ribs 10-12), lean only, trimmed to 1/4" fat, prime, broiled	3 oz	221	24	12	0	0	0	59	68
Small end (ribs 10-12), lean only, trimmed to 1/4" fat, prime, raw	1 oz	57	6	3	0	0	0	18	17
Small end (ribs 10-12), lean only, trimmed to 1/4" fat, prime, roasted	3 oz	258	23	16	0	0	0	64	68
Small end (ribs 10-12), lean only, trimmed to 1/4" fat, select, broiled	3 oz	176	24	7	0	0	0	59	68
Small end (ribs 10-12), lean only, trimmed to 1/4" fat, select, raw	1 oz	40	6	1	0	0	0	18	17
Small end (ribs 10-12), lean only, trimmed to 1/4" fat, select, roasted	3 oz	173	23	7	0	0	0	60	67
Small end (ribs 10-12), lean and fat, trimmed to 1/4" fat, all grades, broiled	3 oz	286	20	19	0	0	0	53	71

Description	Serving Size	Cal	Prot (g)	Fat (g)	Carbs (g)	Net Carb(g)	Fiber (g)	Sod (mg)	Chol (mg)
Small end (ribs 10-12), lean and fat, trimmed to 1/4" fat, all grades, raw	1 oz	84	5	6	0	0	0	15	20
Small end (ribs 10-12), lean and fat, trimmed to 1/4" fat, choice, broiled	3 oz	297	20	20	0	0	0	53	71
Small end (ribs 10-12), lean and fat, trimmed to 1/4" fat, choice, raw	1 oz	89	5	7	0	0	0	15	20
Small end (ribs 10-12), lean and fat, trimmed to 1/4" fat, select, broiled	3 oz	273	20	18	0	0	0	53	71
Small end (ribs 10-12), lean and fat, trimmed to 1/4" fat, select, raw	1 oz	81	5	6	0	0	0	15	20
Small end (ribs 10-12), lean only, trimmed to 1/4" fat, all grades, broiled	3 oz	188	24	8	0	0	0	59	68
Whole (ribs 6-12), lean and fat, trimmed to 1/2" fat, prime, broiled	3 oz	347	18	27	0	0	0	51	73
Whole (ribs 6-12), lean and fat, trimmed to 1/2" fat, prime, raw	1 oz	105	4	9	0	0	0	15	21
Whole (ribs 6-12), lean and fat, trimmed to 1/2" fat, prime, roasted	3 oz	361	18	28	0	0	0	54	73
Whole (ribs 6-12), lean and fat, trimmed to 1/4" fat, all grades, broiled	3 oz	291	19	20	0	0	0	54	70
Whole (ribs 6-12), lean and fat, trimmed to 1/4" fat, all grades, raw	1 oz	89	5	7	0	0	0	15	20
Whole (ribs 6-12), lean and fat, trimmed to 1/4" fat, all grades, roasted	3 oz	304	19	21	0	0	0	54	71
Whole (ribs 6-12), lean and fat, trimmed to 1/4" fat, choice, broiled	3 oz	306	19	22	0	0	0	53	70
Whole (ribs 6-12), lean and fat, trimmed to 1/4" fat, choice, raw	1 oz	94	5	7	0	0	0	15	20
Whole (ribs 6-12), lean and fat, trimmed to 1/4" fat, choice, roasted	3 oz	320	19	23	0	0	0	54	72
Whole (ribs 6-12), lean and fat, trimmed to 1/4" fat, prime, broiled	3 oz	333	18	25	0	0	0	53	72
Whole (ribs 6-12), lean and fat, trimmed to 1/4" fat, prime, raw	1 oz	103	5	8	0	0	0	15	21
Whole (ribs 6-12), lean and fat, trimmed to 1/4" fat, prime, roasted	3 oz	348	19	26	0	0	0	54	72
Whole (ribs 6-12), lean and fat, trimmed to 1/4" fat, select, broiled	3 oz	275	19	19	0	0	0	54	70
Whole (ribs 6-12), lean and fat, trimmed to 1/4" fat, select, raw	1 oz	84	5	6	0	0	0	16	20
Whole (ribs 6-12), lean and fat, trimmed to 1/4" fat, select, roasted	3 oz	286	19	20	0	0	0	54	71

Description	Serving Size	Cal	Prot (g)	Fat (g)	Carbs (g)	Net Carb(g)	Fiber (g)	Sod (mg)	Chol (mg)
Whole (ribs 6-12), lean and fat, trimmed to 1/8" fat, all grades, broiled	3 oz	286	19	20	0	0	0	54	70
Whole (ribs 6-12), lean and fat, trimmed to 1/8" fat, all grades, raw	1 oz	87	5	7	0	0	0	16	20
Whole (ribs 6-12), lean and fat, trimmed to 1/8" fat, all grades, roasted	3 oz	298	19	21	0	0	0	54	71
Whole (ribs 6-12), lean and fat, trimmed to 1/8" fat, choice, broiled	3 oz	299	19	21	0	0	0	54	70
Whole (ribs 6-12), lean and fat, trimmed to 1/8" fat, choice, raw	1 oz	91	5	7	0	0	0	15	20
Whole (ribs 6-12), lean and fat, trimmed to 1/8" fat, choice, roasted	3 oz	310	19	22	0	0	0	54	71
Whole (ribs 6-12), lean and fat, trimmed to 1/8" fat, prime, broiled	3 oz	328	19	24	0	0	0	53	72
Whole (ribs 6-12), lean and fat, trimmed to 1/8" fat, prime, raw	1 oz	101	5	8	0	0	0	15	20
Whole (ribs 6-12), lean and fat, trimmed to 1/8" fat, prime, roasted	3 oz	340	19	25	0	0	0	55	72
Whole (ribs 6-12), lean and fat, trimmed to 1/8" fat, select, broiled	3 oz	268	19	18	0	0	0	54	69
Whole (ribs 6-12), lean and fat, trimmed to 1/8" fat, select, raw	1 oz	82	5	6	0	0	0	16	20
Whole (ribs 6-12), lean and fat, trimmed to 1/8" fat, select, roasted	3 oz	281	20	19	0	0	0	55	71
Whole (ribs 6-12), lean only, trimmed to 1/2" fat, prime, broiled	3 oz	238	22	14	0	0	0	59	70
Whole (ribs 6-12), lean only, trimmed to 1/2" fat, prime, roasted	3 oz	248	23	15	0	0	0	63	69
Whole (ribs 6-12), lean only, trimmed to 1/4" fat, all grades, broiled	3 oz	190	22	9	0	0	0	60	65
Whole (ribs 6-12), lean only, trimmed to 1/4" fat, all grades, raw	1 oz	45	6	2	0	0	0	18	17
Whole (ribs 6-12), lean only, trimmed to 1/4" fat, all grades, roasted	3 oz	195	23	9	0	0	0	61	68
Whole (ribs 6-12), lean only, trimmed to 1/4" fat, choice, broiled	3 oz	201	22	10	0	0	0	60	65
Whole (ribs 6-12), lean only, trimmed to 1/4" fat, choice, raw	1 oz	48	6	2	0	0	0	18	17
Whole (ribs 6-12), lean only, trimmed to 1/4" fat, choice, roasted	3 oz	207	23	10	0	0	0	61	68
Whole (ribs 6-12), lean only, trimmed to 1/4" fat, prime, broiled	3 oz	238	22	14	0	0	0	60	69

Description	Serving Size	Cal	Prot (g)	Fat (g)	Carbs (g)	Net Carb(g)	Fiber (g)	Sod (mg)	Chol (mg)
Whole (ribs 6-12), lean only, trimmed to 1/4" fat, prime, raw	1 oz	58	6	3	0	0	0	18	17
Whole (ribs 6-12), lean only, trimmed to 1/4" fat, prime, roasted	3 oz	248	23	15	0	0	0	63	69
Whole (ribs 6-12), lean only, trimmed to 1/4" fat, select, broiled	3 oz	175	22	8	0	0	0	60	65
Whole (ribs 6-12), lean only, trimmed to 1/4" fat, select, raw	1 oz	42	6	2	0	0	0	18	17
Whole (ribs 6-12), lean only, trimmed to 1/4" fat, select, roasted	3 oz	181	23	8	0	0	0	61	68

Round

BOTTOM ROUND

Description	Serving Size	Cal	Prot (g)	Fat (g)	Carbs (g)	Net Carb(g)	Fiber (g)	Sod (mg)	Chol (mg)
Lean and fat, trimmed to 0" fat, all grades, braised	3 oz	181	26	6	0	0	0	43	82
Lean and fat, trimmed to 0" fat, all grades, roasted	3 oz	160	24	5	0	0	0	56	66
Lean and fat, trimmed to 0" fat, choice, braised	3 oz	193	26	7	0	0	0	43	82
Lean and fat, trimmed to 0" fat, choice, roasted	3 oz	173	24	6	0	0	0	55	66
Lean and fat, trimmed to 0" fat, select, braised	3 oz	171	26	5	0	0	0	43	82
Lean and fat, trimmed to 0" fat, select, roasted	3 oz	150	24	4	0	0	0	56	66
Lean and fat, trimmed to 1/2" fat, prime, braised	3 oz	252	25	14	0	0	0	43	82
Lean and fat, trimmed to 1/2" fat, prime, raw	1 oz	64	6	4	0	0	0	16	18
Lean and fat, trimmed to 1/4" fat, all grades, braised	3 oz	234	24	12	0	0	0	43	82
Lean and fat, trimmed to 1/4" fat, all grades, raw	1 oz	59	6	3	0	0	0	16	18
Lean and fat, trimmed to 1/4" fat, all grades, roasted	3 oz	211	23	11	0	0	0	54	68
Lean and fat, trimmed to 1/4" fat, choice, braised	3 oz	241	24	13	0	0	0	43	82
Lean and fat, trimmed to 1/4" fat, choice, raw	1 oz	62	6	4	0	0	0	16	18
Lean and fat, trimmed to 1/4" fat, choice, roasted	3 oz	221	22	12	0	0	0	54	68
Lean and fat, trimmed to 1/4" fat, select, braised	3 oz	220	25	11	0	0	0	43	82

Description	Serving Size	Cal	Prot (g)	Fat (g)	Carbs (g)	Net Carb(g)	Fiber (g)	Sod (mg)	Chol (mg)
ROUND (continued)									
Lean and fat, trimmed to 1/4" fat, select, raw	1 oz	55	6	3	0	0	0	16	18
Lean and fat, trimmed to 1/4" fat, select, roasted	3 oz	199	23	10	0	0	0	54	68
Lean and fat, trimmed to 1/8" fat, all grades, braised	3 oz	218	25	10	0	0	0	43	82
Lean and fat, trimmed to 1/8" fat, all grades, raw	1 oz	54	6	3	0	0	0	16	18
Lean and fat, trimmed to 1/8" fat, all grades, roasted	3 oz	195	23	9	0	0	0	54	67
Lean and fat, trimmed to 1/8" fat, choice, braised	3 oz	228	25	11	0	0	0	43	82
Lean and fat, trimmed to 1/8" fat, choice, raw	1 oz	57	6	3	0	0	0	16	18
Lean and fat, trimmed to 1/8" fat, choice, roasted	3 oz	205	23	10	0	0	0	54	67
Lean and fat, trimmed to 1/8" fat, select, braised	3 oz	208	25	9	0	0	0	43	82
Lean and fat, trimmed to 1/8" fat, select, raw	1 oz	51	6	3	0	0	0	16	18
Lean and fat, trimmed to 1/8" fat, select, roasted	3 oz	186	23	8	0	0	0	54	67
Lean only, trimmed to 0" fat, all grades, braised	3 oz	173	27	5	0	0	0	43	82
Lean only, trimmed to 0" fat, all grades, roasted	3 oz	156	24	5	0	0	0	56	66
Lean only, trimmed to 0" fat, choice, braised	3 oz	181	27	6	0	0	0	43	82
Lean only, trimmed to 0" fat, choice, roasted	3 oz	164	24	5	0	0	0	56	66
Lean only, trimmed to 0" fat, select, braised	3 oz	163	27	4	0	0	0	43	82
Lean only, trimmed to 0" fat, select, roasted	3 oz	145	24	4	0	0	0	56	66
Lean only, trimmed to 1/2" fat, prime, braised	3 oz	212	27	9	0	0	0	43	82
Lean only, trimmed to 1/2" fat, prime, raw	1 oz	45	6	2	0	0	0	17	17
Lean only, trimmed to 1/4" fat, all grades, braised	3 oz	178	27	6	0	0	0	43	82
Lean only, trimmed to 1/4" fat, all grades, raw	1 oz	41	6	1	0	0	0	17	17

Description	Serving Size	Cal	Prot (g)	Fat (g)	Carbs (g)	Net Carb(g)	Fiber (g)	Sod (mg)	Chol (mg)
Lean only, trimmed to 1/4" fat, all grades, roasted	3 oz	161	24	5	0	0	0	56	66
Lean only, trimmed to 1/4" fat, choice, braised	3 oz	187	27	7	0	0	0	43	82
Lean only, trimmed to 1/4" fat, choice, raw	1 oz	43	6	1	0	0	0	17	17
Lean only, trimmed to 1/4" fat, choice, roasted	3 oz	168	24	6	0	0	0	56	66
Lean only, trimmed to 1/4" fat, select, braised	3 oz	167	27	5	0	0	0	43	82
Lean only, trimmed to 1/4" fat, select, raw	1 oz	39	6	1	0	0	0	17	17
Lean only, trimmed to 1/4" fat, select, roasted	3 oz	152	24	4	0	0	0	56	66
EYE OF ROUND									
Lean and fat, trimmed to 0" fat, all grades, roasted	3 oz	145	24	4	0	0	0	53	59
Lean and fat, trimmed to 0" fat, choice, roasted	3 oz	153	24	4	0	0	0	53	59
Lean and fat, trimmed to 0" fat, select, roasted	3 oz	137	24	3	0	0	0	53	59
Lean and fat, trimmed to 1/2" fat, prime, raw	1 oz	63	6	4	0	0	0	14	17
Lean and fat, trimmed to 1/2" fat, prime, roasted	3 oz	213	23	11	0	0	0	50	61
Lean and fat, trimmed to 1/4" fat, all grades, raw	1 oz	60	6	4	0	0	0	14	17
Lean and fat, trimmed to 1/4" fat, all grades, roasted	3 oz	195	23	9	0	0	0	50	61
Lean and fat, trimmed to 1/4" fat, choice, raw	1 oz	62	6	4	0	0	0	14	17
Lean and fat, trimmed to 1/4" fat, choice, roasted	3 oz	205	23	10	0	0	0	50	61
Lean and fat, trimmed to 1/4" fat, select, raw	1 oz	57	6	3	0	0	0	14	17
Lean and fat, trimmed to 1/4" fat, select, roasted	3 oz	184	23	8	0	0	0	51	61
Lean and fat, trimmed to 1/8" fat, all grades, raw	1 oz	47	6	2	0	0	0	14	16
Lean and fat, trimmed to 1/8" fat, all grades, roasted	3 oz	165	24	6	0	0	0	52	60
Lean and fat, trimmed to 1/8" fat, choice, raw	1 oz	49	6	2	0	0	0	14	16

Description	Serving Size	Cal	Prot (g)	Fat (g)	Carbs (g)	Net Carb(g)	Fiber (g)	Sod (mg)	Chol (mg)
ROUND (continued)									
Lean and fat, trimmed to 1/8" fat, choice, roasted	3 oz	170	24	6	0	0	0	52	60
Lean and fat, trimmed to 1/8" fat, select, raw	1 oz	45	6	2	0	0	0	15	16
Lean and fat, trimmed to 1/8" fat, select, roasted	3 oz	158	24	5	0	0	0	52	60
Lean only, trimmed to 0" fat, all grades, roasted	3 oz	141	25	3	0	0	0	53	59
Lean only, trimmed to 0" fat, choice, roasted	3 oz	149	25	4	0	0	0	53	59
Lean only, trimmed to 0" fat, select, roasted	3 oz	132	25	2	0	0	0	53	59
Lean only, trimmed to 1/2" fat, prime, raw	1 oz	42	6	1	0	0	0	15	15
Lean only, trimmed to 1/2" fat, prime, roasted	3 oz	168	25	6	0	0	0	53	59
Lean only, trimmed to 1/4" fat, all grades, raw	1 oz	37	6	1	0	0	0	15	15
Lean only, trimmed to 1/4" fat, all grades, roasted	3 oz	143	25	3	0	0	0	53	59
Lean only, trimmed to 1/4" fat, choice, raw	1 oz	39	6	1	0	0	0	15	15
Lean only, trimmed to 1/4" fat, choice, roasted	3 oz	149	25	4	0	0	0	53	59
Lean only, trimmed to 1/4" fat, select, raw	1 oz	35	6	1	0	0	0	15	15
Lean only, trimmed to 1/4" fat, select, roasted	3 oz	136	25	3	0	0	0	53	59
FULL CUT									
Lean and fat, trimmed to 1/4" fat, choice, broiled	3 oz	204	23	10	0	0	0	52	68
Lean and fat, trimmed to 1/4" fat, choice, raw	1 oz	58	6	3	0	0	0	15	18
Lean and fat, trimmed to 1/4" fat, select, broiled	3 oz	190	23	8	0	0	0	53	47
Lean and fat, trimmed to 1/4" fat, select, raw	1 oz	54	6	3	0	0	0	15	18
Lean and fat, trimmed to 1/8" fat, choice, broiled	3 oz	200	23	9	0	0	0	53	67
Lean and fat, trimmed to 1/8" fat, choice, raw	1 oz	55	6	3	0	0	0	15	18

Description	Serving Size	Cal	Prot (g)	Fat (g)	Carbs (g)	Net Carb(g)	Fiber (g)	Sod (mg)	Chol (mg)
Lean and fat, trimmed to 1/8" fat, select, broiled	3 oz	185	23	8	0	0	0	53	67
Lean and fat, trimmed to 1/8" fat, select, raw	1 oz	52	6	3	0	0	0	15	18
Lean only, trimmed to 1/4" fat, choice, broiled	3 oz	162	25	5	0	0	0	54	66
Lean only, trimmed to 1/4" fat, choice, raw	1 oz	39	6	1	0	0	0	16	16
Lean only, trimmed to 1/4" fat, select, broiled	3 oz	146	25	4	0	0	0	54	66
Lean only, trimmed to 1/4" fat, select, raw	1 oz	36	6	1	0	0	0	16	16
TIP ROUND									
Lean and fat, trimmed to 0" fat, all grades, roasted	3 oz	162	24	5	0	0	0	54	69
Lean and fat, trimmed to 0" fat, choice, roasted	3 oz	170	24	6	0	0	0	54	70
Lean and fat, trimmed to 0" fat, select, roasted	3 oz	158	24	5	0	0	0	54	69
Lean and fat, trimmed to 1/2" fat, prime, raw	1 oz	63	5	4	0	0	0	16	19
Lean and fat, trimmed to 1/2" fat, prime, roasted	3 oz	241	22	14	0	0	0	52	71
Lean and fat, trimmed to 1/4" fat, all grades, raw	1 oz	57	5	3	0	0	0	16	18
Lean and fat, trimmed to 1/4" fat, all grades, roasted	3 oz	199	23	9	0	0	0	54	70
Lean and fat, trimmed to 1/4" fat, choice, raw	1 oz	60	5	4	0	0	0	16	19
Lean and fat, trimmed to 1/4" fat, choice, roasted	3 oz	210	23	11	0	0	0	53	71
Lean and fat, trimmed to 1/4" fat, prime, raw	1 oz	61	6	4	0	0	0	16	18
Lean and fat, trimmed to 1/4" fat, prime, roasted	3 oz	233	22	13	0	0	0	53	71
Lean and fat, trimmed to 1/4" fat, select, raw	1 oz	53	6	3	0	0	0	16	18
Lean and fat, trimmed to 1/4" fat, select, roasted	3 oz	191	23	9	0	0	0	54	70
Lean and fat, trimmed to 1/8" fat, all grades, raw	1 oz	54	6	3	0	0	0	16	18
Lean and fat, trimmed to 1/8" fat, all grades, roasted	3 oz	186	23	8	0	0	0	54	70

Description	Serving Size	Cal	Prot (g)	Fat (g)	Carbs (g)	Net Carb(g)	Fiber (g)	Sod (mg)	Chol (mg)
ROUND (continued)									
Lean and fat, trimmed to 1/8" fat, choice, raw	1 oz	56	6	3	0	0	0	16	18
Lean and fat, trimmed to 1/8" fat, choice, roasted	3 oz	194	23	9	0	0	0	54	70
Lean and fat, trimmed to 1/8" fat, select, raw	1 oz	50	6	3	0	0	0	16	18
Lean and fat, trimmed to 1/8" fat, select, roasted	3 oz	179	23	7	0	0	0	54	70
Lean only, trimmed to 0" fat, all grades, roasted	3 oz	150	24	4	0	0	0	55	69
Lean only, trimmed to 0" fat, choice, roasted	3 oz	153	24	4	0	0	0	55	69
Lean only, trimmed to 0" fat, select, roasted	3 oz	145	24	4	0	0	0	55	69
Lean only, trimmed to 1/2" fat, prime, roasted	3 oz	181	24	7	0	0	0	55	69
Lean only, trimmed to 1/4" fat, all grades, raw	1 oz	35	6	1	0	0	0	18	17
Lean only, trimmed to 1/4" fat, all grades, roasted	3 oz	157	24	5	0	0	0	55	69
Lean only, trimmed to 1/4" fat, choice, raw	1 oz	37	6	1	0	0	0	18	17
Lean only, trimmed to 1/4" fat, choice, roasted	3 oz	160	24	5	0	0	0	55	69
Lean only, trimmed to 1/4" fat, prime, raw	1 oz	41	6	1	0	0	0	18	17
Lean only, trimmed to 1/4" fat, prime, roasted	3 oz	181	24	7	0	0	0	55	69
Lean only, trimmed to 1/4" fat, select, raw	1 oz	34	6	1	0	0	0	18	17
Lean only, trimmed to 1/4" fat, select, roasted	3 oz	153	24	4	0	0	0	55	69
TOP ROUND									
Lean and fat, trimmed to 0" fat, all grades, braised	3 oz	178	30	4	0	0	0	38	77
Lean and fat, trimmed to 0" fat, choice, braised	3 oz	184	30	5	0	0	0	38	77
Lean and fat, trimmed to 0" fat, select, braised	3 oz	170	30	4	0	0	0	38	77
Lean and fat, trimmed to 1/2" fat, prime, broiled	3 oz	201	26	8	0	0	0	51	72

Description	Serving Size	Cal	Prot (g)	Fat (g)	Carbs (g)	Net Carb(g)	Fiber (g)	Sod (mg)	Chol (mg)
Lean and fat, trimmed to 1/2" fat, prime, raw	1 oz	53	6	3	0	0	0	14	17
Lean and fat, trimmed to 1/4" fat, all grades, braised	3 oz	211	29	8	0	0	0	38	77
Lean and fat, trimmed to 1/4" fat, all grades, broiled	3 oz	184	26	7	0	0	0	51	72
Lean and fat, trimmed to 1/4" fat, all grades, raw	1 oz	50	6	2	0	0	0	14	17
Lean and fat, trimmed to 1/4" fat, choice, braised	3 oz	221	29	9	0	0	0	38	77
Lean and fat, trimmed to 1/4" fat, choice, broiled	3 oz	190	26	7	0	0	0	51	72
Lean and fat, trimmed to 1/4" fat, choice, pan-fried	3 oz	235	28	11	0	0	0	58	82
Lean and fat, trimmed to 1/4" fat, choice, raw	1 oz	51	6	2	0	0	0	14	17
Lean and fat, trimmed to 1/4" fat, prime, broiled	3 oz	195	26	7	0	0	0	51	71
Lean and fat, trimmed to 1/4" fat, prime, raw	1 oz	51	6	2	0	0	0	14	17
Lean and fat, trimmed to 1/4" fat, select, braised	3 oz	199	29	7	0	0	0	38	77
Lean and fat, trimmed to 1/4" fat, select, broiled	3 oz	175	26	6	0	0	0	51	72
Lean and fat, trimmed to 1/4" fat, select, raw	1 oz	46	6	2	0	0	0	14	17
Lean and fat, trimmed to 1/8" fat, all grades, braised	3 oz	202	29	7	0	0	0	38	77
Lean and fat, trimmed to 1/8" fat, all grades, broiled	3 oz	176	26	6	0	0	0	51	72
Lean and fat, trimmed to 1/8" fat, all grades, raw	1 oz	46	6	2	0	0	0	14	17
Lean and fat, trimmed to 1/8" fat, choice, braised	3 oz	213	29	8	0	0	0	38	77
Lean and fat, trimmed to 1/8" fat, choice, broiled	3 oz	184	26	7	0	0	0	51	72
Lean and fat, trimmed to 1/8" fat, choice, pan-fried	3 oz	226	28	10	0	0	0	58	82
Lean and fat, trimmed to 1/8" fat, choice, raw	1 oz	48	6	2	0	0	0	14	17
Lean and fat, trimmed to 1/8" fat, prime, broiled	3 oz	191	27	7	0	0	0	52	71
Lean and fat, trimmed to 1/8" fat, prime, raw	1 oz	49	6	2	0	0	0	14	17

Description	Serving Size	Cal	Prot (g)	Fat (g)	Carbs (g)	Net Carb(g)	Fiber (g)	Sod (mg)	Chol (mg)
ROUND (continued)									
Lean and fat, trimmed to 1/8" fat, select, braised	3 oz	191	29	6	0	0	0	38	77
Lean and fat, trimmed to 1/8" fat, select, broiled	3 oz	167	26	5	0	0	0	51	72
Lean and fat, trimmed to 1/8" fat, select, raw	1 oz	44	6	2	0	0	0	14	17
Lean only, trimmed to 0" fat, all grades, braised	3 oz	169	31	3	0	0	0	38	77
Lean only, trimmed to 0" fat, choice, braised	3 oz	176	31	4	0	0	0	38	77
Lean only, trimmed to 0" fat, select, braised	3 oz	162	31	3	0	0	0	38	77
Lean only, trimmed to 1/2" fat, prime, broiled	3 oz	183	27	6	0	0	0	52	71
Lean only, trimmed to 1/4" fat, all grades, braised	3 oz	174	31	4	0	0	0	38	77
Lean only, trimmed to 1/4" fat, all grades, broiled	3 oz	153	27	3	0	0	0	52	71
Lean only, trimmed to 1/4" fat, all grades, raw	1 oz	36	6	1	0	0	0	15	16
Lean only, trimmed to 1/4" fat, choice, braised	3 oz	181	31	4	0	0	0	38	77
Lean only, trimmed to 1/4" fat, choice, broiled	3 oz	161	27	4	0	0	0	52	71
Lean only, trimmed to 1/4" fat, choice, pan-fried	3 oz	193	30	6	0	0	0	60	82
Lean only, trimmed to 1/4" fat, choice, raw	1 oz	37	6	1	0	0	0	15	16
Lean only, trimmed to 1/4" fat, prime, broiled	3 oz	183	27	6	0	0	0	52	71
Lean only, trimmed to 1/4" fat, prime, raw	1 oz	43	6	1	0	0	0	15	16
Lean only, trimmed to 1/4" fat, select, braised	3 oz	167	31	3	0	0	0	38	77
Lean only, trimmed to 1/4" fat, select, broiled	3 oz	144	27	2	0	0	0	52	71
Lean only, trimmed to 1/4" fat, select, raw	1 oz	34	6	1	0	0	0	15	16

Shank

Description	Serving Size	Cal	Prot (g)	Fat (g)	Carbs (g)	Net Carb(g)	Fiber (g)	Sod (mg)	Chol (mg)
Crosscuts, lean and fat, trimmed to 1/4" fat, choice, raw	3 oz	150	17	7	0	0	0	51	37

Description	Serving Size	Cal	Prot (g)	Fat (g)	Carbs (g)	Net Carb(g)	Fiber (g)	Sod (mg)	Chol (mg)
Crosscuts, lean and fat, trimmed to 1/4" fat, choice, simmered	3 oz	224	26	11	0	0	0	52	68
Crosscuts, lean only, trimmed to 1/4" fat, choice, raw	1 oz	36	6	1	0	0	0	18	11
Crosscuts, lean only, trimmed to 1/4" fat, choice, simmered	3 oz	171	29	5	0	0	0	54	66

Short Loin

PORTERHOUSE STEAK

Description	Serving Size	Cal	Prot (g)	Fat (g)	Carbs (g)	Net Carb(g)	Fiber (g)	Sod (mg)	Chol (mg)
Lean and fat, trimmed to 0" fat, all grades, broiled	3 oz	237	20	14	0	0	0	55	57
Lean and fat, trimmed to 0" fat, USDA choice, broiled	3 oz	241	20	15	0	0	0	55	59
Lean and fat, trimmed to 0" fat, USDA select, broiled	3 oz	227	21	13	0	0	0	55	54
Lean and fat, trimmed to 1/4" fat, all grades, broiled	3 oz	273	19	18	0	0	0	54	62
Lean and fat, trimmed to 1/4" fat, all grades, raw	1 oz	73	5	5	0	0	0	14	18
Lean and fat, trimmed to 1/4" fat, USDA choice, broiled	3 oz	278	19	19	0	0	0	53	64
Lean and fat, trimmed to 1/4" fat, USDA choice, raw	1 oz	73	5	5	0	0	0	15	19
Lean and fat, trimmed to 1/4" fat, USDA select, broiled	3 oz	262	20	17	0	0	0	54	56
Lean and fat, trimmed to 1/4" fat, USDA select, raw	1 oz	63	6	4	0	0	0	15	16
Lean and fat, trimmed to 1/8" fat, all grades, broiled	3 oz	252	20	16	0	0	0	54	60
Lean and fat, trimmed to 1/8" fat, all grades, raw	1 oz	70	5	5	0	0	0	15	18
Lean and fat, trimmed to 1/8" fat, choice, broiled	3 oz	254	20	16	0	0	0	54	63
Lean and fat, trimmed to 1/8" fat, choice, raw	1 oz	73	5	5	0	0	0	15	19
Lean and fat, trimmed to 1/8" fat, select, broiled	3 oz	250	20	16	0	0	0	54	55
Lean and fat, trimmed to 1/8" fat, select, raw	1 oz	63	6	4	0	0	0	15	16
Lean only, trimmed to 0" fat, all grades, broiled	3 oz	183	22	8	0	0	0	59	54
Lean only, trimmed to 0" fat, USDA choice, broiled	3 oz	190	22	9	0	0	0	59	55

Description	Serving Size	Cal	Prot (g)	Fat (g)	Carbs (g)	Net Carb(g)	Fiber (g)	Sod (mg)	Chol (mg)
SHORT LOIN (continued)									
Lean only, trimmed to 0" fat, USDA select, broiled	3 oz	165	23	6	0	0	0	59	49
Lean only, trimmed to 1/4" fat, all grades, broiled	3 oz	180	22	8	0	0	0	59	56
Lean only, trimmed to 1/4" fat, all grades, raw	1 oz	45	6	2	0	0	0	16	16
Lean only, trimmed to 1/4" fat, USDA choice, broiled	3 oz	183	22	8	0	0	0	59	59
Lean only, trimmed to 1/4" fat, USDA choice, raw	1 oz	46	6	2	0	0	0	16	17
Lean only, trimmed to 1/4" fat, USDA select, broiled	3 oz	173	23	7	0	0	0	59	49
Lean only, trimmed to 1/4" fat, USDA select, raw	1 oz	42	6	1	0	0	0	16	14
T-BONE STEAK									
Lean and fat, trimmed to 0" fat, all grades, broiled	3 oz	210	21	12	0	0	0	57	48
Lean and fat, trimmed to 0" fat, USDA choice, broiled	3 oz	217	21	12	0	0	0	57	48
Lean and fat, trimmed to 0" fat, USDA select, broiled	3 oz	194	21	10	0	0	0	58	49
Lean and fat, trimmed to 1/4" fat, all grades, broiled	3 oz	256	20	16	0	0	0	55	54
Lean and fat, trimmed to 1/4" fat, all grades, raw	1 oz	64	5	4	0	0	0	15	16
Lean and fat, trimmed to 1/4" fat, USDA choice, broiled	3 oz	263	20	17	0	0	0	54	57
Lean and fat, trimmed to 1/4" fat, USDA choice, raw	1 oz	67	5	4	0	0	0	15	18
Lean and fat, trimmed to 1/4" fat, USDA select, broiled	3 oz	238	21	14	0	0	0	56	49
Lean and fat, trimmed to 1/4" fat, USDA select, raw	1 oz	56	6	3	0	0	0	15	13
Lean and fat, trimmed to 1/8" fat, all grades, broiled	3 oz	238	21	14	0	0	0	56	53
Lean and fat, trimmed to 1/8" fat, all grades, raw	1 oz	62	5	4	0	0	0	15	16
Lean and fat, trimmed to 1/8" fat, choice, broiled	3 oz	243	20	15	0	0	0	56	55
Lean and fat, trimmed to 1/8" fat, choice, raw	1 oz	66	5	4	0	0	0	15	18

Description	Serving Size	Cal	Prot (g)	Fat (g)	Carbs (g)	Net Carb(g)	Fiber (g)	Sod (mg)	Chol (mg)
Lean and fat, trimmed to 1/8" fat, select, broiled	3 oz	225	21	13	0	0	0	56	48
Lean and fat, trimmed to 1/8" fat, select, raw	1 oz	54	6	3	0	0	0	16	13
Lean only, trimmed to 0" fat, all grades, broiled	3 oz	163	22	6	0	0	0	60	44
Lean only, trimmed to 0" fat, USDA choice, broiled	3 oz	168	22	7	0	0	0	60	44
Lean only, trimmed to 0" fat, USDA select, broiled	3 oz	150	22	5	0	0	0	60	46
Lean only, trimmed to 1/4" fat, all grades, broiled	3 oz	173	23	7	0	0	0	60	48
Lean only, trimmed to 1/4" fat, all grades, raw	1 oz	42	6	2	0	0	0	16	14
Lean only, trimmed to 1/4" fat, USDA choice, broiled	3 oz	174	23	7	0	0	0	60	50
Lean only, trimmed to 1/4" fat, USDA choice, raw	1 oz	44	6	2	0	0	0	16	16
Lean only, trimmed to 1/4" fat, USDA select, broiled	3 oz	168	23	6	0	0	0	60	43
Lean only, trimmed to 1/4" fat, USDA select, raw	1 oz	37	6	1	0	0	0	16	11
TOP LOIN									
Lean and fat, trimmed to 0" fat, all grades, broiled	3 oz	180	24	7	0	0	0	57	65
Lean and fat, trimmed to 0" fat, choice, broiled	3 oz	194	24	8	0	0	0	57	65
Lean and fat, trimmed to 0" fat, select, broiled	3 oz	169	24	6	0	0	0	57	65
Lean and fat, trimmed to 1/2" fat, prime, broiled	3 oz	288	21	20	0	0	0	53	68
Lean and fat, trimmed to 1/2" fat, prime, raw	1 lb	1461	81	114	0	0	0	231	318
Lean and fat, trimmed to 1/4" fat, all grades, broiled	3 oz	244	22	14	0	0	0	54	67
Lean and fat, trimmed to 1/4" fat, choice, broiled	3 oz	253	22	15	0	0	0	54	67
Lean and fat, trimmed to 1/4" fat, choice, raw	1 lb	1179	85	79	0	0	0	240	304
Lean and fat, trimmed to 1/4" fat, prime, broiled	3 oz	275	22	18	0	0	0	54	67

Description	Serving Size	Cal	Prot (g)	Fat (g)	Carbs (g)	Net Carb(g)	Fiber (g)	Sod (mg)	Chol (mg)
SHORT LOIN (continued)									
Lean and fat, trimmed to 1/4" fat, prime, raw	1 lb	1383	83	101	0	0	0	236	313
Lean and fat, trimmed to 1/4" fat, select, broiled	3 oz	226	22	12	0	0	0	54	67
Lean and fat, trimmed to 1/4" fat, select, raw	1 lb	1043	87	65	0	0	0	245	299
Lean and fat, trimmed to 1/8" fat, all grades, broiled	3 oz	228	22	12	0	0	0	54	66
Lean and fat, trimmed to 1/8" fat, all grades, raw	1 lb	1016	88	62	0	0	0	245	295
Lean and fat, trimmed to 1/8" fat, choice, broiled	3 oz	241	22	14	0	0	0	54	67
Lean and fat, trimmed to 1/8" fat, choice, raw	1 lb	1075	88	68	0	0	0	245	299
Lean and fat, trimmed to 1/8" fat, prime, broiled	3 oz	264	22	16	0	0	0	54	67
Lean and fat, trimmed to 1/8" fat, prime, raw	1 lb	1275	86	89	0	0	0	240	304
Lean and fat, trimmed to 1/8" fat, select, broiled	3 oz	215	22	11	0	0	0	55	66
Lean and fat, trimmed to 1/8" fat, select, raw	1 lb	957	89	56	0	0	0	249	295
Lean only, trimmed to 0" fat, all grades, broiled	3 oz	168	24	6	0	0	0	58	65
Lean only, trimmed to 0" fat, choice, broiled	3 oz	178	24	7	0	0	0	58	65
Lean only, trimmed to 0" fat, select, broiled	3 oz	156	24	5	0	0	0	58	65
Lean only, trimmed to 1/2" fat, prime, broiled	3 oz	208	24	10	0	0	0	58	65
Lean only, trimmed to 1/4" fat, all grades, broiled	3 oz	176	24	7	0	0	0	58	65
Lean only, trimmed to 1/4" fat, all grades, raw	1 oz	40	6	1	0	0	0	17	17
Lean only, trimmed to 1/4" fat, choice, broiled	3 oz	182	24	7	0	0	0	58	65
Lean only, trimmed to 1/4" fat, choice, raw	1 oz	43	6	2	0	0	0	17	17
Lean only, trimmed to 1/4" fat, prime, broiled	3 oz	208	24	10	0	0	0	58	65
Lean only, trimmed to 1/4" fat, prime, raw	1 oz	54	6	3	0	0	0	17	17

Description	Serving Size	Cal	Prot (g)	Fat (g)	Carbs (g)	Net Carb(g)	Fiber (g)	Sod (mg)	Chol (mg)
Lean only, trimmed to 1/4" fat, select, broiled	3 oz	164	24	5	0	0	0	58	65
Lean only, trimmed to 1/4" fat, select, raw	1 oz	38	6	1	0	0	0	17	17

Tenderloin

Description	Serving Size	Cal	Prot (g)	Fat (g)	Carbs (g)	Net Carb(g)	Fiber (g)	Sod (mg)	Chol (mg)
Lean and fat, trimmed to 1/2" fat, prime, broiled	3 oz	270	21	17	0	0	0	50	73
Lean and fat, trimmed to 1/2" fat, prime, raw	1 lb	1306	81	97	0	0	0	218	322
Lean and fat, trimmed to 1/2" fat, prime, roasted	3 oz	304	20	21	0	0	0	47	75
Lean only, trimmed to 1/2" fat, prime, broiled	3 oz	197	24	9	0	0	0	54	71
Lean only, trimmed to 1/2" fat, prime, roasted	3 oz	217	23	11	0	0	0	50	73
Lean and fat, trimmed to 0" fat, all grades, broiled	3 oz	200	23	9	0	0	0	53	72
Lean and fat, trimmed to 0" fat, choice, broiled	3 oz	207	23	10	0	0	0	52	72
Lean and fat, trimmed to 0" fat, select, broiled	3 oz	195	23	9	0	0	0	53	72
Lean and fat, trimmed to 1/4" fat, all grades, broiled	3 oz	247	21	14	0	0	0	50	73
Lean and fat, trimmed to 1/4" fat, all grades, raw	1 oz	80	5	6	0	0	0	14	20
Lean and fat, trimmed to 1/4" fat, all grades, raw	1 lb	1102	86	71	0	0	0	240	304
Lean and fat, trimmed to 1/4" fat, all grades, roasted	3 oz	282	20	19	0	0	0	48	73
Lean and fat, trimmed to 1/4" fat, choice, broiled	3 oz	258	21	16	0	0	0	50	73
Lean and fat, trimmed to 1/4" fat, choice, raw	1 oz	82	5	6	0	0	0	14	20
Lean and fat, trimmed to 1/4" fat, choice, roasted	3 oz	288	20	19	0	0	0	55	73
Lean and fat, trimmed to 1/4" fat, prime, broiled	3 oz	269	21	17	0	0	0	50	73
Lean and fat, trimmed to 1/4" fat, prime, raw	1 oz	81	5	6	0	0	0	14	20
Lean and fat, trimmed to 1/4" fat, prime, roasted	3 oz	300	20	20	0	0	0	47	75
Lean and fat, trimmed to 1/4" fat, select, broiled	3 oz	230	22	13	0	0	0	51	73

Description	Serving Size	Cal	Prot (g)	Fat (g)	Carbs (g)	Net Carb(g)	Fiber (g)	Sod (mg)	Chol (mg)
TENDERLOIN (continued)									
Lean and fat, trimmed to 1/4" fat, select, raw	1 oz	79	5	6	0	0	0	14	20
Lean and fat, trimmed to 1/4" fat, select, roasted	3 oz	275	20	18	0	0	0	48	73
Lean and fat, trimmed to 1/8" fat, all grades, broiled	3 oz	239	22	14	0	0	0	51	73
Lean and fat, trimmed to 1/8" fat, all grades, raw	1 oz	77	5	5	0	0	0	14	20
Lean and fat, trimmed to 1/8" fat, all grades, roasted	3 oz	275	20	18	0	0	0	48	72
Lean and fat, trimmed to 1/8" fat, choice, broiled	3 oz	251	22	15	0	0	0	50	73
Lean and fat, trimmed to 1/8" fat, choice, raw	1 oz	79	5	5	0	0	0	14	20
Lean and fat, trimmed to 1/8" fat, choice, roasted	3 oz	281	20	18	0	0	0	55	72
Lean and fat, trimmed to 1/8" fat, prime, broiled	3 oz	262	21	16	0	0	0	50	73
Lean and fat, trimmed to 1/8" fat, prime, raw	1 oz	78	5	5	0	0	0	14	20
Lean and fat, trimmed to 1/8" fat, prime, roasted	3 oz	292	20	19	0	0	0	47	75
Lean and fat, trimmed to 1/8" fat, select, broiled	3 oz	226	22	12	0	0	0	51	73
Lean and fat, trimmed to 1/8" fat, select, raw	1 oz	76	5	5	0	0	0	14	20
Lean and fat, trimmed to 1/8" fat, select, roasted	3 oz	269	20	17	0	0	0	48	72
Lean only, trimmed to 0" fat, all grades, broiled	3 oz	175	24	6	0	0	0	54	71
Lean only, trimmed to 0" fat, choice, broiled	3 oz	180	24	7	0	0	0	54	71
Lean only, trimmed to 0" fat, select, broiled	3 oz	170	24	6	0	0	0	54	71
Lean only, trimmed to 1/4" fat, all grades, roasted	3 oz	189	24	8	0	0	0	52	71
Lean only, trimmed to 1/4" fat, choice, roasted	3 oz	196	24	8	0	0	0	61	71
Lean only, trimmed to 1/4" fat, prime, broiled	3 oz	197	24	9	0	0	0	54	71
Lean only, trimmed to 1/4" fat, prime, raw	1 oz	48	6	2	0	0	0	15	18

Description	Serving Size	Cal	Prot (g)	Fat (g)	Carbs (g)	Net Carb(g)	Fiber (g)	Sod (mg)	Chol (mg)
Lean only, trimmed to 1/4" fat, prime, roasted	3 oz	217	23	11	0	0	0	50	73
Lean only, trimmed to 1/4" fat, select, roasted	3 oz	179	24	7	0	0	0	52	71
Lean, trimmed to 1/4" fat, all grades, broiled	3 oz	179	24	7	0	0	0	54	71
Lean, trimmed to 1/4" fat, all grades, raw	1 oz	45	6	2	0	0	0	15	18
Lean, trimmed to 1/4" fat, choice, broiled	3 oz	189	24	8	0	0	0	54	71
Lean, trimmed to 1/4" fat, choice, raw	1 oz	47	6	2	0	0	0	15	18
Lean, trimmed to 1/4" fat, select, broiled	3 oz	169	24	6	0	0	0	54	71
Lean, trimmed to 1/4" fat, select, raw	1 oz	43	6	2	0	0	0	15	18

Top Sirloin

Description	Serving Size	Cal	Prot (g)	Fat (g)	Carbs (g)	Net Carb(g)	Fiber (g)	Sod (mg)	Chol (mg)
Lean and fat, trimmed to 0" fat, all grades, broiled	3 oz	183	25	7	0	0	0	55	76
Lean and fat, trimmed to 0" fat, choice, broiled	3 oz	195	25	8	0	0	0	54	76
Lean and fat, trimmed to 0" fat, select, broiled	3 oz	166	25	6	0	0	0	55	76
Lean and fat, trimmed to 1/4" fat, all grades, broiled	3 oz	219	24	11	0	0	0	54	77
Lean and fat, trimmed to 1/4" fat, all grades, raw	1 oz	62	5	4	0	0	0	15	19
Lean and fat, trimmed to 1/4" fat, choice, broiled	3 oz	229	23	12	0	0	0	53	77
Lean and fat, trimmed to 1/4" fat, choice, pan-fried	3 oz	277	24	17	0	0	0	60	83
Lean and fat, trimmed to 1/4" fat, choice, raw	1 oz	64	5	4	0	0	0	15	19
Lean and fat, trimmed to 1/4" fat, select, broiled	3 oz	208	24	10	0	0	0	54	77
Lean and fat, trimmed to 1/4" fat, select, raw	1 oz	59	5	3	0	0	0	15	19
Lean and fat, trimmed to 1/8" fat, all grades, broiled	3 oz	211	24	10	0	0	0	54	77
Lean and fat, trimmed to 1/8" fat, all grades, raw	1 oz	58	6	3	0	0	0	15	19
Lean and fat, trimmed to 1/8" fat, choice, broiled	3 oz	220	24	11	0	0	0	54	77
Lean and fat, trimmed to 1/8" fat, choice, pan-fried	3 oz	266	24	16	0	0	0	60	83

Description	Serving Size	Cal	Prot (g)	Fat (g)	Carbs (g)	Net Carb(g)	Fiber (g)	Sod (mg)	Chol (mg)
TOP SIRLOIN (continued)									
Lean and fat, trimmed to 1/8" fat, choice, raw	1 oz	60	5	4	0	0	0	15	19
Lean and fat, trimmed to 1/8" fat, select, broiled	3 oz	204	24	10	0	0	0	54	77
Lean and fat, trimmed to 1/8" fat, select, raw	1 oz	55	6	3	0	0	0	15	19
Lean only, trimmed to 0" fat, all grades, broiled	3 oz	162	26	5	0	0	0	56	76
Lean only, trimmed to 0" fat, choice, broiled	3 oz	170	26	6	0	0	0	56	76
Lean only, trimmed to 0" fat, select, broiled	3 oz	153	26	4	0	0	0	56	76
Lean only, trimmed to 1/4" fat, all grades, broiled	3 oz	166	26	5	0	0	0	56	76
Lean only, trimmed to 1/4" fat, all grades, raw	1 oz	37	6	1	0	0	0	16	17
Lean only, trimmed to 1/4" fat, choice, broiled	3 oz	172	26	6	0	0	0	56	76
Lean only, trimmed to 1/4" fat, choice, pan-fried	3 oz	202	28	8	0	0	0	65	84
Lean only, trimmed to 1/4" fat, choice, raw	1 oz	39	6	1	0	0	0	16	17
Lean only, trimmed to 1/4" fat, select, broiled	3 oz	158	26	4	0	0	0	56	76
Lean only, trimmed to 1/4" fat, select, raw	1 oz	35	6	1	0	0	0	16	17

Variety Meats & By-Products

Description	Serving Size	Cal	Prot (g)	Fat (g)	Carbs (g)	Net Carb(g)	Fiber (g)	Sod (mg)	Chol (mg)
Brain, pan-fried	3 oz	167	11	9	0	0	0	134	1696
Brain, raw	1 oz	36	3	1	0	0	0	29	474
Brain, simmered	3 oz	136	9	6	0	0	0	102	1746
Heart, raw	1 oz	33	5	1	1	1	0	18	40
Heart, simmered	3 oz	149	24	4	0	0	0	54	164
Kidneys, raw	1 oz	30	5	1	1	1	0	51	81
Kidneys, simmered	3 oz	122	22	2	1	1	0	114	329
Liver, braised	3 oz	137	21	3	3	3	0	60	331
Liver, pan-fried	3 oz	184	23	5	7	7	0	90	410
Liver, raw	1 oz	41	6	1	2	2	0	21	100
Lungs, braised	3 oz	102	17	2	0	0	0	86	235
Lungs, raw	1 oz	26	5	1	0	0	0	56	69
Mechanically separated beef, raw	1 oz	78	4	6	0	0	0	16	59

Description	Serving Size	Cal	Prot (g)	Fat (g)	Carbs (g)	Net Carb(g)	Fiber (g)	Sod (mg)	Chol (mg)
Pancreas, braised	3 oz	230	23	13	0	0	0	51	223
Pancreas, raw	1 oz	67	4	5	0	0	0	19	58
Spleen, braised	3 oz	123	21	2	0	0	0	48	295
Spleen, raw	1 oz	30	5	1	0	0	0	24	75
Suet, raw	1 oz	242	0	25	0	0	0	2	19
Thymus, braised	3 oz	271	19	19	0	0	0	99	250
Thymus, raw	1 oz	67	3	5	0	0	0	27	63
Tongue, raw	1 oz	64	4	4	1	1	0	20	25
Tongue, simmered	3 oz	241	19	16	0	0	0	51	91
Tripe, raw	1 oz	28	4	1	0	0	0	13	27

Description	Serving Size	Cal	Prot (g)	Fat (g)	Carbs (g)	Net Carb(g)	Fiber (g)	Sod (mg)	Chol (mg)
Alcoholic Beverages									
BEER									
Light	1 fl oz	8	0	0	0	0	0	1	0
Light	1 can	99	1	0	5	5	0	11	0
Regular	1 fl oz	12	0	0	1	1	0	1	0
Regular	1 can	146	1	0	13	12	1	18	0
COCKTAILS									
Daiquiri, canned	1 can	259	0	0	32	32	0	83	0
Daiquiri, prepared-from-recipe	1 cocktail	112	0	0	4	4	0	3	0
Pina colada, canned	1 can	526	1	16	61	61	0	158	0
Pina colada, prepared-from-recipe	1 cocktail	252	1	2	32	31	0	8	0
Tequila sunrise, canned	1 can	232	1	0	24	24	0	120	0
Whiskey sour mix, bottled	1 fl oz	26	0	0	7	7	0	32	0
Whiskey sour mix, bottled, with added potassium and sodium	1 fl oz	27	0	0	7	7	0	11	0
Whiskey sour mix, powder	1 packet	64	0	0	16	16	0	46	0
Whiskey sour, canned	1 can	249	0	0	28	28	0	92	0
Whiskey sour, prepared	1 portion	158	0	0	14	14	0	66	0
Whiskey sour, prepared with water, whiskey and powder mix	1 packet	169	0	0	16	16	0	47	0
LIQUOR									
Creme de menthe, 72 proof	1 fl oz	125	0	0	14	14	0	2	0
Distilled, all (gin, rum, vodka, whiskey) 100 proof	1 fl oz	82	0	0	0	0	0	0	0
Distilled, all (gin, rum, vodka, whiskey) 80 proof	1 fl oz	64	0	0	0	0	0	0	0
Distilled, all (gin, rum, vodka, whiskey) 86 proof	1 fl oz	70	0	0	0	0	0	0	0
Distilled, all (gin, rum, vodka, whiskey) 90 proof	1 fl oz	73	0	0	0	0	0	0	0
Distilled, all (gin, rum, vodka, whiskey) 94 proof	1 fl oz	76	0	0	0	0	0	0	0
Distilled, gin, 90 proof	1 fl oz	73	0	0	0	0	0	1	0
Distilled, rum, 80 proof	1 fl oz	64	0	0	0	0	0	0	0
Distilled, vodka, 80 proof	1 fl oz	64	0	0	0	0	0	0	0
Distilled, whiskey, 86 proof	1 fl oz	70	0	0	0	0	0	0	0
Liqueur, coffee with cream, 34 proof	1 fl oz	0	0	0	0	0	0	2	0
Liqueur, coffee, 53 proof	1 fl oz	102	1	5	6	6	0	29	5
Liqueur, coffee, 63 proof	1 fl oz	107	0	0	11	11	0	3	0

Description	Serving Size	Cal	Prot (g)	Fat (g)	Carbs (g)	Net Carb(g)	Fiber (g)	Sod (mg)	Chol (mg)
ALCOHOLIC BEVERAGES (continued)									
WINE									
All	1 fl oz	21	0	0	0	0	0	2	0
Dessert, dry	1 fl oz	37	0	0	1	1	0	3	0
Dessert, sweet	1 fl oz	45	0	0	3	3	0	3	0
Non-alcoholic	1 fl oz	2	0	0	0	0	0	2	0
Red	1 fl oz	21	0	0	1	1	0	1	0
Rose	1 fl oz	21	0	0	0	0	0	1	0
White	1 fl oz	20	0	0	0	0	0	1	0

Carbonated Beverages

Description	Serving Size	Cal	Prot (g)	Fat (g)	Carbs (g)	Net Carb(g)	Fiber (g)	Sod (mg)	Chol (mg)
Chocolate-flavored soda	1 can	207	0	0	53	53	0	433	0
Club soda	1 can	0	0	0	0	0	0	100	0
Cola	1 can	202	0	0	51	51	0	20	0
Cola, contains caffeine	1 can	202	0	0	51	51	0	20	0
Cream soda	1 can	252	0	0	66	66	0	59	0
Ginger ale	1 can	166	0	0	42	42	0	34	0
Grape soda	1 can	160	0	0	42	42	0	56	0
Lemon-lime soda	1 can	196	0	0	51	51	0	54	0
Low calorie, cola or pepper-type, with aspartame, contains caffeine	1 packet	119	2	3	24	23	1	207	0
Low calorie, cola or pepper-types, with sodium saccharin, contains caffeine	1 can	0	0	0	0	0	0	76	0
Low calorie, cola, with aspartame, without caffeine	1 can	5	0	0	0	0	0	28	0
Low calorie, other than cola or pepper, without caffeine	1 can	0	0	0	0	0	0	21	0
Low calorie, other than cola or pepper, with aspartame, with caffeine	1 can	0	0	0	0	0	0	21	0
Low calorie, other than cola or pepper, with sodium saccharin, without caffeine	1 can	0	0	0	0	0	0	57	0
Orange soda	1 can	238	0	0	61	61	0	60	0
Pepper-type, contains caffeine	1 can	201	0	0	51	51	0	49	0
Root beer	1 can	202	0	0	52	52	0	64	0
Tonic water	1 can	166	0	0	43	43	0	20	0

Chocolate Milk

Description	Serving Size	Cal	Prot (g)	Fat (g)	Carbs (g)	Net Carb(g)	Fiber (g)	Sod (mg)	Chol (mg)
Carob-flavor beverage mix, powder	1 tbsp	45	0	0	11	10	1	12	0
Carob-flavor beverage mix, powder, prepared with whole milk	1 cup	195	8	8	23	22	1	133	33

Description	Serving Size	Cal	Prot (g)	Fat (g)	Carbs (g)	Net Carb(g)	Fiber (g)	Sod (mg)	Chol (mg)
Chocolate syrup	1 tbsp	52	0	0	12	12	0	14	0
Chocolate syrup, prepared with whole milk	1 cup	231	9	8	34	33	1	155	34
Chocolate syrup, with added nutrition	1 tbsp	46	0	0	12	12	0	29	0
Chocolate syrup, with added nutrition , prepared with milk	1 cup	197	8	8	24	23	0	147	34
Chocolate-flavor beverage mix for milk, powder, without added nutrients	1 portion	75	1	1	20	18	1	45	0
Chocolate-flavor beverage mix, powder, prepared with whole milk	1 cup	226	9	8	31	30	1	165	32

Cocoa

NESTLE, CARNATION

Description	Serving Size	Cal	Prot (g)	Fat (g)	Carbs (g)	Net Carb(g)	Fiber (g)	Sod (mg)	Chol (mg)
Hot Cocoa Mix With Marshmallows	1 envelope	112	1	1	24	24	1	96	2
No Sugar Added Hot Cocoa Mix	1 envelope	55	4	0	8	8	1	142	3
Rich Chocolate Hot Cocoa Mix	1 envelope	112	1	1	24	24	1	102	2
ALBA Cocoa mix, no sugar added, powder	1 envelope	61	5	1	11	10	0	214	2
Cocoa mix, powder	1 serving	102	3	1	22	22	0	143	1
Cocoa mix, powder, prepared with water	1 fl oz	103	3	1	22	20	2	148	2
Cocoa mix, with added nutrition, powder	1 packet	120	2	3	24	23	1	201	1
Cocoa mix, with aspartame, powder, prepared from item 14196	1 packet	48	4	0	8	8	0	173	2
SWISS MISS cocoa mix, with aspartame, low calorie, powder	1 envelope	48	4	0	9	8	0	98	1

Coffee

GENERAL FOODS INTERNATIONAL COFFEES

Description	Serving Size	Cal	Prot (g)	Fat (g)	Carbs (g)	Net Carb(g)	Fiber (g)	Sod (mg)	Chol (mg)
Cafe Francais Flavored Instant Coffee, powder	1 serving	62	1	1	7	7	0	93	0
French Vanilla Cafe Flavored Instant Coffee, powder	1 serving	65	0	1	10	10	0	56	0
Sugar Free Fat Free Low Calorie French Vanilla Cafe Flavored Instant Coffee, with aspartame and acesulfame potassium sweetener, powder	1 serving	25	0	0	5	5	0	65	0
Sugar Free Fat Free Low Calorie Suisse Mocha Flavored Instant Coffee, with aspartame and acesulfame potassium sweetener, powder	1 serving	24	0	0	5	4	1	36	0

Description	Serving Size	Cal	Prot (g)	Fat (g)	Carbs (g)	Net Carb(g)	Fiber (g)	Sod (mg)	Chol (mg)
COFFEE (continued)									
Suisse Mocha Flavored Instant Coffee, powder	1 serving	57	0	1	9	9	0	33	0
Brewed from grounds, prepared with water	1 cup	5	0	0	1	1	0	5	0
Brewed from grounds, prepared with water, decaffeinated	1 cup	5	0	0	1	1	0	5	0
Instant, decaffeinated, powder	1 tsp	4	0	0	1	1	0	0	0
Instant, decaffeinated, powder, prepared with water	6 fl oz	4	0	0	1	1	0	5	0
Instant, regular, powder	1 tsp	2	0	0	0	0	0	0	0
Instant, regular, prepared with water	1 fl oz	1	0	0	0	0	0	1	0
Instant, with chicory, powder	1 tsp	6	0	0	1	1	0	5	0
Instant, with chicory, prepared with water	6 fl oz	7	0	0	1	1	0	11	0

Coffee Substitutes

Description	Serving Size	Cal	Prot (g)	Fat (g)	Carbs (g)	Net Carb(g)	Fiber (g)	Sod (mg)	Chol (mg)
Cereal grain beverage, powder	1 tsp	8	0	0	2	2	0	2	0
Cereal grain beverage, powder, prepared with whole milk	6 fl oz	120	6	6	10	10	0	91	24
Cereal grain beverage, prepared with water	1 cup	12	0	0	2	2	0	10	0

Fruit Drinks & Juice

Description	Serving Size	Cal	Prot (g)	Fat (g)	Carbs (g)	Net Carb(g)	Fiber (g)	Sod (mg)	Chol (mg)
ACEROLA									
Acerola juice, raw	1 cup	56	1	1	12	11	1	7	0
APPLE									
Apple juice, canned or bottled, unsweetened, with added ascorbic acid	1 cup	117	0	0	29	29	0	7	0
Apple juice, canned or bottled, unsweetened, without added ascorbic acid	1 cup	117	0	0	29	29	0	7	0
Apple juice, frozen concentrate, unsweetened, diluted with 3 volume water without added ascorbic acid	1 cup	112	0	0	28	27	0	17	0
Apple juice, frozen concentrate, unsweetened, diluted with 3 volume water, with added ascorbic acid	1 cup	112	0	0	28	27	0	17	0
Apple juice, frozen concentrate, unsweetened, undiluted, with added ascorbic acid	1 can	350	1	0	87	N.A.	N.A.	53	0

Description	Serving Size	Cal	Prot (g)	Fat (g)	Carbs (g)	Net Carb(g)	Fiber (g)	Sod (mg)	Chol (mg)
Apple juice, frozen concentrate, unsweetened, undiluted, without added ascorbic acid	1 can	350	1	0	87	86	1	53	0
CONTINENTAL MILLS, Alpine Spiced Cider instant apple flavor drink mix, powder	1 pouch	83	0	0	21	N.A.	N.A.	0	0
APRICOT									
Apricot nectar, canned, with added ascorbic acid	1 cup	141	1	0	36	35	2	8	0
Apricot nectar, canned, without added ascorbic acid	1 cup	141	1	0	36	35	2	8	0
CRANBERRY									
Cranberry juice cocktail, bottled	1 cup	144	0	0	36	36	0	5	0
Cranberry juice cocktail, bottled, low calorie, with calcium, saccharin and corn sweetener	1 cup	45	0	0	11	11	0	7	0
Cranberry juice cocktail, frozen concentrate, prepared with water	1 cup	138	0	0	35	35	0	8	0
Cranberry-apple juice drink, bottled	1 cup	164	0	0	42	42	0	5	0
Cranberry-apricot juice drink, bottled	1 cup	157	0	0	40	39	0	5	0
Cranberry-grape juice drink, bottled	1 cup	137	0	0	34	34	0	7	0
FRUIT PUNCH									
Fruit punch drink, frozen concentrate	1 fl oz	56	0	0	14	14	0	3	0
Fruit punch drink, frozen concentrate, prepared with water	1 cup	114	0	0	29	29	0	10	0
Fruit punch drink, with added nutrients, canned	1 cup	117	0	0	30	29	0	55	0
Fruit punch juice drink, frozen concentrate	1 fl oz	62	0	0	15	15	0	4	0
Fruit punch juice drink, frozen concentrate, prepared with water	1 cup	124	0	0	30	30	0	12	0
Fruit punch-flavor drink, powder, without added sodium	2 tbsp	97	0	0	25	25	0	11	0
Fruit punch-flavor drink, powder, without added sodium, prepared with water	1 cup	97	0	0	25	25	0	10	0
Fruit-flavored thirst quencher beverage, low calorie	1 cup	26	0	0	7	7	0	84	0
GRAPE									
Grape drink, canned	1 cup	113	0	0	29	29	0	15	0
Grape juice drink, canned	1 cup	125	0	0	32	32	0	3	0

Description	Serving Size	Cal	Prot (g)	Fat (g)	Carbs (g)	Net Carb(g)	Fiber (g)	Sod (mg)	Chol (mg)
FRUIT DRINKS & JUICE (continued)									
Grape juice, canned or bottled, unsweetened, without added vitamin C	1 cup	154	1	0	38	38	0	8	0
Grape juice, frozen concentrate, sweetened, diluted with 3 volume water, with added vitamin C	1 cup	128	0	0	32	32	0	5	0
Grape juice, frozen concentrate, sweetened, undiluted, with added vitamin C	1 can	387	1	0	96	95	1	15	0
GRAPEFRUIT									
Grapefruit juice, pink, raw	1 cup	96	1	0	23	N.A.	N.A.	2	0
Grapefruit juice, white, canned, sweetened	1 cup	115	1	0	28	28	0	5	0
Grapefruit juice, white, canned, unsweetened	1 cup	94	1	0	22	22	0	2	0
Grapefruit juice, white, frozen concentrate, unsweetened, diluted with 3 volume water	1 cup	101	1	0	24	24	0	2	0
Grapefruit juice, white, frozen concentrate, unsweetened, undiluted	1 can	302	4	0	72	71	1	6	0
Grapefruit juice, white, raw	1 cup	96	1	0	23	22	0	2	0
KRAFT									
CAPRI SUN ALL NATURAL Juice Drink Fruit Punch, ready-to-drink	1 serving	99	0	0	26	26	0	21	0
COUNTRY TIME Lemonade Mix, with vitamin C	1 portion	64	0	0	18	N.A.	N.A.	13	0
COUNTRY TIME Sugar Free Pink Lemonade Mix, with vitamin C	1 portion	5	0	0	2	N.A.	N.A.	0	0
CRYSTAL LIGHT Sugar Free Low Calorie Soft Drink Mix Lemonade, with aspartame and acesulfame potassium sweetener, powder	1 serving	5	0	0	0	0	0	1	0
KOOL-AID BURSTS Soft Drink Tropical Punch, ready-to-drink	1 serving	90	0	0	24	24	0	29	0
KOOL-AID SPLASH Soft Drink Grape Berry Punch, ready-to-drink	1 serving	116	0	0	31	31	0	35	0
KOOL-AID Sugar Free Mix, with aspartame and vitamin C, cherry flavor	1/8 envelope	3	0	0	1	N.A.	N.A.	5	0
KOOL-AID Sugar Sweetened Soft Drink Mix Tropical Punch, powder	1 serving	64	0	0	16	16	0	2	0
KOOL-AID Unsweetened Soft Drink Mix Tropical Punch, powder	1 serving	1	0	0	0	0	0	15	0

Description	Serving Size	Cal	Prot (g)	Fat (g)	Carbs (g)	Net Carb(g)	Fiber (g)	Sod (mg)	Chol (mg)
LEMON									
Lemon juice, canned or bottled	1 cup	51	1	0	16	15	1	51	0
Lemon juice, frozen, unsweetened, single strength	1 cup	54	1	0	16	15	1	2	0
Lemon juice, raw	1 cup	61	1	0	21	20	1	2	0
LEMON-LIME									
GATORADE Lemon Lime Flavor Mix, powder	3/4 scoop	58	0	0	15	N.A.	N.A.	96	0
LEMONADE									
Frozen concentrate, pink	1 fl oz	66	0	0	17	17	0	1	0
Frozen concentrate, pink, prepared with water	1 cup	99	0	0	26	26	0	7	0
Frozen concentrate, white	1 fl oz	66	0	0	17	17	0	1	0
Frozen concentrate, white, prepared with water	1 cup	99	0	0	26	26	0	7	0
Lemonade-flavor drink, powder	1 cup	902	0	0	230	230	0	98	0
Lemonade-flavor drink, powder, prepared with water	1 cup	112	0	0	29	29	0	19	0
Low calorie, with aspartame, powder	1 packet	40	0	0	10	10	0	1	0
Low calorie, with aspartame, powder, prepared with water	1 cup	5	0	0	1	1	0	7	0
Powder	1 cup	820	0	0	215	215	0	50	0
Powder, prepared with water	1 cup	103	0	0	27	27	0	13	0
LIME									
Lime juice, canned or bottled, unsweetened	1 cup	52	1	0	16	15	1	39	0
Lime juice, raw	1 cup	66	1	0	22	21	1	2	0
LIMEADE									
Limeade, frozen concentrate	1 fl oz	68	0	0	18	18	0	0	0
Limeade, frozen concentrate, prepared with water	1 cup	101	0	0	27	27	0	5	0
MIXED FRUIT									
Citrus fruit juice drink, frozen concentrate	1 fl oz	57	0	0	14	14	0	1	0
Citrus fruit juice drink, frozen concentrate, prepared with water	1 cup	114	1	0	29	29	0	7	0
Orange and apricot juice drink, canned	1 cup	128	1	0	32	32	0	5	0
Orange-grapefruit juice, canned, unsweetened	1 cup	106	1	0	25	25	0	7	0

Description	Serving Size	Cal	Prot (g)	Fat (g)	Carbs (g)	Net Carb(g)	Fiber (g)	Sod (mg)	Chol (mg)
FRUIT DRINKS & JUICE (continued)									
Pineapple and grapefruit juice drink, canned	1 cup	118	1	0	29	29	0	35	0
Pineapple and orange juice drink, canned	1 cup	125	3	0	30	29	0	8	0
ORANGE									
Orange drink, breakfast type, with juice and pulp, frozen concentrate	1 fl oz	56	0	0	14	14	0	9	0
Orange drink, breakfast type, with juice and pulp, frozen concentrate, prepared with water	1 cup	113	0	0	28	28	0	25	0
Orange drink, canned	1 cup	126	0	0	32	32	0	40	0
Orange juice, California, chilled, includes from concentrate	1 cup	110	2	0	25	N.A.	N.A.	2	0
Orange juice, canned, unsweetened	1 cup	105	1	0	25	24	0	5	0
Orange juice, chilled, includes from concentrate	1 cup	110	2	0	25	25	0	2	0
Orange juice, frozen concentrate, unsweetened, diluted with 3 volume water	1 cup	112	2	0	27	26	0	2	0
Orange juice, frozen concentrate, unsweetened, undiluted	1 cup	452	7	0	108	106	2	9	0
Orange juice, raw	1 cup	112	2	0	26	25	0	2	0
Orange-flavor drink, breakfast type, low calorie, powder	1 fl oz	117	0	0	16	16	0	3	0
Orange-flavor drink, breakfast type, powder	1 serving	88	0	0	22	22	0	2	0
Orange-flavor drink, breakfast type, powder, prepared with water	1 cup	114	0	0	29	29	0	12	0
Orange-flavor drink, breakfast type, with pulp, frozen concentrate	1 fl oz	61	0	0	15	15	0	8	0
Orange-flavor drink, breakfast type, with pulp, frozen concentrate, prepared with water	1 cup	122	0	0	30	30	0	22	0
Orange-flavor drink, KRAFT, TANG Drink Mix	2 tbsp	92	0	0	25	25	0	2	0
Orange-flavor drink, KRAFT, TANG SUGAR FREE Low Calorie Drink Mix	1 portion	5	0	0	2	2	0	2	0
PASSION-FRUIT									
Passion-fruit juice, purple, raw	1 cup	126	1	0	34	33	0	15	0
Passion-fruit juice, yellow, raw	1 cup	148	2	0	36	35	0	15	0

Description	Serving Size	Cal	Prot (g)	Fat (g)	Carbs (g)	Net Carb(g)	Fiber (g)	Sod (mg)	Chol (mg)
PAPAYA									
Papaya nectar, canned	1 cup	143	0	0	36	35	2	13	0
PEACH									
Peach nectar, canned, with added ascorbic acid	1 cup	134	1	0	35	33	1	17	0
Peach nectar, canned, without added ascorbic acid	1 cup	134	1	0	35	33	1	17	0
PEAR									
Pear nectar, canned, with added ascorbic acid	1 cup	150	0	0	39	38	2	10	0
Pear nectar, canned, without added ascorbic acid	1 cup	150	0	0	39	38	2	10	0
PINEAPPLE									
Pineapple juice, canned, unsweetened, without added ascorbic acid	1 cup	140	1	0	34	34	1	3	0
Pineapple juice, canned, with added ascorbic acid, unsweetened	1 cup	140	1	0	34	34	1	3	0
Pineapple juice, frozen concentrate, unsweetened, diluted with 3 volume water	1 cup	130	1	0	32	31	1	3	0
Pineapple juice, frozen concentrate, unsweetened, undiluted	1 can	387	3	0	96	94	2	6	0
PRUNE									
Prune juice, canned	1 cup	182	2	0	45	42	3	10	0
TANGERINE									
Tangerine juice, canned, sweetened	1 cup	125	1	0	30	29	0	2	0
Tangerine juice, frozen concentrate, sweetened, diluted with 3 volume water	1 cup	111	1	0	27	N.A.	N.A.	2	0
Tangerine juice, frozen concentrate, sweetened, undiluted	1 can	345	3	0	83	82	1	6	0
Tangerine juice, raw	1 cup	106	1	0	25	24	0	2	0

Gelatin

Description	Serving Size	Cal	Prot (g)	Fat (g)	Carbs (g)	Net Carb(g)	Fiber (g)	Sod (mg)	Chol (mg)
Gelatin, drinking, orange-flavor, powder	1 packet	66	6	0	11	11	0	29	0
Gelatin, drinking, orange-flavor, powder, prepared with water	1 packet	67	6	0	10	10	0	33	0
NABISCO, KNOX DRINKING GELATIN, with aspartame, low calorie, powder	1 envelope	41	7	0	3	N.A.	N.A.	18	0

Description	Serving Size	Cal	Prot (g)	Fat (g)	Carbs (g)	Net Carb(g)	Fiber (g)	Sod (mg)	Chol (mg)
Malt Beverages									
Malt beverage	1 cup	142	1	0	32	32	0	31	0
Malted drink mix, chocolate, powder	1 serving	79	1	1	18	18	0	53	1
Malted drink mix, chocolate, powder, prepared with whole milk	1 cup	228	9	8	30	30	0	172	34
Malted drink mix, chocolate, with added nutrients, powder	1 cup	279	4	3	66	65	1	463	4
Malted drink mix, chocolate, with added nutrients, powder, prepared with whole milk	1 cup	225	9	8	29	29	0	244	34
Malted drink mix, natural, powder	1 serving	87	2	2	16	16	0	104	4
Malted drink mix, natural, powder, prepared with whole milk	1 cup	236	10	9	27	27	0	223	37
Malted drink mix, natural, with added nutrients, powder	1 serving	80	2	1	17	17	0	85	4
Malted drink mix, natural, with added nutrients, powder, prepared with whole milk	1 cup	231	10	8	28	28	0	204	34
Milk Drinks									
Dairy drink mix, chocolate, reduced calorie, with aspartame, powder	1 packet	63	5	1	11	10	0	166	2
Dairy drink mix, chocolate, reduced calorie, with aspartame, powder, prepared with water	6 fl oz	63	5	1	11	10	0	171	2
Eggnog-flavor mix, powder	2 tsp	111	0	0	28	27	1	44	7
Eggnog-flavor mix, powder, prepared with whole milk	1 cup	261	8	8	39	38	1	163	33
Rice beverage, RICE DREAM, canned	1 cup	120	0	2	25	25	0	86	0
Shake, fast food, chocolate	1 cup	211	6	6	34	33	1	161	22
Shake, fast food, strawberry	10 fl oz	320	10	8	53	52	1	235	31
Shake, fast food, vanilla	1 cup	184	6	5	30	29	1	136	18
Strawberry-flavor beverage mix, powder	1 serving	85	0	0	22	22	0	8	0
Strawberry-flavor beverage mix, powder, prepared with whole milk	1 cup	234	8	8	33	33	0	128	32
Teas									
Herb, chamomile, brewed	1 cup	2	0	0	0	0	0	2	0
Herb, other than chamomile, brewed	1 cup	2	0	0	0	0	0	2	0
Instant, sweetened with sodium saccharin, lemon-flavored, powder	2 tsp	5	0	0	1	1	0	17	0

Description	Serving Size	Cal	Prot (g)	Fat (g)	Carbs (g)	Net Carb(g)	Fiber (g)	Sod (mg)	Chol (mg)
Instant, sweetened with sodium saccharin, lemon-flavored, prepared	1 cup	5	0	0	1	1	0	24	0
Instant, sweetened with sugar, lemon-flavored, with added ascorbic acid, powder	1 cup	701	1	0	178	178	0	9	0
Instant, sweetened with sugar, lemon-flavored, with added ascorbic acid, powder, prepared	1 cup	88	0	0	22	22	0	8	0
Instant, sweetened with sugar, lemon-flavored, without added ascorbic acid, powder	1 cup	701	1	0	178	178	0	9	0
Instant, sweetened with sugar, lemon-flavored, without added ascorbic acid, powder, decaffeinated	1 cup	701	1	0	178	178	0	9	0
Instant, sweetened with sugar, lemon-flavored, without added ascorbic acid, powder, prepared	1 cup	88	0	0	22	22	0	8	0
Instant, unsweetened, lemon-flavored, powder	1 tsp	4	0	0	1	1	0	7	0
Instant, unsweetened, lemon-flavored, powder, prepared	1 cup	5	0	0	1	1	0	14	0
Instant, unsweetened, powder	1 tsp	2	0	0	0	0	0	1	0
Instant, unsweetened, powder, prepared	1 cup	2	0	0	0	0	0	7	0
KRAFT, CRYSTAL LIGHT Sugar Free Low Calorie Iced Tea Mix, with aspartame, powder	1 serving	3	0	0	0	0	0	2	0
NESTLE, NESTEA Ice Tea, Lemon Flavor, ready-to-drink	1 cup	89	0	0	20	20	0	0	0
Plain, brewed	1 cup	2	0	0	1	1	0	7	0

Vegetable Juice

Description	Serving Size	Cal	Prot (g)	Fat (g)	Carbs (g)	Net Carb(g)	Fiber (g)	Sod (mg)	Chol (mg)
Clam and tomato juice, canned	1 fl oz	14	0	0	3	3	0	109	0
Tomato juice, canned, with salt added	1 cup	41	2	0	10	9	1	877	0
Tomato juice, canned, without salt added	1 cup	41	2	0	10	8	2	24	0
Vegetable juice cocktail, canned	1 cup	46	2	0	11	9	2	653	0
Carrot juice, canned	1 cup	94	2	0	22	20	2	68	0

Description	Serving Size	Cal	Prot (g)	Fat (g)	Carbs (g)	Net Carb(g)	Fiber (g)	Sod (mg)	Chol (mg)
Bread Crumbs									
Dry, grated, plain	1 cup	427	14	5	78	70	3	931	0
Dry, grated, plain	1 oz	112	4	1	21	70	1	244	0
Dry, grated, seasoned	1 cup	440	17	3	84	66	5	3180	1
Dry, grated, seasoned	1 oz	104	4	1	20	66	1	751	0
White, commercially prepared (includes soft bread crumbs)	1 cup, crumbs	120	4	1	22	47	1	242	0
White, commercially prepared, low sodium no salt	1 cup, crumbs	120	4	1	22	47	1	12	0
White, commercially prepared, toasted	1 cup, crumbs	132	4	2	24	52	1	266	0
Breading									
KRAFT FOODS, SHAKE 'N' BAKE ORIGINAL RECIPE, Coating for Pork, dry	1 serving	106	2	0	22	N.A.	N.A.	795	0
Croutons									
Plain	1 cup	122	4	2	22	68	2	209	0
Seasoned	1 cup	186	4	7	25	59	2	495	3
HIDDEN VALLEY RANCH, SALAD CRISPINS Italian Style, Parmesan	1 serving	30	1	1	5	N.A.	N.A.	80	0
PEPPERIDGE FARM Classic Style, seasoned	1 serving	33	1	0	4	N.A.	N.A.	97	0
White, commercially prepared (includes soft bread crumbs)	1 cup, cubes	93	3	1	17	47	1	188	0
White, commercially prepared, low sodium no salt	1 cup, cubes	93	3	1	17	47	1	9	0
White, commercially prepared, toasted	1 cup, cubes	123	4	1	23	52	1	249	0
Hush Puppies									
Hush puppies, prepared from recipe	1 oz	96	2	4	13	43	1	189	13
Rolls									
DINNER									
Egg	1 roll	107	3	2	18	48	1	191	18
Oat bran	1 roll	78	3	1	13	36	1	136	0
Plain, commercially prepared (includes brown-and-serve)	1 roll	129	4	3	22	47	1	224	0
Plain, prepared from recipe, made with low fat (2%) milk	1 large	136	4	3	23	52	1	178	15
Rye	1 medium	103	4	1	19	48	2	321	0
Wheat	1 roll	77	2	2	13	42	1	96	0

Description	Serving Size	Cal	Prot (g)	Fat (g)	Carbs (g)	Net Carb(g)	Fiber (g)	Sod (mg)	Chol (mg)
ROLLS (continued)									
Whole-wheat	1 roll	359	12	6	69	44	10	645	0
HAMBURGER OR HOTDOG									
Mixed-grain	1 roll	113	4	2	19	41	2	197	0
Plain	1 roll	123	4	2	22	48	1	241	0
Reduced-calorie	1 roll	84	4	1	18	36	3	190	0
SWEET ROLLS									
Cheese	1 roll	238	5	11	29	43	1	236	50
Cinnamon, commercially prepared with raisins	1 large	309	5	13	42	49	2	318	55
Cinnamon, refrigerated dough with frosting	1 roll	100	2	3	15	N.A.	N.A.	230	0
Cinnamon, refrigerated dough with frosting, baked	1 roll	109	2	4	17	N.A.	N.A.	250	0
PILLSBURY Cinnamon Rolls with Icing, refrigerated dough	1 serving	150	2	1	24	N.A.	N.A.	334	0
French	1 roll	105	3	1	19	47	1	231	0
Hard (includes Kaiser)	1 roll	167	6	2	30	50	1	310	0
WONDER Hamburger Rolls	1 serving	117	3	2	22	48	1	256	0

Stuffing

Description	Serving Size	Cal	Prot (g)	Fat (g)	Carbs (g)	Net Carb(g)	Fiber (g)	Sod (mg)	Chol (mg)
BEST FOODS, BROWNBERRY Sage and Onion Stuffing Mix, dry	1 serving	255	9	3	47	65	4	1126	0
Cornbread, dry mix	1 oz	110	3	1	22	62	4	364	0
Cornbread, dry mix, prepared	1 oz	51	1	2	6	19	1	129	0
CPC FOOD SERVICE, OROWEAT Seasoned Dressing Mix, dry	1 serving	107	4	0	22	67	1	284	0
Dry mix	1 oz	109	3	1	22	73	1	451	0
Dry mix, prepared	1 oz	50	1	2	6	19	1	154	0
KRAFT, STOVE TOP Stuffing Mix Chicken Flavor	1 serving	107	4	0	20	71	1	429	1

Tacos & Tortillas

Description	Serving Size	Cal	Prot (g)	Fat (g)	Carbs (g)	Net Carb(g)	Fiber (g)	Sod (mg)	Chol (mg)
Taco shells, baked	1 large	98	2	4	13	55	2	77	0
Taco shells, baked, without added salt	1 medium	61	1	3	8	55	1	2	0
Tortillas, ready-to-bake or -fry, corn	1 tortilla	58	1	1	12	41	1	42	0
Tortillas, ready-to-bake or -fry, corn, without added salt	1 tortilla	58	1	1	12	41	1	3	0
Tortillas, ready-to-bake or -fry, flour	1 tortilla	104	3	2	18	52	1	153	0

Description	Serving Size	Cal	Prot (g)	Fat (g)	Carbs (g)	Net Carb(g)	Fiber (g)	Sod (mg)	Chol (mg)
Banana, prepared from recipe, made with margarine	1 oz	92	1	3	15	54	0	86	12
Boston brown, canned	1 slice	88	2	0	19	39	2	284	0
Bread sticks, plain	1 stick	21	1	0	3	65	0	33	0
CAMPIONE D'ITALIA FOODS, CAMPIONE Garlic Bread, frozen	1 serving	101	2	1	12	40	1	154	0
Cornbread, dry mix, (includes corn muffin mix)	1 oz	119	2	3	20	63	2	315	1
Cornbread, dry mix, prepared	1 oz	89	2	3	14	46	1	221	17
Cornbread, prepared from recipe, made with low fat (2%) milk	1 oz	75	2	2	12	N.A.	N.A.	187	11
Cracked-wheat	1 oz	74	2	1	14	44	2	153	0
Egg	1 slice	115	4	2	19	46	1	197	20
Egg, toasted	1 slice	117	4	2	19	50	1	200	21
French or Vienna (includes sourdough)	1 slice	175	6	2	33	49	2	390	0
French or Vienna, toasted (includes sourdough)	1 slice	176	6	2	33	53	2	390	0
Indian (Navajo), fried	1 piece	526	11	14	85	52	3	1112	0
Irish soda, prepared from recipe	1 oz	82	2	1	16	53	1	113	5
Italian	1 slice	81	3	1	15	47	1	175	0
Mixed-grain (includes whole-grain, 7-grain)	1 slice	80	3	1	15	40	2	156	0
Mixed-grain, toasted (includes whole-grain, 7-grain)	1 slice	79	3	1	15	44	2	154	0
Oat bran	1 slice	71	3	1	12	35	1	122	0
Oat bran, toasted	1 slice	70	3	1	12	39	1	121	0
Oatmeal	1 slice	73	2	1	13	45	1	162	0
Oatmeal, toasted	1 slice	73	2	1	13	48	1	163	0
PEPPERIDGE FARM Crusty Italian Bread, Garlic	1 serving	186	4	8	21	N.A.	N.A.	200	6
PILLSBURY, Crusty French Loaf, refrigerated dough	1 serving	154	6	1	29	N.A.	N.A.	389	0
Pita, white	1 pita	165	5	0	33	54	1	322	0
Pita, whole-wheat	1 pita	170	6	1	35	48	5	340	0
Protein (includes gluten)	1 slice	47	2	0	8	41	1	104	0
Protein, toasted (includes gluten)	1 slice	46	2	0	8	45	1	102	0
Pumpernickel	1 slice	65	2	1	12	41	2	174	0
Pumpernickel, toasted	1 slice	80	3	1	15	45	2	214	0
Raisin	1 slice	88	3	1	17	48	1	125	0
Raisin, toasted	1 slice	86	2	1	17	52	1	123	0

Description	Serving Size	Cal	Prot (g)	Fat (g)	Carbs (g)	Net Carb(g)	Fiber (g)	Sod (mg)	Chol (mg)
BREADS (continued)									
Reduced-calorie, oat bran	1 slice	46	2	1	9	29	3	81	0
Reduced-calorie, oat bran, toasted	1 slice	45	2	1	9	35	3	79	0
Reduced-calorie, oatmeal	1 slice	48	2	1	10	N.A.	N.A.	89	0
Reduced-calorie, rye	1 slice	47	2	0	9	29	3	93	0
Reduced-calorie, wheat	1 slice	46	2	0	10	32	3	118	0
Reduced-calorie, white	1 slice	48	2	1	10	35	2	104	0
Rice bran	1 slice	66	2	1	12	39	1	119	0
Rice bran, toasted	1 slice	66	2	1	12	42	1	120	0
Rye	1 slice	83	3	1	15	43	2	211	0
Rye, toasted	1 slice	82	3	1	15	47	2	210	0
Wheat (includes wheat berry)	1 slice	65	2	1	12	43	1	133	0
Wheat bran	1 slice	89	3	1	17	44	1	175	0
Wheat germ	1 slice	73	3	1	14	46	1	155	0
Wheat germ, toasted	1 slice	73	3	1	14	52	1	155	0
Wheat, toasted (includes wheat berry)	1 slice	65	2	1	12	46	1	132	0
White, commercially prepared, toasted, low sodium no salt	1 slice	67	2	1	13	N.A.	N.A.	7	0
White, prepared from recipe, made with low fat (2%) milk	1 slice	120	3	2	21	48	1	151	1
White, prepared from recipe, made with nonfat dry milk	1 slice	121	3	1	24	52	1	148	0
Whole-wheat, commercially prepared	1 slice	69	3	1	13	39	2	148	0
Whole-wheat, commercially prepared, toasted	1 slice	69	3	1	13	44	2	148	0
Whole-wheat, prepared from recipe	1 slice	128	4	2	24	45	3	159	0
Whole-wheat, prepared from recipe, toasted	1 slice	128	4	2	24	50	3	160	0

Description	Serving Size	Cal	Prot (g)	Fat (g)	Carbs (g)	Net Carb(g)	Fiber (g)	Sod (mg)	Chol (mg)
Bagels									
LENDER'S									
Bagel Shop Blueberry Bagels	1 bagel	264	11	1	53	51	2	427	0
Big'N Crusty Blueberry Bagel	1 serving	214	8	1	46	52	2	409	0
Premium Refrigerated Blueberry Bagels	1 bagel	209	8	1	43	50	2	409	0
Cinnamon-raisin	1 bagel	156	6	1	31	53	1	184	0
Egg	1 bagel	158	6	1	30	51	1	288	14
Oat bran	1 bagel	145	6	1	30	50	2	289	0
Plain (includes onion, poppy, sesame)	1 bagel	157	6	1	30	51	1	304	0
Biscuits									
PILLSBURY									
Buttermilk Biscuits, Artificial Flavor, refrigerated dough	1 serving	154	5	1	30	N.A.	N.A.	547	0
GRANDS Buttermilk Biscuits, refrigerated dough	1 serving	195	4	2	25	N.A.	N.A.	605	0
HUNGRY JACK Buttermilk Biscuits, Artificial Flavor, refrigerated dough	1 serving	108	2	4	14	N.A.	N.A.	343	0
MARTHA WHITE'S Buttermilk Biscuit Mix, dry	1 biscuit	171	3	5	26	N.A.	N.A.	504	0
Mixed grain, refrigerated dough	1 biscuit	116	3	2	21	N.A.	N.A.	295	0
Plain or buttermilk, commercially baked	1 biscuit	127	2	5	17	47	0	368	0
Plain or buttermilk, dry mix	1 cup	488	9	17	72	61	2	1455	2
Plain or buttermilk, dry mix, prepared	1 oz	95	2	3	14	47	1	271	1
Plain or buttermilk, prepared from recipe	1 biscuit	358	7	16	45	43	2	586	3
Plain or buttermilk, refrigerated dough, higher fat	1 biscuit	95	2	4	13	42	0	332	0
Plain or buttermilk, refrigerated dough, higher fat, baked	1 biscuit	93	2	4	13	46	0	325	0
Plain or buttermilk, refrigerated dough, lower fat	1 biscuit	59	2	1	11	46	0	287	0
Plain or buttermilk, refrigerated dough, lower fat, baked	1 biscuit	63	2	1	12	54	0	305	0
Cereals (Cold)									
GENERAL MILLS									
APPLE CINNAMON CHEERIOS	3/4 cup	118	2	1	25	78	2	150	0
BASIC 4	1 cup	201	4	3	42	70	3	323	0
BERRY BERRY KIX	3/4 cup	120	1	1	26	87	0	185	0

Description	Serving Size	Cal	Prot (g)	Fat (g)	Carbs (g)	Net Carb (g)	Fiber (g)	Sod (mg)	Chol (mg)
CEREALS (COLD) (continued)									
BOO BERRY	1 cup	116	1	0	27	90	0	214	0
BRAN CHEX	1 cup	156	5	1	39	64	8	345	0
CHEERIOS	1 cup	110	3	1	23	67	3	284	0
CINNAMON TOAST CRUNCH	3/4 cup	124	2	2	24	74	2	210	0
COCOA PUFFS	1 cup	119	1	1	27	88	0	181	0
COOKIE CRISP	1 cup	120	2	1	26	86	0	207	0
CORN CHEX	1 cup	113	2	0	26	84	1	289	0
COUNT CHOCULA	1 cup	117	1	1	26	87	0	209	0
Country Corn Flakes	1 cup	114	2	0	26	85	0	284	0
FIBER ONE	1/2 cup	62	3	0	24	33	14	143	0
FRANKENBERRY	1 cup	117	1	0	27	90	0	209	0
FROSTED WHEATIES	3/4 cup	110	2	0	26	83	2	211	0
GOLDEN GRAHAMS	3/4 cup	116	2	1	26	83	1	275	0
HONEY NUT CHEERIOS	1 cup	115	3	1	24	76	2	259	0
HONEY NUT CHEX	3/4 cup	116	2	1	26	87	0	224	0
HONEY NUT CLUSTERS	1 cup	213	5	3	43	71	4	239	0
KABOOM	1 1/4 cup	118	3	1	24	76	2	275	0
KIX	1 1/3 cup	114	2	0	26	84	1	263	0
LUCKY CHARMS	1 cup	116	2	1	25	80	1	203	0
MULTI-BRAN CHEX	1 cup	129	2	3	24	77	1	130	0
Multi-Grain CHEERIOS	1 cup	108	3	1	24	72	3	201	0
NATURE VALLEY LOW FAT FRUIT GRANOLA	2/3 cup	212	5	2	44	73	3	205	0
OATMEAL CRISP WITH ALMONDS	1 cup	219	6	4	42	68	4	250	0
OATMEAL CRISP WITH APPLES	1 cup	205	4	1	46	76	4	282	0
Oatmeal Raisin Crisp	1 cup	204	4	2	44	73	4	224	0
RAISIN NUT BRAN	1 cup	209	5	3	41	66	5	246	0
REESE'S PUFFS	3/4 cup	129	3	3	23	75	0	177	0
RICE CHEX	1 cup	178	4	0	46	70	8	486	0
Team CHEERIOS	1 cup	113	2	1	25	78	2	224	0
TOTAL Corn Flakes	1 1/3 cup	112	2	0	26	83	1	203	0
TOTAL Raisin Bran	1 cup	178	4	1	43	69	5	240	0
TRIX	1 cup	122	1	2	26	84	1	197	0
WHEAT CHEX	1 cup	104	3	1	24	70	3	269	0
WHEATIES	1 cup	110	3	1	24	72	2	222	0
WHEATIES Raisin Bran	1 cup	191	4	0	44	74	3	285	0
Whole Grain TOTAL	3/4 cup	105	3	0	24	71	3	199	0

Description	Serving Size	Cal	Prot (g)	Fat (g)	Carbs (g)	Net Carb(g)	Fiber (g)	Sod (mg)	Chol (mg)
HEARTLAND NATURAL									
Plain	1 cup	499	12	16	79	62	7	293	0
With Coconut	1 cup	463	11	16	71	61	7	213	0
With Raisins	1 cup	468	11	14	76	64	6	226	0
KELLOGG'S									
ALL-BRAN BRAN BUDS	1/3 cup	83	3	1	24	40	12	200	0
ALL-BRAN Original	1/2 cup	79	4	1	23	44	10	61	0
ALL-BRAN WITH EXTRA FIBER	1/2 cup	53	4	1	23	25	15	127	0
APPLE CINNAMON SQUARES MINI-WHEATS	3/4 cup	182	4	1	44	72	5	20	0
APPLE JACKS	1 cup	116	1	0	27	88	1	134	0
APPLE RAISIN CRISP	1 cup	185	3	0	47	77	4	373	0
APPLE-CINNAMON RICE KRISPIES	3/4 cup	112	2	0	27	88	0	223	0
BLUEBERRY SQUARES MINI-WHEATS	3/4 cup	182	4	1	44	71	5	20	0
CINNAMIN MINI BUNS	3/4 cup	115	1	1	27	87	1	208	0
COCOA FROSTED FLAKES	3/4 cup	120	1	0	28	89	0	208	0
COCOA KRISPIES	3/4 cup	120	2	1	27	87	0	210	0
Complete Oat Bran Flakes	3/4 cup	109	4	1	23	64	4	270	0
Complete Wheat Bran Flakes	3/4 cup	95	3	1	23	64	5	226	0
Corn Flakes	1 cup	102	2	0	24	84	1	298	0
CORN POPS	1 cup	115	6	0	22	69	1	250	0
CRACKLIN' OAT BRAN	3/4 cup	225	5	7	40	61	7	195	0
CRISPIX	1 cup	108	2	0	25	84	1	240	0
DOUBLE DIP CRUNCH	3/4 cup	115	1	0	27	90	0	176	0
FROOT LOOPS	1 cup	117	1	1	26	86	1	141	0
FROSTED BRAN	3/4 cup	101	2	0	25	74	3	206	0
FROSTED FLAKES	1 cup	118	1	0	28	90	0	123	0
FROSTED FLAKES	3/4 cup	119	1	0	28	89	1	200	0
FROSTED MINI-WHEATS, bite size	1 cup	187	5	1	45	71	6	2	0
FROSTED MINI-WHEATS, original	1 cup	173	5	1	42	72	5	2	0
FROSTED RICE KRISPIES	3/4 cup	113	1	0	27	89	0	219	0
FRUITY MARSHMALLOW KRISPIES	3/4 cup	113	1	0	27	89	0	179	0
HEALTHY CHOICE Multi-Grain Flakes	1 cup	104	3	0	25	75	3	174	0
HEALTHY CHOICE Toasted Brown Sugar Squares	1 1/4 cup	189	5	1	45	73	5	2	0
HEALTHY CHOICE, Almond Crunch with Raisins	1 cup	198	5	2	43	70	5	215	0
HONEY CRUNCH CORN FLAKES	3/4 cup	115	2	1	26	83	1	216	0

Description	Serving Size	Cal	Prot (g)	Fat (g)	Carbs (g)	Net Carb(g)	Fiber (g)	Sod (mg)	Chol (mg)
CEREALS (COLD) (continued)									
JUST RIGHT Fruit & Nut	1 cup	193	4	2	44	76	3	266	0
Low Fat Granola with Raisins	2/3 cup	202	5	3	44	73	3	124	0
Low Fat Granola without Raisins	1/2 cup	213	5	3	44	74	3	135	0
MUESLIX	2/3 cup	200	4	3	40	67	4	160	0
MUESLIX APPLE & ALMOND CRUNCH	3/4 cup	211	5	5	41	66	5	270	0
NUT & HONEY CRUNCH	1 1/4 cup	223	4	2	46	82	1	370	0
NUTRI-GRAIN WHEAT	3/4 cup	101	3	1	24	67	4	221	0
POP-TARTS CRUNCH FROSTED STRAWBERRY	3/4 cup	118	1	1	27	89	0	114	0
PRODUCT 19	1 cup	110	3	0	25	80	1	216	0
RAISIN BRAN	1 cup	186	6	1	47	64	8	354	0
RAISIN MINI-WHEATS	3/4 cup	187	4	1	43	69	5	3	0
RAZZLE DAZZLE RICE KRISPIES	3/4 cup	108	1	0	25	90	0	166	0
RICE KRISPIES	1 1/4 cup	117	2	0	27	87	0	291	0
RICE KRISPIES TREATS Cereal	3/4 cup	120	1	2	26	85	0	190	0
SMACKS	3/4 cup	103	2	1	24	84	1	51	0
SMART START Cereal	1 cup	183	3	1	43	81	2	313	0
SPECIAL K	1 cup	54	1	0	12	86	0	1	0
STRAWBERRY MINI-WHEATS	1 cup	187	4	1	43	70	5	17	0
TEMPTATIONS, FRENCH VANILLA ALMOND	3/4 cup	119	2	2	25	80	1	207	0
MALT-O-MEAL									
BERRY COLOSSAL CRUNCH	3/4 cup	120	1	1	26	83	1	220	0
COLOSSAL CRUNCH	3/4 cup	120	1	1	26	83	1	230	0
CORN BURSTS	1 cup	118	1	0	29	91	0	122	0
Crispy Rice	1 cup	125	2	0	29	86	0	320	0
MARSHMALLOW MATEYS	1 cup	115	2	1	25	79	1	211	0
TOASTY O'S	1 cup	112	3	2	22	66	3	284	0
TOOTIE FRUITIES	1 cup	125	2	1	28	85	1	149	0
POST									
100% BRAN Cereal	1/3 cup	83	4	0	23	50	8	121	0
BANANA NUT CRUNCH Cereal	1 cup	249	5	1	44	67	4	253	0
BLUEBERRY MORNING Cereal	1 1/4 cup	211	4	0	43	75	2	266	0
Bran Flakes	3/4 cup	96	3	1	24	63	5	220	0
Cocoa PEBBLES Cereal	3/4 cup	115	1	1	25	86	0	157	0
Frosted ALPHA-BITS Cereal	1 cup	130	3	0	27	79	1	212	0

Description	Serving Size	Cal	Prot (g)	Fat (g)	Carbs (g)	Net Carb(g)	Fiber (g)	Sod (mg)	Chol (mg)
Frosted Shredded Wheat Bite Size Cereal	1 cup	183	4	0	44	74	5	10	0
FRUIT & FIBRE Dates, Raisins & Walnuts Cereal	1 cup	212	4	0	42	67	5	280	0
Fruity PEBBLES Cereal	3/4 cup	108	1	0	24	87	0	158	0
GOLDEN CRISP Cereal	3/4 cup	107	1	0	25	91	0	41	0
GRAPE-NUTS Cereal	1/2 cup	208	6	0	47	73	5	354	0
GRAPE-NUTS Flakes	3/4 cup	106	3	0	24	73	3	140	0
GREAT GRAINS Crunchy Pecan Cereal	2/3 cup	216	5	1	38	64	4	214	0
GREAT GRAINS Raisin, Date & Pecan Cereal	2/3 cup	204	4	1	40	66	4	156	0
HONEY BUNCHES OF OATS Honey Roasted Cereal	3/4 cup	118	2	0	25	77	1	193	0
HONEY BUNCHES OF OATS with Almonds Cereal	3/4 cup	126	2	0	24	74	1	187	0
HONEYCOMB Cereal	1/3 cup	115	2	0	26	86	1	215	0
Marshmallow ALPHA-BITS Cereal	1 cup	115	2	0	25	85	0	206	0
OREO O'S Cereal	3/4 cup	112	1	0	22	74	1	128	0
RAISIN BRAN	1 cup	187	5	0	46	65	8	360	0
SHREDDED WHEAT	2 biscuits	156	5	0	38	71	5	3	0
THE ORIGINAL SHREDDED WHEAT 'N BRAN Cereal	1 1/4 cup	197	7	0	47	67	8	3	0
THE ORIGINAL SHREDDED WHEAT SPOON SIZE Cereal	1 cup	167	5	0	41	72	6	3	0
TOASTIES Corn Flakes	1 cup	101	2	0	24	82	1	266	0
QUAKER									
100% Natural Cereal with oats, honey, and raisins	1/2 cup	218	5	7	36	63	4	11	1
100% Natural Granola Oats and Honey	1/2 cup	213	5	8	33	61	4	13	0
APPLE ZAPS	3/4 cup	118	1	1	27	86	1	132	0
CAP'N CRUNCH	3/4 cup	107	1	1	23	82	1	208	0
CAP'N CRUNCH with CRUNCHBERRIES	3/4 cup	104	1	1	22	83	1	190	0
CAP'N CRUNCH'S PEANUT BUTTER CRUNCH	3/4 cup	112	2	2	22	77	1	204	0
CINNAMON OATMEAL SQUARES	1 cup	232	8	2	47	71	5	266	0
COCOA BLASTS	1 cup	129	1	1	29	86	1	133	0
CORN BLASTS	1 cup	133	1	2	28	83	1	240	0
CRUNCHY BRAN	3/4 cup	90	2	1	23	66	5	253	0
FRUITANGY OH!S	1 cup	122	2	1	27	85	1	152	0

Description	Serving Size	Cal	Prot (g)	Fat (g)	Carbs (g)	Net Carb(g)	Fiber (g)	Sod (mg)	Chol (mg)
CEREALS (COLD) (continued)									
HONEY GRAHAM OH!S	3/4 cup	112	1	2	23	82	1	178	0
Honey Nut Heaven	1 cup	191	5	2	39	73	3	166	0
KING VITAMAN	1 1/2 cup	120	2	1	26	80	1	260	0
KRETSCHMER Honey Crunch Wheat Germ	1 2/3 tbsp	52	4	1	8	48	1	2	0
Low Fat 100% Natural Granola with Raisins	1/2 cup	195	4	3	40	75	3	129	1
MARSHMALLOW SAFARI	3/4 cup	119	2	2	25	80	1	192	0
Oat Bran Cereal	1 1/4 cup	213	9	3	41	62	6	205	0
OAT CINNAMON LIFE	1 cup	122	2	2	24	79	1	248	0
OAT LIFE, plain	3/4 cup	121	3	1	25	72	2	174	0
OATMEAL SQUARES	1 cup	216	7	2	43	70	4	263	0
Puffed Rice	1 1/4 cup	124	2	0	29	85	0	354	0
Puffed Wheat	1 1/4 cup	55	2	0	11	67	1	1	0
RALSTON									
SUGAR FROSTED FLAKES	1 cup	149	2	0	34	88	1	247	0
GENERIC CEREALS									
Crispy rice	1 cup	111	2	0	25	87	0	206	0
Frosted Flakes	3/4 cup	117	1	0	28	87	1	281	0
Granola, homemade	1 cup	570	18	28	65	43	13	29	0
HONEYBRAN	1 cup	119	3	1	29	71	4	202	0
JUST RIGHT with Crunchy Nuggets	1 cup	204	4	1	46	79	3	338	0
LIFE, Cinnamon Oat	1 cup	190	4	2	40	75	3	220	0
Rice, puffed, fortified	1 cup	56	1	0	13	88	0	0	0
Rice, puffed, presweetened, fruit flavored, single brand	1 cup	173	2	0	41	91	0	284	0
SUGAR SPARKLED FLAKES, corn	1 cup	146	2	0	35	90	0	215	0
SUN COUNTRY Granola with Almonds	1/2 cup	266	7	6	38	62	3	19	0
SUN COUNTRY GRANOLA, RAISIN & DATE	1/2 cup	135	3	3	22	66	2	8	0
SWEET CRUNCH/QUISP	1 cup	109	1	1	23	83	1	194	0
TASTEEOS	1 cup	94	3	1	19	69	3	183	0
WAFFELOS	1 cup	122	2	0	26	N.A.	N.A.	125	0
Wheat germ, toasted, plain	1 cup	432	33	11	56	37	15	5	0
Wheat, puffed, fortified	1 cup	44	2	0	10	75	1	0	0
Wheat, shredded, plain, sugar and salt free	1 biscuit	80	3	0	19	72	3	0	0

Description	Serving Size	Cal	Prot (g)	Fat (g)	Carbs (g)	Net Carb (g)	Fiber (g)	Sod (mg)	Chol (mg)
Cereals (Hot)									
CREAM OF RICE									
Cooked with water, with salt	1 cup	127	2	0	28	11	0	422	0
Cooked with water, without salt	1 cup	127	2	0	28	11	0	2	0
Dry	1 tbsp	38	1	0	8	82	0	1	0
CREAM OF WHEAT									
Instant, dry	1 tbsp	42	1	0	9	72	0	2	0
Instant, prepared with water, with salt, (wheat)	1 cup	154	4	0	32	12	3	364	0
Instant, prepared with water, without salt	1 cup	154	4	0	32	12	3	7	0
Mix 'n' eat, apple, banana and maple flavored, dry	1 packet	132	2	0	29	79	1	241	0
Mix 'n' eat, apple, banana and maple flavored, prepared	1 packet	132	2	0	29	19	0	242	0
Mix 'n' eat, plain, prepared with water	1 packet	102	3	0	21	15	0	241	0
Mix 'n' eat, plain, dry	1 packet	102	3	0	21	73	1	241	0
Quick, cooked with water, with salt	1 cup	129	4	0	27	11	1	464	0
Quick, cooked with water, without salt	1 cup	129	4	0	27	11	1	139	0
Quick, dry	1 tbsp	40	1	0	8	72	0	43	0
Regular, cooked with water, with salt, (wheat)	1 cup	133	4	0	28	10	2	336	0
Regular, cooked with water, without salt	1 cup	133	4	0	28	10	2	3	0
Regular, dry	1 tbsp	39	1	0	8	73	0	1	0
MALTEX									
MALTEX, cooked with water, with salt	1 cup	179	6	0	40	15	3	189	0
MALTEX, cooked with water, without salt	1 cup	179	6	1	40	15	3	10	0
MALTEX, dry	1/4 cup	134	4	1	29	73	2	6	0
MALT-O-MEAL									
Chocolate, dry	1 tbsp	38	1	0	8	N.A.	N.A.	1	0
Plain and chocolate, cooked with water, with salt	1 cup	122	4	0	26	10	1	324	0
Plain and chocolate, cooked with water, without salt	1 cup	122	4	0	26	10	1	2	0
Plain, dry	1 tbsp	38	1	0	8	N.A.	N.A.	1	0
QUAKER									
Corn grits, instant, butter flavor, dry	1 packet	101	2	1	21	70	1	323	0

Description	Serving Size	Cal	Prot (g)	Fat (g)	Carbs (g)	Net Carb(g)	Fiber (g)	Sod (mg)	Chol (mg)
CEREALS (HOT) (continued)									
Corn grits, instant, cheddar cheese flavor, dry	1 packet	102	2	1	21	69	1	522	1
Corn grits, instant, cheddar cheese flavor, prepared with water	1 packet	20	0	0	4	13	0	102	0
Corn grits, instant, country bacon (imitation bacon bits), prepared with water	1 packet	94	3	0	21	14	1	331	0
Corn grits, instant, plain, dry	1 packet	96	2	0	22	74	1	305	0
Corn grits, instant, plain, prepared with water	1 cup	159	4	0	37	14	2	517	0
Corn grits, instant, with imitation bacon bits, dry	1 packet	98	3	0	22	72	1	341	0
Corn grits, instant, with imitation ham bits, dry	1 packet	95	3	0	21	70	1	493	0
Corn grits, instant, with imitation ham bits, prepared with water	1 packet	92	3	0	20	13	1	510	0
Creamy Wheat, farina, dry	1/4 cup	154	5	0	33	73	1	1	0
MOTHER'S Oat Bran, dry	1/2 cup	146	7	3	25	49	6	2	0
MultiGrain Oatmeal, dry	1/2 cup	133	5	1	29	61	5	1	0
Oatmeal, instant, apples and cinnamon, dry	1 packet	128	3	1	27	70	3	121	0
Oatmeal, instant, apples and cinnamon, prepared with boiling water	1 packet	125	3	1	26	16	3	121	0
Oatmeal, instant, low sodium, dry	1 packet	103	4	2	18	57	3	78	0
Oatmeal, instant, maple and brown sugar, dry	1 packet	160	4	2	33	70	3	240	0
Oatmeal, instant, maple and brown sugar, prepared with boiling water	1 packet	153	4	2	31	19	3	234	0
Oatmeal, instant, POWER RANGERS fruit punch flavor, dry	1 packet	149	4	2	31	70	3	165	0
Oatmeal, instant, raisins, dates and walnuts, dry	1 packet	135	3	2	27	67	2	237	0
QUICK 'N HEARTY, apple spice	1 packet	166	4	2	35	71	3	306	0
QUICK 'N HEARTY, brown sugar cinnamon	1 packet	155	4	2	31	68	3	255	0
QUICK 'N HEARTY, cinnamon double raisin	1 packet	169	4	2	35	68	3	275	0
QUICK 'N HEARTY, honey bran	1 packet	151	4	2	31	68	3	253	0
QUICK 'N HEARTY, regular flavor	1 packet	106	4	2	19	57	2	153	0
RALSTON									
Cooked with water, with salt	1 cup	134	6	0	28	9	6	476	0

Description	Serving Size	Cal	Prot (g)	Fat (g)	Carbs (g)	Net Carb(g)	Fiber (g)	Sod (mg)	Chol (mg)
Cooked with water, without salt	1 cup	134	6	1	28	9	6	5	0
Dry	1/4 cup	102	4	0	22	59	4	3	0
ROMAN MEAL									
Plain, cooked with water, with salt	1 cup	147	7	0	33	10	8	198	0
Plain, cooked with water, without salt	1 cup	147	7	0	33	10	8	2	0
Plain, dry	1 tbsp	19	1	0	4	54	1	0	0
With Oats, cooked with water, with salt	1 cup	170	7	0	34	11	8	540	0
With Oats, cooked with water, without salt	1 cup	170	7	0	34	11	7	10	0
WHEATENA									
Cooked with water	1 cup	136	5	1	29	9	7	5	0
Cooked with water, with salt	1 cup	136	5	0	29	9	7	578	0
Dry	1/4 cup	125	5	1	26	63	4	5	0
Corn grits, white, regular and quick, cooked with water, with salt	1 cup	145	3	0	31	13	0	540	0
Corn grits, white, regular and quick, cooked with water, without salt	1 cup	145	3	0	31	13	0	0	0
Corn grits, white, regular and quick, dry	1 tbsp	36	1	0	8	78	0	0	0
Corn grits, yellow, regular and quick, cooked with water, without salt	1 cup	145	3	0	31	13	0	0	0
Corn grits, yellow, regular and quick, cooked with water, without salt	1 cup	145	3	0	31	13	0	0	0
Corn grits, yellow, regular and quick, dry	1 tbsp	36	1	0	8	78	0	0	0
Farina, cooked with water, with salt,	1 cup	117	3	0	25	9	3	767	0
Farina, cooked with water, without salt	1 cup	117	3	0	25	9	3	0	0
Farina, dry	1 tbsp	40	1	0	9	76	0	0	0
MAYPO, cooked with water, with salt	1 cup	170	6	0	32	11	6	259	0
MAYPO, cooked with water, without salt	1 cup	170	6	2	32	11	6	10	0
MAYPO, dry	1/2 cup	181	6	0	34	61	5	9	0
Oats, instant, fortified, plain, dry	1 packet	103	4	1	18	53	3	283	0
Oats, instant, fortified, plain, prepared with water	1 cup, cooked	138	6	2	24	9	4	377	0
Oats, instant, fortified, with bran and raisins, dry	1 packet	158	5	0	30	N.A.	N.A.	247	0
Oats, instant, fortified, with bran and raisins, prepared with water	1 packet	158	5	0	30	13	5	248	0

Description	Serving Size	Cal	Prot (g)	Fat (g)	Carbs (g)	Net Carb(g)	Fiber (g)	Sod (mg)	Chol (mg)
CEREALS (HOT) (continued)									
Oats, instant, fortified, with cinnamon and spice, dry	1 packet	172	4	2	36	71	3	288	0
Oats, instant, fortified, with cinnamon and spice, prepared with water	1 cup	264	7	2	52	20	4	418	0
Oats, instant, fortified, with raisins and spice, dry	1 packet	154	4	2	32	68	3	247	0
Oats, instant, fortified, with raisins and spice, prepared with water	1 cup	245	6	2	48	19	3	343	0
Oats, regular and quick and instant, cooked with water, with salt	1 cup	145	6	2	25	9	4	374	0
Oats, regular and quick and instant, cooked with water, without salt	1 cup	145	6	2	25	9	4	2	0
Oats, regular and quick and instant, not fortified, dry	1/3 cup	104	4	1	18	56	3	1	0
Whole wheat hot natural cereal, cooked with water, with salt	1 cup	150	5	0	33	12	4	564	0
Whole wheat hot natural cereal, cooked with water, without salt	1 cup	150	5	1	33	12	4	0	0
Whole wheat hot natural cereal, dry	1/3 cup	106	3	0	23	66	3	1	0

English Muffins

Description	Serving Size	Cal	Prot (g)	Fat (g)	Carbs (g)	Net Carb(g)	Fiber (g)	Sod (mg)	Chol (mg)
BEST FOODS, THOMAS' English Muffins, plain	1 serving	132	5	4	26	N.A.	N.A.	210	0
Mixed-grain (includes granola)	1 muffin	155	6	1	31	44	2	275	0
Mixed-grain, toasted (includes granola)	1 muffin	156	6	1	31	47	2	276	0
Raisin-cinnamon (includes apple-cinnamon)	1 muffin	139	4	1	28	46	2	255	0
Raisin-cinnamon, toasted (includes apple-cinnamon)	1 muffin	137	4	1	28	50	2	253	0
Wheat	1 muffin	127	5	1	26	40	3	218	0
Wheat, toasted	1 muffin	126	5	1	25	44	3	216	0
Whole-wheat	1 muffin	134	6	1	27	34	4	420	0
Whole-wheat, toasted	1 muffin	135	6	1	27	37	4	422	0

French Toast

Description	Serving Size	Cal	Prot (g)	Fat (g)	Carbs (g)	Net Carb(g)	Fiber (g)	Sod (mg)	Chol (mg)
French toast, frozen, ready-to-heat	1 piece	126	4	3	19	31	1	292	48
French toast, prepared from recipe, made with low fat (2%) milk	1 slice	149	5	6	16	N.A.	N.A.	311	75

Description	Serving Size	Cal	Prot (g)	Fat (g)	Carbs (g)	Net Carb(g)	Fiber (g)	Sod (mg)	Chol (mg)
Muffins									
GENERAL MILLS									
BETTY CROCKER Wild Blueberry Muffin Mix, dry	1 serving	128	2	1	26	N.A.	N.A.	186	0
GOLD MEDAL Imitation Blueberry Muffin Mix, dry	1 serving	127	1	2	24	N.A.	N.A.	205	0
GENERIC MUFFINS									
Artificial Blueberry Muffin Mix, dry	1 muffin	126	1	2	24	N.A.	N.A.	236	0
Blueberry, commercially prepared	1 muffin	30	1	1	5	45	0	49	3
Blueberry, dry mix	1 package	1303	17	33	225	N.A.	N.A.	1951	0
Blueberry, prepared from recipe, made with low fat (2%) milk	1 muffin	162	4	6	23	N.A.	N.A.	251	21
Blueberry, toaster-type	1 muffin	103	2	3	18	52	1	158	2
Blueberry, toaster-type, toasted	1 muffin	103	2	3	18	55	1	158	2
CONTINENTAL MILLS, KRUSTEAZ Almond Poppyseed Muffin Mix, Artificially Flavored, dry	1 serving	167	2	1	30	N.A.	N.A.	242	0
Corn, commercially prepared	1 muffin	174	3	4	29	48	2	297	15
Corn, dry mix, prepared	1 oz	91	2	3	14	47	1	225	18
Corn, prepared from recipe, made with low fat (2%) milk	1 muffin	180	4	7	25	N.A.	N.A.	333	24
Corn, toaster-type	1 muffin	114	2	4	19	56	1	142	4
MARTHA WHITE'S Artificial Blueberry Muffin Mix	1 serving	162	2	2	30	N.A.	N.A.	343	0
Oat bran	1 muffin	154	4	4	28	44	3	224	0
Wheat bran, dry mix	1 oz	112	2	3	21	N.A.	N.A.	198	0
Wheat bran, toaster-type with raisins	1 muffin	106	2	3	19	45	3	178	6
Wheat bran, toaster-type with raisins, toasted	1 muffin	106	2	3	19	47	3	179	3
Pancakes & Waffles									
CONTINENTAL MILLS, KRUSTEAZ Buttermilk Mini Pancakes, frozen, ready to microwave	1 serving	116	4	1	22	N.A.	N.A.	290	0
KELLOGG'S									
EGGO Golden Oat Waffles	1 waffle, round	69	2	1	13	34	1	135	0
EGGO Lowfat Blueberry Nutri-Grain Waffles	1 waffle, round	73	2	1	15	39	1	207	0
EGGO Lowfat Homestyle Waffles	1 round waffle, (4" dia) (inc.frozen)	83	2	1	15	43	0	155	9

Description	Serving Size	Cal	Prot (g)	Fat (g)	Carbs (g)	Net Carb(g)	Fiber (g)	Sod (mg)	Chol (mg)
PANCAKES & WAFFLES (continued)									
EGGO Lowfat Nutri-Grain Waffles	1 waffle, round	71	2	1	14	37	1	215	0
EGGO, Banana Bread Waffles	1 serving	212	5	7	32	39	2	280	0

Pancakes

Description	Serving Size	Cal	Prot (g)	Fat (g)	Carbs (g)	Net Carb(g)	Fiber (g)	Sod (mg)	Chol (mg)
Plain, frozen, ready-to-heat (includes buttermilk)	1 pancake	82	2	1	16	42	1	183	3
Blueberry, prepared from recipe	1 pancake	84	2	3	11	N.A.	N.A.	157	21
Buckwheat, dry mix, incomplete	1 oz	96	3	1	20	63	2	393	0
Buttermilk, prepared from recipe	1 pancake	86	3	3	11	N.A.	N.A.	198	22
Plain, dry mix, complete (includes buttermilk)	1 oz	107	3	1	20	69	1	344	6
Pancakes, plain, dry mix, complete, prepared	1 pancake	74	2	1	14	35	0	239	5
Plain, dry mix, incomplete (includes buttermilk)	1 oz	101	3	0	21	68	2	371	0
Plain, dry mix, incomplete, prepared	1 pancake	83	3	3	11	27	1	192	27
Plain, prepared from recipe	1 pancake	86	2	3	11	N.A.	N.A.	167	22
Special dietary, dry mix	1 oz	99	3	0	21	N.A.	N.A.	129	0
Whole-wheat, dry mix, incomplete	1 oz	98	4	0	20	N.A.	N.A.	402	0
Whole-wheat, dry mix, incomplete, prepared	1 pancake	92	4	3	13	27	1	252	27

Waffles

Description	Serving Size	Cal	Prot (g)	Fat (g)	Carbs (g)	Net Carb(g)	Fiber (g)	Sod (mg)	Chol (mg)
AUNT JEMIMA Original Waffles, frozen	1 serving	197	5	2	30	N.A.	N.A.	563	12
Plain, frozen, ready-to-heat (includes buttermilk)	1 waffle, square	88	2	3	14	36	1	262	11
Plain, frozen, ready-to-heat, toasted (includes buttermilk)	1 waffle, round	87	2	2	13	38	1	260	8
Plain, prepared from recipe	1 waffle, round	218	6	10	25	N.A.	N.A.	383	52

Toaster Pastries

KELLOGG'S

Description	Serving Size	Cal	Prot (g)	Fat (g)	Carbs (g)	Net Carb(g)	Fiber (g)	Sod (mg)	Chol (mg)
LOW FAT POP TARTS, Blueberry	1 pastry	192	2	3	40	75	1	222	0
LOW FAT POP TARTS, Cherry	1 pastry	192	2	3	40	75	1	222	0
LOW FAT POP TARTS, Frosted apple cinnamon	1 pastry	191	2	3	40	76	1	206	0
LOW FAT POP TARTS, Frosted brown sugar cinnamon	1 pastry	188	2	3	39	77	1	210	0
LOW FAT POP TARTS, Frosted chocolate fudge	1 pastry	190	3	3	40	75	1	249	0

Description	Serving Size	Cal	Prot (g)	Fat (g)	Carbs (g)	Net Carb(g)	Fiber (g)	Sod (mg)	Chol (mg)
LOW FAT POP TARTS, Frosted strawberry	1 pastry	191	2	3	40	76	1	201	0
LOW FAT POP TARTS, Strawberry	1 pastry	192	2	3	40	75	1	220	0
POP TARTS, Apple cinnamon	1 pastry	205	2	5	37	71	1	174	0
POP TARTS, Blueberry	1 pastry	212	2	7	36	67	1	207	0
POP TARTS, Brown sugar cinnamon	1 pastry	219	3	9	32	63	1	214	0
POP TARTS, Cherry	1 pastry	204	2	5	37	70	1	220	0
POP TARTS, Frosted blueberry	1 pastry	203	2	5	37	71	1	207	0
POP TARTS, Frosted brown sugar cinnamon	1 pastry	211	3	7	34	67	1	185	0
POP TARTS, Frosted cherry	1 pastry	204	2	5	37	71	1	220	0
POP TARTS, Frosted chocolate fudge	1 pastry	201	3	5	37	71	1	203	0
POP TARTS, Frosted chocolate vanilla creme	1 pastry	203	3	5	37	70	1	229	0
POP TARTS, Frosted grape	1 pastry	203	2	5	38	71	1	198	0
POP TARTS, Frosted raspberry	1 pastry	205	2	6	37	71	1	211	0
POP TARTS, Frosted strawberry	1 pastry	203	2	5	38	71	1	169	0
POP TARTS, Frosted wild berry	1 pastry	210	2	5	39	72	1	168	0
POP TARTS, Frosted Wild Watermelon	1 pastry	210	2	5	39	72	1	168	0
POP TARTS, Milk chocolate	1 pastry	205	3	6	36	67	1	227	0
POP TARTS, S'mores	1 pastry	204	3	5	36	68	1	199	0
POP TARTS, Strawberry	1 pastry	205	2	6	37	70	1	185	0
Pop-Tarts Pastry Swirls, Apple Cinnamon Danish	1 pastry	256	3	11	37	58	1	190	0
Pop-Tarts Pastry Swirls, Cheese Danish	1 pastry	252	3	11	37	59	0	180	1
Pop Tarts Pastry Swirls, Strawberry Danish	1 pastry	254	3	11	37	58	1	170	0
GENERIC TOASTER PASTRIES									
FRANCHISE ASSOCIATES, HOWARD JOHNSON'S TOASTEES, Blueberry Toaster Muffins, frozen, ready to eat	1 pastry	235	5	2	32	N.A.	N.A.	408	21
Toaster pastries, brown-sugar-cinnamon	1 pastry	206	3	7	34	67	1	212	0
Toaster pastries, fruit (includes apple, blueberry, cherry, strawberry)	1 pastry	204	2	5	37	69	1	218	0

Description	Serving Size	Cal	Prot (g)	Fat (g)	Carbs (g)	Net Carb(g)	Fiber (g)	Sod (mg)	Chol (mg)
Fudge									
Chocolate marshmallow, with nuts, prepared-by-recipe	1 piece	96	1	4	15	67	0	21	5
Chocolate, prepared-from-recipe	1 piece	65	0	1	14	79	0	11	2
Chocolate, with nuts, prepared-from-recipe	1 piece	81	1	3	14	72	0	11	3
Vanilla with nuts	1 piece	62	0	2	11	75	0	9	2
Vanilla, prepared-from-recipe	1 piece	59	0	1	13	82	0	11	3
Candy Bars & Other Candies									
100 GRAND Bar	1 bar	200	2	8	30	69	1	89	8
5TH AVENUE Candy Bar	1 bar	280	5	12	38	64	1	94	3
AFTER EIGHT Mints	1 piece	29	0	1	6	75	0	1	0
ALMOND JOY Candy Bar	1 bar	93	1	5	12	54	1	29	1
BABY RUTH Bar	1 bar	164	3	8	22	62	1	77	1
BUTTERFINGER Bar	1 bar	216	6	8	30	63	1	89	0
Butterscotch	1 piece	24	0	0	6	95	0	22	1
CARAMELLO Candy Bar	1 bar	213	3	10	29	62	1	62	12
Caramels	1 piece	39	0	1	8	76	0	25	1
Caramels, chocolate-flavor roll	1 piece	25	0	0	6	87	0	6	0
Carob	1 oz	153	2	8	16	52	1	30	1
CHUNKY Bar	1 bar	173	3	10	20	52	2	19	4
Confectioner's coating, butterscotch	1 cup, chips	916	4	46	114	67	0	151	0
Confectioner's coating, peanut butter	1 cup, chips	835	31	47	75	37	14	420	0
Confectioner's coating, white	1 cup, chips	916	10	50	101	59	0	153	36
CRUNCH Bar and Dessert Topping	1 bar	209	2	10	26	63	1	53	5
DEMET'S TURTLES Candy	1 package	825	11	45	99	55	4	160	37
E.J. BRACH'S, BRACH'S STAR BRITES Peppermint Mints	3 pieces	59	0	0	15	N.A.	N.A.	6	0
Fondant, prepared-from-recipe	1 piece	57	0	0	15	93	0	6	0
Fudge, cake-type (includes trolley cakes)	1 cookie	73	1	1	16	76	1	40	0
GOOBERS Chocolate Covered Peanuts	1 package	200	5	12	19	43	2	16	4
Gumdrops, starch jelly pieces	1 cup	703	0	0	180	99	0	80	0
Hard	1 piece	24	0	0	6	98	0	2	0
HERSHEY'S GOLDEN ALMOND SOLITAIRES	1 package	444	9	29	37	43	3	44	10
HERSHEY'S POT OF GOLD Almond Bar	1 package	448	10	30	36	41	4	52	12
Jellybeans	10 small	40	0	0	10	93	0	3	0

Description	Serving Size	Cal	Prot (g)	Fat (g)	Carbs (g)	Net Carb(g)	Fiber (g)	Sod (mg)	Chol (mg)
CANDY BARS & OTHER CANDY (continued)									
Jellybeans	10 large	104	0	0	26	93	0	7	0
KIT KAT Wafer Bar	1 bar	216	3	10	27	62	1	32	3
KRACKEL Chocolate Bar	1 bar	218	3	12	25	59	1	57	8
M&M MARS, 3 MUSKETEERS Bar	1 bar	96	1	3	18	75	0	45	3
M&M MARS, MARS Almond Bar	1 bar	234	4	11	31	61	1	85	9
M&M MARS, MARS MILKY WAY Bar	1 bar	97	1	3	16	70	0	55	3
M&M MARS, SKITTLES Original Bite Size Candies	1 cup	830	0	8	186	91	0	33	0
M&M MARS, SNICKERS Bar	1 bar	273	5	14	34	57	1	152	7
M&M MARS, STARBURST Fruit Chews	1 package	166	0	3	35	85	0	24	0
M&M MARS, TWIX Caramel Cookie Bars	1 package	284	3	13	37	64	1	110	3
M&M MARS, TWIX Peanut Butter Cookie Bars	1 package	286	5	16	28	49	2	147	3
M&M's Milk Chocolate Candies	1 cup	1023	9	43	148	69	5	127	29
M&M's Mini Milk Chocolate Candies	1 serving	209	2	10	28	64	1	29	6
M&M's Peanut Chocolate Candies	1 cup	877	16	43	103	57	6	82	15
Marshmallows	1 cup	159	1	0	41	81	0	24	0
Milk chocolate	1 cup, chips	862	12	50	99	56	6	138	37
Milk chocolate coated peanuts	10 pieces	208	5	13	20	45	2	16	4
Milk chocolate coated raisins	10 pieces	39	0	1	7	64	0	4	0
Milk chocolate, with almonds	1 bar	231	4	14	23	47	3	33	8
Milk chocolate, with rice cereal	1 bar	223	3	11	29	60	1	65	9
MOUNDS Candy Bar	1 bar	91	1	5	11	53	1	28	0
MR. GOODBAR Chocolate Bar	1 bar	398	8	23	38	48	3	109	6
OH HENRY! Bar	1 bar	246	6	9	37	61	2	135	5
Peanut bar	1 bar	209	6	13	19	42	2	62	0
Peanut brittle, prepared-from-recipe	1 oz	128	2	5	20	67	1	128	4
RAISINETS Chocolate Covered Raisins	10 pieces	41	0	2	7	66	1	4	0
REESE'S Peanut Butter Cups	1 miniature	38	1	2	4	51	0	22	0
REESE'S Peanut Butter Cups	1 package	243	5	13	25	51	1	143	2
REESE'S PIECES Candy	1/4 cup	231	6	10	29	59	1	69	1
REESE'S PIECES Candy	10 pieces	39	1	2	5	59	0	12	0
ROLO Caramels in Milk Chocolate	1 roll	202	2	9	26	53	0	86	9
Semisweet chocolate	1 cup, chips	805	7	48	106	57	10	18	0
Semisweet chocolate, made with butter	1 cup, chips	811	7	48	108	58	10	19	31
Sesame crunch	1 oz	147	3	9	14	42	2	47	0

Description	Serving Size	Cal	Prot (g)	Fat (g)	Carbs (g)	Net Carb(g)	Fiber (g)	Sod (mg)	Chol (mg)
SKOR Toffee Bar	1 bar	217	2	13	23	56	1	108	20
SPECIAL DARK Chocolate Bar	1 bar	226	2	13	25	56	2	3	0
Sweet chocolate	1 oz	143	1	9	17	54	2	5	0
Sweet chocolate coated fondant	1 patty	157	1	4	34	79	1	11	0
SYMPHONY Milk Chocolate Bar	1 bar	232	3	0	24	56	1	39	9
TWIZZLERS CHERRY BITES	22 pieces	139	1	0	31	77	1	85	0
TWIZZLERS Strawberry Twists Candy	1 package	237	2	0	55	76	1	175	0
WHATCHAMACALLIT Candy Bar	1 bar	214	4	9	29	58	1	99	5
WILLY WONKA'S EVERLASTING GOBSTOPPERS Jawbreakers	6 pieces	59	0	0	15	N.A.	N.A.	1	0
YORK Peppermint Pattie	1 patty	55	0	1	11	78	0	3	0

Description	Serving Size	Cal	Prot (g)	Fat (g)	Carbs (g)	Net Carb(g)	Fiber (g)	Sod (mg)	Chol (mg)
Barley									
Pearled, cooked	1 cup	193	4	1	44	24	6	5	0
Pearled, raw	1 cup	704	20	2	155	62	31	18	0
Regular	1 cup	651	23	3	135	56	32	22	0
Bran									
Corn bran, crude	1 cup	170	6	1	65	0	65	5	0
Oat bran, cooked	1 cup	88	7	2	25	9	6	2	0
Oat bran, raw	1 cup	231	16	6	62	51	14	4	0
Rice bran, crude	1 cup	373	16	23	59	29	25	6	0
Wheat bran, crude	1 cup	125	9	2	37	22	25	1	0
Buckwheat									
Groats, roasted, cooked	1 cup	155	6	1	33	17	5	7	0
Groats, roasted, dry	1 cup	567	19	4	123	65	17	18	0
Regular	1 cup	583	23	5	122	62	17	2	0
Bulgur									
Cooked	1 cup	151	6	0	34	14	8	9	0
Dry	1 cup	479	17	1	106	58	26	24	0
Corn									
White	1 cup	606	16	7	123	N.A.	N.A.	58	0
Yellow	1 cup	606	16	7	123	N.A.	N.A.	58	0
Couscous									
Cooked	1 cup	176	6	0	36	22	2	8	0
Dry	1 cup	650	22	1	134	72	9	17	0
Flour									
Arrowroot flour	1 cup	457	0	0	113	85	4	3	0
Barley malt flour	1 cup	585	17	3	127	71	12	18	0
Buckwheat flour, whole-groat	1 cup	402	15	3	85	61	12	13	0
Corn flour, degermed, yellow	1 cup	473	7	1	104	81	2	1	0
Corn flour, masa	1 cup	416	11	4	87	67	11	6	0
Corn flour, masa, yellow	1 cup	416	11	4	87	63	15	6	0
Corn flour, whole-grain, white	1 cup	422	8	4	90	67	11	6	0
Corn flour, whole-grain, yellow	1 cup	422	8	4	90	63	16	6	0
Rice flour, brown	1 cup	574	11	4	121	72	7	13	0
Rice flour, white	1 cup	578	9	2	127	78	4	0	0

Description	Serving Size	Cal	Prot (g)	Fat (g)	Carbs (g)	Net Carb(g)	Fiber (g)	Sod (mg)	Chol (mg)
FLOUR (continued)									
Rye flour, dark	1 cup	415	18	2	88	46	29	1	0
Rye flour, light	1 cup	374	9	1	82	66	15	2	0
Rye flour, medium	1 cup	361	10	1	79	63	15	3	0
Triticale flour, whole-grain	1 cup	439	17	2	95	59	19	3	0
Wheat flour, white, all-purpose	1 cup	455	13	1	95	74	3	3	0
Wheat flour, white, all-purpose, self-rising	1 cup	443	12	1	93	72	3	1588	0
Wheat flour, white, bread	1 cup	495	16	2	99	70	3	3	0
Wheat flour, white, cake	1 cup	496	11	1	107	76	2	3	0
Wheat flour, white, tortilla mix	1 cup	450	11	11	75	N.A.	N.A.	751	0
Wheat flour, whole-grain	1 cup	407	16	2	87	60	15	6	0

Germ

Description	Serving Size	Cal	Prot (g)	Fat (g)	Carbs (g)	Net Carb(g)	Fiber (g)	Sod (mg)	Chol (mg)
Wheat germ, crude	1 cup	414	27	10	60	39	15	14	0

Hominy

Description	Serving Size	Cal	Prot (g)	Fat (g)	Carbs (g)	Net Carb(g)	Fiber (g)	Sod (mg)	Chol (mg)
Canned, white	1 cup	119	2	1	24	12	4	347	0
Canned, yellow	1 cup	115	2	1	23	12	4	336	0

Macaroni

Description	Serving Size	Cal	Prot (g)	Fat (g)	Carbs (g)	Net Carb(g)	Fiber (g)	Sod (mg)	Chol (mg)
Elbow, cooked	1 cup	197	7	1	40	27	2	1	0
Elbow, dry	1 cup	390	13	1	78	72	3	7	0
Elbow, whole-wheat, cooked	1 cup	174	7	1	37	24	4	4	0
Elbow, whole-wheat, dry	1 cup	365	15	1	79	67	9	8	0
Small shells, protein-fortified, cooked	1 cup	189	10	0	36	29	2	6	0
Small shells, protein-fortified, dry	1 cup	349	18	1	63	65	2	7	0
Spiral, cooked	1 cup	189	6	1	38	27	2	1	0
Spiral, dry	1 cup	312	11	1	63	72	2	6	0
Spiral, vegetable, cooked	1 cup	172	6	0	36	22	6	8	0
Spiral, vegetable, dry	1 cup	308	11	1	63	71	4	36	0

Meal

Description	Serving Size	Cal	Prot (g)	Fat (g)	Carbs (g)	Net Carb(g)	Fiber (g)	Sod (mg)	Chol (mg)
Cornmeal, degermed, white and yellow	1 cup	505	12	2	107	70	10	4	0
Cornmeal, self-rising, bolted, plain, white and yellow	1 cup	407	10	4	86	64	8	1521	0
Cornmeal, self-rising, bolted, with wheat flour added, white and yellow	1 cup	592	14	4	125	67	11	2242	0
Cornmeal, self-rising, degermed, white and yellow	1 cup	490	12	2	103	68	10	1860	0
Cornmeal, whole-grain, white and yellow	1 cup	442	10	4	94	70	9	43	0

Description	Serving Size	Cal	Prot (g)	Fat (g)	Carbs (g)	Net Carb(g)	Fiber (g)	Sod (mg)	Chol (mg)
Millet									
Cooked	1 cup	207	6	2	41	22	2	3	0
Raw	1 cup	756	22	7	146	64	17	10	0
Noodles									
Chinese, chow mein	1 cup	237	4	13	26	54	2	198	0
Chinese, chow mein	1 1/2 oz	227	4	13	25	54	2	189	0
Egg, cooked	1 cup	213	8	2	40	24	2	11	53
Egg, cooked, with added salt	1 cup	213	8	2	40	24	2	264	53
Egg, dry	1 cup	145	5	1	27	68	1	8	36
Egg, spinach, cooked	1 cup	211	8	2	39	22	4	19	53
Egg, spinach, dry	1 cup	145	6	1	27	64	3	27	36
Japanese, soba, cooked	1 cup	113	6	0	24	N.A.	N.A.	68	0
Japanese, soba, dry	2 oz	192	8	0	43	N.A.	N.A.	451	0
Japanese, somen, cooked	1 cup	231	7	0	48	N.A.	N.A.	283	0
Japanese, somen, dry	2 oz	203	6	0	42	70	2	1049	0
Rice noodles, cooked	1 cup	192	2	0	44	24	2	33	0
Pasta									
SPAGHETTI									
Cooked, with added salt	1 cup	197	7	1	40	27	2	140	0
Cooked, without added salt	1 cup	197	7	1	40	27	2	1	0
Dry	2 oz	211	7	1	43	72	1	4	0
Protein-fortified, cooked	1 cup	230	11	0	44	30	2	7	0
Protein-fortified, dry	2 oz	213	12	1	37	63	1	5	0
Spinach, cooked	1 cup	182	6	1	37	N.A.	N.A.	20	0
Spinach, dry	2 oz	212	8	1	43	64	6	21	0
Whole-wheat, cooked	1 cup	174	7	1	37	22	6	4	0
Whole-wheat, dry	2 oz	198	8	1	43	N.A.	N.A.	5	0
GENERIC PASTA									
Corn pasta, cooked	1 cup	176	4	1	39	23	7	0	0
Corn pasta, dry	1 cup	375	8	2	83	68	12	3	0
Fresh-refrigerated, plain, as purchased	4 1/2 oz	369	14	2	70	N.A.	N.A.	33	93
Fresh-refrigerated, plain, cooked	2 oz	75	3	0	14	N.A.	N.A.	3	19
Fresh-refrigerated, spinach, as purchased	4 1/2 oz	370	14	2	71	N.A.	N.A.	35	93
Fresh-refrigerated, spinach, cooked	2 oz	74	3	0	14	N.A.	N.A.	3	19
Homemade, made with egg, cooked	2 oz	74	3	1	13	N.A.	N.A.	47	23
Homemade, made without egg, cooked	2 oz	71	2	0	14	N.A.	N.A.	42	0

Description	Serving Size	Cal	Prot (g)	Fat (g)	Carbs (g)	Net Carb(g)	Fiber (g)	Sod (mg)	Chol (mg)
Rice									
Brown, long-grain, cooked	1 cup	216	5	2	45	21	4	10	0
Brown, long-grain, raw	1 cup	685	15	5	143	74	6	13	0
Brown, medium-grain, cooked	1 cup	218	5	1	46	22	4	2	0
Brown, medium-grain, raw	1 cup	688	14	5	145	73	6	8	0
White, glutinous, cooked	1 cup	169	4	0	37	20	2	9	0
White, glutinous, raw	1 cup	685	13	1	151	79	5	13	0
White, long-grain, parboiled, cooked	1 cup	200	4	0	43	24	1	5	0
White, long-grain, parboiled, dry	1 cup	686	13	1	151	80	3	9	0
White, long-grain, precooked or instant, enriched, dry	1 cup	360	7	0	79	82	2	6	0
White, long-grain, precooked or instant, enriched, prepared	1 cup	162	3	0	35	21	1	5	0
White, long-grain, regular, cooked	1 cup	205	4	0	45	28	1	2	0
White, long-grain, regular, cooked, with salt	1 cup	205	4	0	45	28	1	604	0
White, long-grain, regular, raw	1 cup	675	13	1	148	79	2	9	0
White, medium-grain, cooked	1 cup	242	4	0	53	28	1	0	0
White, medium-grain, raw, enriched	1 cup	702	13	1	155	78	3	2	0
White, short-grain, cooked	1 cup	242	4	0	53	N.A.	N.A.	0	0
White, short-grain, raw	1 cup	716	13	1	158	76	6	2	0
White, with pasta, cooked	1 cup	246	5	5	43	19	5	1147	2
White, with pasta, dry	1 cup	600	15	3	123	N.A.	N.A.	3042	3
Wild rice, cooked	1 cup	166	7	1	35	20	3	5	0
Wild rice, raw	1 cup	571	24	2	120	69	10	11	0
Rye									
Regular	1 cup	566	25	3	118	55	25	10	0
Semolina									
Semolina	1 cup	601	21	1	122	69	7	2	0
Sorghum									
Sorghum	1 cup	651	22	5	143	N.A.	N.A.	12	0
Wheat									
Wheat, durum	1 cup	651	26	3	137	N.A.	N.A.	4	0
Wheat, hard red spring	1 cup	632	30	3	131	56	23	4	0
Wheat, hard red winter	1 cup	628	24	2	137	59	23	4	0
Wheat, hard white	1 cup	657	22	2	146	N.A.	N.A.	4	0

Description	Serving Size	Cal	Prot (g)	Fat (g)	Carbs (g)	Net Carb(g)	Fiber (g)	Sod (mg)	Chol (mg)
Wheat, soft red winter	1 cup	556	17	2	125	62	21	3	0
Wheat, soft white	1 cup	571	18	2	127	63	21	3	0
Wheat, sprouted	1 cup	214	8	1	46	41	1	17	0
Amaranth	1 cup	729	28	12	129	51	30	41	0
Cornstarch	1 cup	488	0	0	117	90	1	12	0
Oats	1 cup	607	26	9	103	56	17	3	0
Quinoa	1 cup	636	22	8	117	63	10	36	0
Tapioca, pearl, dry	1 cup	544	0	0	135	88	1	2	0

Description	Serving Size	Cal	Prot (g)	Fat (g)	Carbs (g)	Net Carb(g)	Fiber (g)	Sod (mg)	Chol (mg)
Ice Cream Topping									
Butterscotch or caramel	2 tbsp	103	1	0	27	65	0	143	0
Marshmallow cream	1 oz	91	0	0	22	79	0	14	0
NESTLE, BUNCHA CRUNCH Dessert Topping	1 serving	103	1	5	13	64	0	46	3
NESTLE, RAINBOW MORSEL Dessert Topping	1 serving	68	1	3	10	69	1	0	0
Nuts in syrup	2 tbsp	167	2	8	22	52	1	17	0
Pineapple	2 tbsp	106	0	0	28	65	0	26	0
Strawberry	2 tbsp	107	0	0	28	65	0	9	0
Jams, Jellies, & Preserves									
Fruit butters, apple	1 tbsp	29	0	0	7	41	0	1	0
Jams and preserves	1 packet	39	0	0	10	68	0	4	0
Jellies	1 tbsp	54	0	0	13	69	0	5	0
Marmalade, orange	1 tbsp	49	0	0	13	66	0	11	0
Pectin, unsweetened, dry mix	1 package	163	0	0	45	82	4	100	0
POLANER ALL-FRUIT Strawberry Spread	1 tbsp	42	0	0	10	N.A.	N.A.	4	0
Pop, with added ascorbic acid	1 bar	37	0	0	10	19	0	6	0
Sugars & Sweeteners									
Honey	1 tbsp	64	0	0	17	82	0	1	0
Molasses	1 tbsp	53	0	0	14	69	0	7	0
Molasses, blackstrap	1 tbsp	47	0	0	12	61	0	11	0
NUTRASWEET or EQUAL	1 tsp	12	0	0	3	86	0	0	0
NUTRASWEET or EQUAL	1 packet	4	0	0	1	86	0	0	0
Sugars, brown	1 cup	827	0	0	214	97	0	86	0
Sugars, granulated	1 tsp	16	0	0	4	100	0	0	0
Sugars, maple	1 tsp	11	0	0	3	91	0	0	0
Sugars, powdered	1 cup	467	0	0	119	100	0	1	0
Sugars, powdered	1 tbsp	31	0	0	8	100	0	0	0
Syrups									
Chocolate, fudge-type	1 cup	1064	14	25	191	60	9	1052	6
Chocolate, HERSHEY'S Genuine Chocolate Flavored Lite Syrup	2 tbsp	50	1	0	12	31	1	48	0
Corn, dark	1 tbsp	56	0	0	15	77	0	31	0
Corn, high-fructose	1 tbsp	53	0	0	14	76	0	0	0
Corn, light	1 tbsp	56	0	0	15	77	0	24	0

Description	Serving Size	Cal	Prot (g)	Fat (g)	Carbs (g)	Net Carb(g)	Fiber (g)	Sod (mg)	Chol (mg)
SYRUPS (continued)									
Malt	1 tbsp	76	1	0	17	71	0	8	0
Maple	1 tbsp	52	0	0	13	67	0	2	0
Sorghum	1 tbsp	61	0	0	16	75	0	2	0
Table blends, cane and 15% maple	1 tbsp	56	0	0	15	75	0	21	0
Table blends, corn, refiner, and sugar	1 tbsp	64	0	0	17	84	0	14	0
Table blends, pancake	1 tbsp	57	0	0	15	76	0	17	0
Table blends, pancake, reduced-calorie	1 tbsp	25	0	0	7	44	0	30	0
Table blends, pancake, with 2% maple	1 tbsp	53	0	0	14	70	0	12	0
Table blends, pancake, with 2% maple, with added potassium	1 tbsp	53	0	0	14	70	0	12	0
Table blends, pancake, with butter	1 tbsp	59	0	0	15	74	0	20	1

Description	Serving Size	Cal	Prot (g)	Fat (g)	Carbs (g)	Net Carb(g)	Fiber (g)	Sod (mg)	Chol (mg)
Butter									
Oil, anhydrous	1 tbsp	112	0	13	0	0	0	0	33
Oil, anhydrous	1 cup	1796	1	204	0	0	0	4	525
Salted	1 tbsp	102	0	12	0	0	0	117	31
Salted	1 cup	1628	2	184	0	0	0	1875	497
Unsalted	1 tbsp	102	0	12	0	0	0	2	31
Unsalted	1 cup	1628	2	184	0	0	0	25	497
Whipped, with salt	1 tbsp	67	0	8	0	0	0	78	21
Whipped, with salt	1 cup	1083	1	122	0	0	0	1249	331
Cheese									
Blue	1 cubic inch	61	4	5	0	0	0	241	13
Blue	1 oz	100	6	8	1	1	0	395	21
Brick	1 cup, shredded	419	26	34	3	3	0	633	106
Brick	1 cup, diced	490	31	39	4	4	0	739	124
Brie	1 cup, sliced	481	30	40	1	1	0	906	144
Brie	1 cup, melted	802	50	66	1	1	0	1510	240
Camembert	1 oz	85	6	7	0	0	0	239	20
Camembert	1 cup	738	49	60	1	1	0	2071	177
Caraway	1 oz	107	7	8	1	1	0	196	26
Cheddar	1 cup, melted	983	61	81	3	3	0	1515	256
Cheddar	1 cup, diced	532	33	44	2	2	0	820	139
Cheese fondue	1/2 cup	247	15	15	4	4	0	143	49
Cheese fondue	1 cup	492	31	29	8	8	0	284	97
Cheese sauce, prepared from recipe	2 tbsp	59	3	4	2	2	0	148	11
Cheese sauce, prepared from recipe	1 cup	479	25	36	13	13	0	1198	92
Cheese spread, pasteurized process, American, with di sodium phosphate	1 jar	412	23	30	12	12	0	2308	78
Cheese spread, pasteurized process, American, with di sodium phosphate	1 oz	82	5	6	2	2	0	461	16
Cheese spread, pasteurized process, American, without di sodium phosphate	1 cup	708	40	52	21	21	0	3282	134
Cheese spread, pasteurized process, American, without di sodium phosphate	1 cup, diced	406	23	30	12	12	0	1883	77
Cheese substitute, mozzarella	1 oz	70	3	3	7	7	0	194	0
Cheese substitute, mozzarella	1 cup, shredded	280	13	14	27	27	0	774	0

Description	Serving Size	Cal	Prot (g)	Fat (g)	Carbs (g)	Net Carb(g)	Fiber (g)	Sod (mg)	Chol (mg)
CHEESE (continued)									
Cheshire	1 oz	110	7	9	1	1	0	198	29
Colby	1 cup, shredded	445	27	36	3	3	0	683	107
Colby	1 cup, diced	520	31	42	3	3	0	797	125
Cold pack, American	1 package	751	45	56	19	19	0	2193	145
Cold pack, American	1 oz	94	6	7	2	2	0	274	18
Cottage cheese, creamed, large or small curd	1 cup, large curd	216	26	9	6	6	0	851	32
Cottage cheese, creamed, large or small curd	4 oz	116	14	5	3	3	0	458	17
Cottage cheese, creamed, with fruit	4 oz	140	11	4	15	15	0	458	12
Cottage cheese, creamed, with fruit	1 cup	280	22	8	30	30	0	915	25
Cottage cheese, lowfat, 1% milkfat	4 oz	81	14	1	3	3	0	459	5
Cottage cheese, lowfat, 1% milkfat	1 cup	163	28	2	6	6	0	918	9
Cottage cheese, lowfat, 2% milkfat	4 oz	102	16	2	4	4	0	459	9
Cottage cheese, lowfat, 2% milkfat	1 cup	203	31	4	8	8	0	918	18
Cottage cheese, nonfat, uncreamed, dry, large or small curd	4 oz	96	20	0	2	2	0	15	8
Cottage cheese, nonfat, uncreamed, dry, large or small curd	1 cup	123	25	1	3	3	0	19	10
Cream cheese	1 tbsp	51	1	5	0	0	0	43	16
Cream cheese	1 cup	810	18	81	6	6	0	687	255
Edam	1 package	707	49	55	3	3	0	1911	176
Edam	1 oz	101	7	8	0	0	0	274	25
Feta	1 oz	75	4	6	1	1	0	316	25
Feta	1 cup, crumbled	396	21	32	6	6	0	1674	134
Fontina	1 cup, shredded	420	28	34	2	2	0	864	125
Fontina	1 cup, diced	513	34	41	2	2	0	1056	153
Gjetost	1 package	1058	22	67	97	97	0	1362	213
Gjetost	1 oz	132	3	8	12	12	0	170	27
Goat, hard type	1 oz	128	9	10	1	1	0	98	30
Goat, semisoft type	1 oz	103	6	8	1	1	0	146	22
Goat, soft type	1 oz	76	5	6	0	0	0	104	13
Gouda	1 package	705	49	54	4	4	0	1622	226
Gouda	1 oz	101	7	8	1	1	0	232	32

Description	Serving Size	Cal	Prot (g)	Fat (g)	Carbs (g)	Net Carb(g)	Fiber (g)	Sod (mg)	Chol (mg)
Gruyere	1 cup, shredded	446	32	35	0	0	0	363	119
Gruyere	1 cup, diced	545	39	43	0	0	0	444	145
KRAFT CHEEZ WHIZ LIGHT Pasteurized Process Cheese Product	2 tbsp	75	6	3	6	6	0	597	12
KRAFT CHEEZ WHIZ Pasteurized Process Cheese Sauce	2 tbsp	91	4	7	3	3	0	541	25
KRAFT FREE Singles American Nonfat Pasteurized Process Cheese Product	1 slice	31	5	0	2	2	0	273	3
KRAFT VELVEETA LIGHT Reduced Fat Pasteurized Process Cheese Product	1 oz	62	5	3	3	3	0	444	12
KRAFT VELVEETA Pasteurized Process Cheese Spread	1 oz	85	5	6	3	3	0	420	22
Limburger	1 oz	93	6	8	0	0	0	227	26
Limburger	1 cup	438	27	37	1	1	0	1072	121
Low-fat, cheddar or colby	1 cup, shredded	195	28	8	2	2	0	692	24
Low-fat, cheddar or colby	1 cup, diced	228	32	9	3	3	0	808	28
Low-sodium, cheddar or colby	1 cup, shredded	450	28	37	2	2	0	24	113
Low-sodium, cheddar or colby	1 cup, diced	525	32	43	3	3	0	28	132
Mexican, queso anejo	1 oz	106	6	8	1	1	0	321	30
Mexican, queso anejo	1 cup, crumbled	492	28	40	6	6	0	1493	139
Mexican, queso asadero	1 cup, shredded	402	26	32	3	3	0	740	119
Mexican, queso asadero	1 cup, diced	470	30	37	4	4	0	865	139
Mexican, queso chihuahua	1 cup, shredded	423	24	34	6	6	0	697	119
Mexican, queso chihuahua	1 cup, diced	494	28	39	7	7	0	814	139
Monterey	1 cup, shredded	421	28	34	1	1	0	606	101
Monterey	1 cup, diced	492	32	40	1	1	0	708	117
Mozzarella, part skim milk	1 oz	72	7	5	1	1	0	132	16
Mozzarella, part skim milk, low moisture	1 cup, shredded	316	31	19	4	4	0	597	61
Mozzarella, part skim milk, low moisture	1 cup, diced	370	36	23	4	4	0	697	71
Mozzarella, whole milk	1 oz	80	6	6	1	1	0	106	22
Mozzarella, whole milk	1 cup, shredded	315	22	24	2	2	0	418	87
Mozzarella, whole milk, low moisture	1 cubic inch	56	4	4	0	0	0	73	16
Mozzarella, whole milk, low moisture	1 oz	90	6	7	1	1	0	118	25

Description	Serving Size	Cal	Prot (g)	Fat (g)	Carbs (g)	Net Carb(g)	Fiber (g)	Sod (mg)	Chol (mg)
CHEESE (continued)									
Muenster	1 cup, shredded	416	26	34	1	1	0	710	108
Muenster	1 cup, diced	486	31	40	1	1	0	829	127
Neufchatel	1 package	221	8	20	2	2	0	339	65
Neufchatel	1 oz	74	3	7	1	1	0	113	22
Parmesan, grated	1 tbsp	23	2	2	0	0	0	93	4
Parmesan, grated	1 cup	456	42	30	4	4	0	1862	79
Parmesan, hard	1 cubic inch	40	4	3	0	0	0	165	7
Parmesan, hard	1 oz	111	10	7	1	1	0	454	19
Parmesan, shredded	1 tbsp	21	2	1	0	0	0	85	4
Pasteurized process, American, with di sodium phosphate	1 cup, melted	915	54	76	4	4	0	3489	229
Pasteurized process, American, with di sodium phosphate	1 cup, diced	525	31	44	2	2	0	2002	132
Pasteurized process, American, with di sodium phosphate	1 package	745	45	56	17	17	0	3623	145
Pasteurized process, American, with di sodium phosphate	1 oz	93	6	7	2	2	0	452	18
Pasteurized process, American, without di sodium phosphate	1 oz	93	6	7	2	2	0	337	18
Pasteurized process, American, without di sodium phosphate	1 cubic inch	66	4	5	0	0	0	114	16
Pasteurized process, American, without di sodium phosphate	1 cup	371	22	28	8	8	0	1344	72
Pasteurized process, American, without di sodium phosphate	1 oz	106	6	9	0	0	0	184	27
Pasteurized process, pimento	1 cup, melted	915	54	76	4	4	0	3484	229
Pasteurized process, pimento	1 cup, diced	525	31	44	2	2	0	1999	132
Pasteurized process, Swiss	1 package	733	50	55	10	10	0	3523	186
Pasteurized process, Swiss	1 oz	92	6	7	1	1	0	440	23
Pasteurized process, Swiss, with di sodium phosphate	1 cup, shredded	377	28	28	2	2	0	1548	96
Pasteurized process, Swiss, with di sodium phosphate	1 cup, diced	468	35	35	3	3	0	1918	119
Pasteurized process, Swiss, without di sodium phosphate	1 cubic inch	60	4	4	0	0	0	122	15
Pasteurized process, Swiss, without di sodium phosphate	1 oz	95	7	7	1	1	0	193	24

Description	Serving Size	Cal	Prot (g)	Fat (g)	Carbs (g)	Net Carb(g)	Fiber (g)	Sod (mg)	Chol (mg)
Port du salut	1 cup, shredded	398	27	32	1	1	0	603	139
Port du salut	1 cup, diced	465	31	37	1	1	0	705	162
Provolone	1 oz	100	7	8	1	1	0	248	20
Provolone	1 cup, diced	463	34	35	3	3	0	1156	91
Ricotta, part skim milk	1 oz	39	3	2	1	1	0	35	9
Ricotta, part skim milk	1 cup	339	28	19	13	13	0	308	76
Ricotta, whole milk	1/2 cup	216	14	16	4	4	0	104	63
Ricotta, whole milk	1 cup	428	28	32	7	7	0	207	125
Romano	1/2 package	550	45	38	5	5	0	1704	148
Romano	1 oz	110	9	8	1	1	0	340	29
Roquefort	1 package	314	18	26	2	2	0	1538	77
Roquefort	1 oz	105	6	9	1	1	0	513	26
Swiss	1 cup, melted	917	69	67	8	8	0	634	224
Swiss	1 cup, diced	496	38	36	4	4	0	343	121
Tilsit	1 package	578	41	44	3	3	0	1280	173
Tilsit	1 oz	96	7	7	1	1	0	213	29

Dessert Topping

Description	Serving Size	Cal	Prot (g)	Fat (g)	Carbs (g)	Net Carb(g)	Fiber (g)	Sod (mg)	Chol (mg)
Powdered	1 portion	8	0	1	1	1	0	2	0
Powdered	1 1/2 oz	245	2	17	22	22	0	52	0
Powdered, 1 1/2 ounce prepared with 1/2 cup milk	1 tbsp	8	0	0	1	1	0	3	0
Powdered, 1 1/2 ounce prepared with 1/2 cup milk	1 cup	151	3	10	13	13	0	53	8
Pressurized	1 tbsp	11	0	1	1	1	0	2	0
Pressurized	1 cup	185	1	16	11	11	0	43	0
Semi solid, frozen	1 tbsp	13	0	1	1	1	0	1	0
Semi solid, frozen	1 cup	239	1	19	17	17	0	19	0

Eggs

Description	Serving Size	Cal	Prot (g)	Fat (g)	Carbs (g)	Net Carb(g)	Fiber (g)	Sod (mg)	Chol (mg)
Substitute, frozen	1/4 cup	96	7	7	2	2	0	119	1
Substitute, frozen	1 cup	384	27	27	8	8	0	478	5
Substitute, liquid	1 tbsp	13	2	1	0	0	0	28	0
Substitute, liquid	1 cup	211	30	8	2	2	0	444	3
Substitute, powder	.7 oz	88	11	3	4	4	0	158	113
Substitute, powder	.35 oz	44	5	1	2	2	0	79	57
Duck, whole, fresh, raw	1 egg	130	9	10	1	1	0	102	619
Goose, whole, fresh, raw	1 egg	266	20	19	2	2	0	199	1227

Description	Serving Size	Cal	Prot (g)	Fat (g)	Carbs (g)	Net Carb(g)	Fiber (g)	Sod (mg)	Chol (mg)
EGGS (continued)									
Quail, whole, fresh, raw	1 egg	14	1	1	0	0	0	13	76
Turkey, whole, fresh, raw	1 egg	135	11	9	1	1	0	119	737
White, dried, flakes, glucose reduced	1/2 lb	797	175	0	9	9	0	2624	0
White, dried, powder, glucose reduced	1 tbsp	53	12	0	1	1	0	173	0
White, dried, powder, glucose reduced	1 cup	402	88	0	5	5	0	1325	0
White, raw, fresh	1 large	17	4	0	0	0	0	55	0
White, raw, fresh	1 cup	122	26	0	3	3	0	399	0
Whole, cooked, fried	1 large	92	6	7	1	1	0	162	211
Whole, cooked, hard-boiled	1 tbsp	13	1	1	0	0	0	11	36
Whole, cooked, hard-boiled	1 cup, chopped	211	17	14	2	2	0	169	577
Whole, cooked, omelet	1 large	93	6	7	1	1	0	165	214
Whole, cooked, omelet	1 tbsp	23	2	2	0	0	0	41	53
Whole, cooked, poached	1 large	75	6	5	1	1	0	140	212
Whole, cooked, scrambled	1 tbsp	23	2	2	0	0	0	38	48
Whole, cooked, scrambled	1 cup	365	24	27	5	5	0	616	774
Whole, dried	1 tbsp	30	2	2	0	0	0	26	86
Whole, dried	1 cup	505	40	35	4	4	0	445	1458
Whole, dried, stabilized, glucose reduced	1 tbsp	31	2	2	0	0	0	27	101
Whole, dried, stabilized, glucose reduced	1 cup	523	41	37	2	2	0	466	1714
Whole, raw, fresh	1 extra large	86	7	6	1	1	0	73	247
Whole, raw, fresh	1 cup	362	30	24	3	3	0	306	1033
Yolk, dried	1 tbsp	27	1	2	0	0	0	5	93
Yolk, dried	1 cup	446	23	37	2	2	0	90	1564
Yolk, raw, fresh	1 large	59	3	5	0	0	0	7	213
Yolk, raw, fresh	1 cup	870	41	75	4	4	0	104	3113

Cream

Description	Serving Size	Cal	Prot (g)	Fat (g)	Carbs (g)	Net Carb(g)	Fiber (g)	Sod (mg)	Chol (mg)
Fluid, half and half	1 tbsp	20	0	2	1	1	0	6	6
Fluid, half and half	1 cup	315	7	28	10	10	0	99	90
Fluid, heavy whipping	1 cup, fluid	821	5	88	7	7	0	90	326
Fluid, heavy whipping	1 cup	412	2	44	3	3	0	45	164

Description	Serving Size	Cal	Prot (g)	Fat (g)	Carbs (g)	Net Carb(g)	Fiber (g)	Sod (mg)	Chol (mg)
Fluid, light (coffee cream or table cream)	1 tbsp	29	0	3	1	1	0	6	10
Fluid, light (coffee cream or table cream)	1 cup	468	6	46	9	9	0	96	158
Fluid, light whipping	1 cup, fluid	698	5	74	7	7	0	81	265
Fluid, light whipping	1 cup	350	3	37	4	4	0	41	133
Substitute, liquid, with hydrogenated vegetable oil and soy protein	1 fl oz	41	0	3	3	3	0	24	0
Substitute, liquid, with hydrogenated vegetable oil and soy protein	1 cup	326	2	24	27	27	0	190	0
Substitute, liquid, with lauric acid oil and sodium caseinate	1/2 cup	163	1	12	14	14	0	95	0
Substitute, liquid, with lauric acid oil and sodium caseinate	1 container	20	0	1	2	2	0	12	0
Substitute, powdered	1 tsp	11	0	1	1	1	0	4	0
Substitute, powdered	1 cup	513	5	33	52	52	0	170	0
Whipped, cream topping, pressurized	1 tbsp	8	0	1	0	0	0	4	2
Whipped, cream topping, pressurized	1 cup	154	2	13	7	7	0	78	46

Milk

Description	Serving Size	Cal	Prot (g)	Fat (g)	Carbs (g)	Net Carb(g)	Fiber (g)	Sod (mg)	Chol (mg)
Buttermilk, dried	1 tbsp	25	2	0	3	3	0	34	4
Buttermilk, dried	1 cup	464	41	7	59	59	0	620	83
Buttermilk, fluid, cultured, lowfat	1 fl oz	12	1	0	1	1	0	32	1
Buttermilk, fluid, cultured, lowfat	1 cup	98	8	2	12	12	0	257	10
Canned, condensed, sweetened	1 fl oz	123	3	3	21	21	0	49	13
Canned, condensed, sweetened	1 cup	982	24	27	166	166	0	389	104
Canned, evaporated, nonfat	1 fl oz	25	2	0	4	4	0	37	1
Canned, evaporated, nonfat	1 cup	200	19	1	29	29	0	294	10
Canned, evaporated, with added vitamin A	1/2 cup	169	9	10	13	13	0	134	37
Canned, evaporated, with added vitamin A	1 fl oz	42	2	2	3	3	0	33	9
Canned, evaporated, without added vitamin A	1 fl oz	42	2	2	3	3	0	33	9
Canned, evaporated, without added vitamin A	1 cup	338	17	19	25	25	0	267	73
Chocolate beverage, hot cocoa, homemade	1 fl oz	24	1	1	4	3	0	16	2
Chocolate beverage, hot cocoa, homemade	1 cup	193	10	6	29	27	2	128	20
Chocolate, fluid, commercial	1 fl oz	26	1	1	3	3	0	19	4

Description	Serving Size	Cal	Prot (g)	Fat (g)	Carbs (g)	Net Carb(g)	Fiber (g)	Sod (mg)	Chol (mg)
Milk (continued)									
Chocolate, fluid, commercial	1 cup	208	8	8	26	24	2	150	30
Chocolate, fluid, commercial, lowfat	1 quart	630	32	10	104	99	5	610	30
Chocolate, fluid, commercial, lowfat	1 cup	158	8	3	26	25	1	153	8
Chocolate, fluid, commercial, reduced fat	1 fl oz	22	1	1	3	3	0	19	2
Chocolate, fluid, commercial, reduced fat	1 cup	180	8	5	26	25	1	150	18
Dry, nonfat, calcium reduced	1/4 lb	400	40	0	59	59	0	2576	2
Dry, nonfat, calcium reduced	1 oz	100	10	0	15	15	0	646	1
Dry, nonfat, instant, with added vitamin A	1 envelope	326	32	1	47	47	0	500	16
Dry, nonfat, instant, with added vitamin A	1 cup	243	24	0	35	35	0	373	12
Dry, nonfat, instant, without added vitamin A	1 envelope	326	32	1	47	47	0	500	16
Dry, nonfat, instant, without added vitamin A	1 cup	243	24	0	35	35	0	373	12
Dry, nonfat, regular, with added vitamin A	1/4 cup	109	11	0	16	16	0	161	6
Dry, nonfat, regular, with added vitamin A	1 cup	434	43	1	62	62	0	642	24
Dry, nonfat, regular, without added vitamin A	1/4 cup	109	11	0	16	16	0	161	6
Dry, nonfat, regular, without added vitamin A	1 cup	434	43	1	62	62	0	642	24
Dry, whole	1/4 cup	159	8	9	12	12	0	119	31
Dry, whole	1 cup	635	34	34	49	49	0	475	124
Eggnog	1 fl oz	43	1	2	4	4	0	17	19
Eggnog	1 cup	343	10	19	34	34	0	137	150
Filled, fluid, with blend of hydrogenated vegetable oils	1 quart	615	33	34	46	46	0	556	20
Filled, fluid, with blend of hydrogenated vegetable oils	1 cup	154	8	8	12	12	0	139	5
Filled, fluid, with lauric acid oil	1 fl oz	19	1	1	1	1	0	17	1
Filled, fluid, with lauric acid oil	1 cup	154	8	8	12	12	0	139	5
Goat, fluid	1 fl oz	21	1	1	1	1	0	15	3
Goat, fluid	1 cup	168	9	10	11	11	0	122	27
Human, mature, fluid	1 fl oz	22	0	1	2	2	0	5	4
Human, mature, fluid	1 cup	172	3	11	17	17	0	42	34

Description	Serving Size	Cal	Prot (g)	Fat (g)	Carbs (g)	Net Carb(g)	Fiber (g)	Sod (mg)	Chol (mg)
Low sodium, fluid	1 fl oz	19	1	1	1	1	0	1	4
Low sodium, fluid	1 cup	149	8	8	11	11	0	7	34
Lowfat, fluid, 1% milkfat, protein-fortified, with added vitamin A	1 quart	472	39	12	54	54	0	571	39
Lowfat, fluid, 1% milkfat, protein-fortified, with added vitamin A	1 cup	118	10	3	14	14	0	143	10
Lowfat, fluid, 1% milkfat, with added nonfat milk solids and vitamin A	1 quart	421	34	10	49	49	0	510	39
Lowfat, fluid, 1% milkfat, with added nonfat milk solids and vitamin A	1 cup	105	9	2	12	12	0	127	10
Lowfat, fluid, 1% milkfat, with added vitamin A	1 fl oz	13	1	0	1	1	0	16	1
Lowfat, fluid, 1% milkfat, with added vitamin A	1 cup	102	8	3	12	12	0	124	10
Nonfat, fluid, protein fortified, with added vitamin A	1 quart	403	39	2	55	55	0	581	20
Nonfat, fluid, protein fortified, with added vitamin A	1 cup	101	10	1	14	14	0	145	5
Nonfat, fluid, with added nonfat milk solids and vitamin A (fat free or skim)	1 fl oz	11	1	0	2	2	0	16	1
Nonfat, fluid, with added nonfat milk solids and vitamin A (fat free or skim)	1 cup	91	9	1	12	12	0	130	5
Nonfat, fluid, with added vitamin A (fat free or skim)	1 fl oz	11	1	0	1	1	0	16	1
Nonfat, fluid, with added vitamin A (fat free or skim)	1 cup	86	8	0	12	12	0	127	5
Nonfat, fluid, without added vitamin A (fat free or skim)	1 quart	343	33	2	48	48	0	510	20
Nonfat, fluid, without added vitamin A (fat free or skim)	1 cup	86	8	0	12	12	0	127	5
Producer, fluid, 3.7% milkfat	1 quart	625	32	36	45	45	0	478	137
Producer, fluid, 3.7% milkfat	1 cup	156	8	9	11	11	0	120	34
Reduced fat, fluid, 2% milkfat, protein-fortified, with added vitamin A	1 quart	551	39	19	54	54	0	581	79
Reduced fat, fluid, 2% milkfat, protein-fortified, with added vitamin A	1 cup	138	10	5	14	14	0	145	20

Description	Serving Size	Cal	Prot (g)	Fat (g)	Carbs (g)	Net Carb(g)	Fiber (g)	Sod (mg)	Chol (mg)
Milk (continued)									
Reduced fat, fluid, 2% milkfat, with added nonfat milk solids and vitamin A	1 quart	500	34	19	49	49	0	510	78
Reduced fat, fluid, 2% milkfat, with added nonfat milk solids and vitamin A	1 cup	125	9	5	12	12	0	127	20
Reduced fat, fluid, 2% milkfat, with added nonfat milk solids, without added vitamin A	1 quart	549	39	19	54	54	0	578	78
Reduced fat, fluid, 2% milkfat, with added nonfat milk solids, without added vitamin A	1 cup	137	10	5	13	13	0	145	20
Reduced fat, fluid, 2% milkfat, with added vitamin A	1 fl oz	15	1	1	1	1	0	15	2
Reduced fat, fluid, 2% milkfat, with added vitamin A	1 cup	122	8	5	12	12	0	122	20
Shakes, thick chocolate	1 container	357	9	8	63	63	1	333	33
Shakes, thick chocolate	1 fl oz	34	1	1	6	6	0	31	3
Shakes, thick vanilla	1 container	351	12	9	56	56	0	297	38
Shakes, thick vanilla	1 fl oz	32	1	1	5	5	0	27	3
Sheep, fluid	1 quart	1058	59	69	53	53	0	431	265
Sheep, fluid	1 cup	265	15	17	13	13	0	108	66
Substitutes, fluid with hydrogenated vegetable oils	1 fl oz	19	1	1	2	2	0	24	0
Substitutes, fluid with hydrogenated vegetable oils	1 cup	149	4	8	15	15	0	190	0
Substitutes, fluid, with lauric acid oil	1 quart	595	17	33	60	60	0	761	0
Substitutes, fluid, with lauric acid oil	1 cup	149	4	8	15	15	0	190	0
Whole, 3 1/4% milkfat	1 tbsp	9	1	1	1	1	0	7	2
Whole, 3 1/4% milkfat	1 cup	149	8	8	11	11	0	120	34

Sour Cream

Description	Serving Size	Cal	Prot (g)	Fat (g)	Carbs (g)	Net Carb(g)	Fiber (g)	Sod (mg)	Chol (mg)
KRAFT BREAKSTONE'S FREE Fat Free Sour Cream	2 tbsp	29	2	0	5	5	0	23	3
KRAFT BREAKSTONE'S Reduced Fat Sour Cream	2 tbsp	47	1	4	2	2	0	18	16
Sour cream, cultured	1 tbsp	26	0	3	1	1	0	6	5
Sour cream, cultured	1 cup	492	7	48	10	10	0	122	101
Sour cream, imitation, cultured	1 oz	59	1	6	2	2	0	29	0
Sour cream, imitation, cultured	1 cup	478	6	45	15	15	0	235	0

Description	Serving Size	Cal	Prot (g)	Fat (g)	Carbs (g)	Net Carb(g)	Fiber (g)	Sod (mg)	Chol (mg)
Sour cream, reduced fat, cultured	1 tbsp	20	0	2	1	1	0	6	6
Sour cream, reduced fat, cultured	1 cup	327	7	29	10	10	0	99	94
Sour dressing, non-butterfat, cultured, filled cream-type	1 tbsp	21	0	2	1	1	0	6	1
Sour dressing, non-butterfat, cultured, filled cream-type	1 cup	418	8	39	11	11	0	113	12

Whey

Description	Serving Size	Cal	Prot (g)	Fat (g)	Carbs (g)	Net Carb(g)	Fiber (g)	Sod (mg)	Chol (mg)
Whey, acid, dried	1 tbsp	10	0	0	2	2	0	28	0
Whey, acid, dried	1 cup	193	7	0	42	42	0	552	2
Whey, acid, fluid	1 quart	236	7	1	50	50	0	472	10
Whey, acid, fluid	1 cup	59	2	0	13	13	0	118	2
Whey, sweet, dried	1 tbsp	26	1	0	6	6	0	81	0
Whey, sweet, dried	1 cup	512	19	2	108	108	0	1565	9
Whey, sweet, fluid	1 quart	266	8	4	51	51	0	531	20
Whey, sweet, fluid	1 cup	66	2	1	13	13	0	133	5

Yogurt

Description	Serving Size	Cal	Prot (g)	Fat (g)	Carbs (g)	Net Carb(g)	Fiber (g)	Sod (mg)	Chol (mg)
KRAFT BREYERS LIGHT N' LIVELY Lowfat Yogurt (1% Milkfat)	1 container	135	4	1	27	27	0	56	11
KRAFT BREYERS LIGHT Nonfat Yogurt (with Aspartame and Fructose Sweeteners	1 container	125	8	0	22	22	0	102	11
KRAFT BREYERS Lowfat Yogurt (1% Milkfat)	1 container	218	9	2	41	41	0	118	20
KRAFT BREYERS Smooth & Creamy Lowfat Yogurt (1% Milkfat)	1 container	232	9	2	45	44	1	125	20
Yogurt, fruit, low fat, 10 grams protein per 8 ounce	1 container	173	7	2	32	32	0	99	7
Yogurt, fruit, low fat, 10 grams protein per 8 ounce	1 cup	250	11	3	47	47	0	142	10
Yogurt, fruit, low fat, 11 grams protein per 8 ounce	1/2 container	119	5	2	21	21	0	73	7
Yogurt, fruit, low fat, 11 grams protein per 8 ounce	1 container	238	11	3	42	42	0	148	14
Yogurt, fruit, low fat, 9 grams protein per 8 ounce	1 container	124	5	1	23	23	0	66	6
Yogurt, fruit, low fat, 9 grams protein per 8 ounce	1 cup	243	10	3	46	46	0	130	12
Yogurt, plain, low fat, 12 grams protein per 8 ounce	1 container	143	12	4	16	16	0	159	14
Yogurt, plain, low fat, 12 grams protein per 8 ounce	1 cup	154	13	4	17	17	0	172	15

Description	Serving Size	Cal	Prot (g)	Fat (g)	Carbs (g)	Net Carb(g)	Fiber (g)	Sod (mg)	Chol (mg)
YOGURT (continued)									
Yogurt, plain, skim milk, 13 grams protein per 8 ounce	1 container	127	13	0	17	17	0	175	5
Yogurt, plain, skim milk, 13 grams protein per 8 ounce	1 cup	137	14	0	19	19	0	189	5
Yogurt, plain, whole milk, 8 grams protein per 8 ounce	1 container	138	8	7	11	11	0	104	30
Yogurt, plain, whole milk, 8 grams protein per 8 ounce	1 cup	149	9	8	11	11	0	113	32
Yogurt, vanilla, low fat, 11 grams protein per 8 ounce	1 container	193	11	3	31	31	0	150	11
Yogurt, vanilla, low fat, 11 grams protein per 8 ounce	1 cup	208	12	3	34	34	0	162	12

Description	Serving Size	Cal	Prot (g)	Fat (g)	Carbs (g)	Net Carb(g)	Fiber (g)	Sod (mg)	Chol (mg)
Brownies									
Commercially prepared	1 square	227	3	9	36	62	1	175	10
Prepared from recipe	1 brownie	112	1	7	12	N.A.	N.A.	82	18
Cakes & Frostings									
CAKE									
Angelfood, commercially prepared	1 piece	73	2	0	16	56	0	212	0
Angelfood, dry mix, prepared	1 piece	129	3	0	29	58	0	255	0
Boston cream pie, commercially prepared	1 piece	232	2	7	39	41	1	132	34
Cheesecake, commercially prepared	1 piece	257	4	16	20	25	0	166	44
Cheesecake prepared from mix, no-bake type	1 piece	271	5	12	35	34	2	376	29
Cherry fudge with chocolate frosting	1 piece	187	2	8	27	37	1	160	30
Chocolate, commercially prepared with chocolate frosting	1 piece	235	3	10	35	52	2	214	27
Chocolate, prepared from recipe without frosting	1 piece	340	5	14	51	52	2	299	55
Coffeecake, cheese	1 piece	258	5	11	34	43	1	258	65
Coffeecake, cinnamon with crumb topping, commercially prepared	1 individual	238	4	12	27	45	1	200	18
Coffeecake, cinnamon with crumb topping, dry mix, prepared	1 piece	178	3	5	30	52	1	236	27
Coffeecake, creme-filled with chocolate frosting	1 piece	298	5	9	48	52	2	291	62
Coffeecake, fruit	1 piece	156	3	5	26	49	1	193	4
Fruitcake, commercially prepared	1 piece	139	1	4	26	58	2	116	2
GENERAL MILLS, BETTY CROCKER SUPERMOIST PARTY CAKE, SWIRL Cake Mix, dry	1 serving	178	2	1	35	N.A.	N.A.	266	0
GENERAL MILLS, BETTY CROCKER SUPERMOIST Yellow Cake Mix, dry	1 serving	178	2	1	35	N.A.	N.A.	289	0
Gingerbread, prepared from recipe	1 piece	263	3	11	36	N.A.	N.A.	242	24
MARTHA WHITE'S Chewy Fudge Brownie Mix, dry	1 serving	114	1	0	23	N.A.	N.A.	138	0
PILLSBURY, Traditional Fudge Brownie Mix, dry	1 serving	132	1	1	23	N.A.	N.A.	88	0
Pineapple upside-down, prepared from recipe	1 piece	367	4	13	58	50	1	367	25
Pound, commercially prepared, butter	1 piece	110	2	5	14	48	0	113	63

Description	Serving Size	Cal	Prot (g)	Fat (g)	Carbs (g)	Net Carb(g)	Fiber (g)	Sod (mg)	Chol (mg)
CAKES & FROSTING (continued)									
Pound, commercially prepared, other than all butter	1 piece	110	1	5	15	51	0	113	16
Snack cakes, creme-filled, chocolate with frosting	1 cupcake	188	2	7	30	60	0	213	9
Snack cakes, creme-filled, sponge	1 cake	155	1	4	27	63	0	155	7
Snack cakes, cupcakes, chocolate, with frosting, low-fat	1 cupcake	131	2	1	29	63	2	178	0
Sponge, commercially prepared	1 piece	110	2	1	23	61	0	93	39
Sponge, prepared from recipe	1 piece	187	5	2	36	N.A.	N.A.	144	107
White, prepared from recipe with coconut frosting	1 piece	399	5	11	71	62	1	318	1
White, prepared from recipe without frosting	1 piece	264	4	9	42	56	1	242	1
Yellow, commercially prepared, with chocolate frosting	1 piece	243	2	10	35	54	1	216	35
Yellow, commercially prepared, with vanilla frosting	1 piece	239	2	9	38	58	0	220	35
Yellow, prepared from recipe without frosting	1 piece	245	4	9	36	52	0	233	37
FROSTING									
Chocolate, creamy, dry mix, prepared with butter	1/12 container	160	0	4	30	70	1	63	10
Chocolate, creamy, dry mix, prepared with margarine	1/12 container	161	0	4	30	70	1	69	0
Chocolate, creamy, ready-to-eat	1/12 container	151	0	6	24	63	0	70	0
Coconut-nut, ready-to-eat	1/12 container	157	1	9	20	51	1	74	0
Cream cheese-flavor, ready-to-eat	1/12 container	157	0	6	25	67	0	90	0
Gláze, prepared-from-recipe	1 recipe	1174	2	24	240	73	0	307	7
Sour cream-flavor, ready-to-eat	1/12 container	157	0	6	26	67	0	78	0
Vanilla, creamy, dry mix	1/12 container	139	0	0	32	94	0	4	0
Vanilla, creamy, dry mix, prepared with butter	1/12 container	182	0	7	30	71	0	90	10
Vanilla, creamy, dry mix, prepared with margarine	1/12 container	182	0	7	30	71	0	95	0
Vanilla, creamy, ready-to-eat	1/12 container	159	0	6	26	69	0	34	0
White, fluffy, dry mix	1/12 container	63	0	0	16	95	0	40	0
White, fluffy, dry mix, prepared with water	1/12 container	63	0	0	16	63	0	41	0

Description	Serving Size	Cal	Prot (g)	Fat (g)	Carbs (g)	Net Carb(g)	Fiber (g)	Sod (mg)	Chol (mg)
Croissants									
Apple	1 croissant	145	4	5	21	35	1	156	18
Butter	1 croissant	115	2	5	13	43	1	211	19
Cheese	1 croissant	174	4	8	20	44	1	233	24
Doughnuts									
Cake-type, chocolate, sugared or glazed	1 doughnut	250	3	11	34	55	1	204	34
Cake-type, plain (includes unsugared, old-fashioned)	1 doughnut	219	3	11	26	48	1	284	19
Cake-type, plain, chocolate-coated or frosted	1 doughnut	133	1	8	13	46	1	120	17
Cake-type, plain, sugared or glazed	1 doughnut	192	2	10	23	49	1	181	14
Cake-type, wheat, sugared or glazed	1 doughnut	101	2	5	12	40	1	99	6
French crullers, glazed	1 cruller	169	1	7	24	58	0	141	5
Yeast-leavened, glazed, enriched (includes honey buns)	1 doughnut	52	1	3	6	43	0	44	1
Yeast-leavened, with creme filling	1 doughnut	307	5	18	26	29	1	263	20
Yeast-leavened, with jelly filling	1 doughnut	289	5	15	33	38	1	249	22
Gelatin Desserts									
JELL-O BRAND									
Sugar-Free Low Calorie Gelatin Dessert, with aspartame and acesulfame potassium sweetener, powder	1 serving	8	1	0	0	5	0	57	0
Sugar Free Low Calorie Gelatin Snacks Strawberry, with aspartame and acesulfame potassium sweetener, ready-to-eat	1 serving	7	1	0	0	0	0	45	0
Dry mix	1 package	324	7	0	77	90	0	216	0
Dry mix	1 portion	81	2	0	19	90	0	54	0
Dry mix, prepared with water	1 package	319	6	0	76	14	0	227	0
Dry mix, prepared with water	1/2 cup	80	2	0	19	14	0	57	0
Dry mix, reduced calorie, with aspartame	1 tbsp	31	5	0	3	33	0	195	0
Dry mix, reduced calorie, with aspartame	1 package	35	6	0	3	33	0	217	0
Dry mix, reduced calorie, with aspartame, no added sodium	1 tbsp	31	5	0	3	33	0	14	0
Dry mix, reduced calorie, with aspartame, prepared with water	1/2 cup	8	1	0	1	1	0	56	0

Description	Serving Size	Cal	Prot (g)	Fat (g)	Carbs (g)	Net Carb(g)	Fiber (g)	Sod (mg)	Chol (mg)
GELETAN DESSERTS (continued)									
Dry mix, reduced calorie, with aspartame, prepared with water	1 package	33	5	0	3	1	0	225	0
Dry mix, with added ascorbic acid, sodium-citrate and salt	1 package	324	7	0	77	90	0	417	0
Dry mix, with added ascorbic acid, sodium-citrate and salt	1 portion	81	2	0	19	90	0	105	0
Dry powder, unsweetened	1 envelope	23	6	0	0	0	0	14	0

Pastries

Description	Serving Size	Cal	Prot (g)	Fat (g)	Carbs (g)	Net Carb(g)	Fiber (g)	Sod (mg)	Chol (mg)
Cream puffs, prepared from recipe, shell (includes eclair)	1 eclair	174	4	12	11	22	0	267	94
Cream puffs, prepared from recipe, shell, with custard filling	1 cream puff	335	9	19	30	22	1	443	174
Danish pastry, cheese	1 pastry	266	6	15	26	36	1	320	11
Danish pastry, cinnamon	1 large	572	10	30	63	43	2	527	30
Danish pastry, fruit (includes apple, cinnamon, raisin, lemon, raspberry, strawberry)	1 large	527	8	24	68	46	3	503	162
Danish pastry, lemon	1 pastry	263	4	7	34	46	1	251	28
Danish pastry, nut (includes almond, raisin nut, cinnamon nut)	1 pastry	280	5	15	30	44	1	236	30
Danish pastry, raspberry	1 pastry	263	4	7	34	46	1	251	28
Eclairs, custard-filled with chocolate glaze, prepared from recipe	1 cream puff	293	7	16	27	24	1	377	142
HEINZ, WEIGHT WATCHERS Chocolate Eclairs, frozen	1 eclair, frozen	140	2	1	23	38	1	186	30
Phyllo dough	1 oz	85	2	2	15	51	1	137	0
Phyllo dough	1 sheet	57	1	1	10	51	0	92	0
Puff pastry, frozen, ready-to-bake	1 oz	156	2	10	13	44	0	71	0
Puff pastry, frozen, ready-to-bake	1 shell	259	3	17	21	44	1	117	0
Puff pastry, frozen, ready-to-bake, baked	1 oz	158	2	10	13	44	0	72	0
Puff pastry, frozen, ready-to-bake, baked	1 sheet	1367	18	90	112	44	4	620	0

Pies

PIE CRUST

Description	Serving Size	Cal	Prot (g)	Fat (g)	Carbs (g)	Net Carb(g)	Fiber (g)	Sod (mg)	Chol (mg)
Cookie-type, prepared from recipe, chocolate wafer, chilled	1 crust	1128	11	65	121	53	3	1499	2
Cookie-type, prepared from recipe, chocolate wafer, chilled	1 piece	142	1	8	15	53	0	188	0

Description	Serving Size	Cal	Prot (g)	Fat (g)	Carbs (g)	Net Carb(g)	Fiber (g)	Sod (mg)	Chol (mg)
Cookie-type, prepared from recipe, graham cracker, baked	1 pie shell	1037	9	49	137	64	3	1199	0
Cookie-type, prepared from recipe, graham cracker, chilled	1 piece	145	1	7	19	62	0	168	0
Cookie-type, prepared from recipe, vanilla wafer, chilled	1 crust	935	7	59	88	50	0	906	69
Standard-type, dry mix	1 oz	147	2	8	15	N.A.	N.A.	213	0
Standard-type, dry mix	1 package	1471	20	85	148	N.A.	N.A.	2139	0
Standard-type, dry mix, prepared, baked	1 piece	100	1	6	10	49	0	146	0
Standard-type, frozen, ready-to-bake	1 piece	73	1	4	7	43	0	92	0
Standard-type, frozen, ready-to-bake, baked	1 piece	82	1	5	8	49	0	104	0
Standard-type, prepared from recipe, baked	1 piece	121	1	8	11	46	0	125	0
Standard-type, prepared from recipe, unbaked	1 piece	113	1	7	10	39	1	116	0
PIE FILLING									
Apple, canned	1/8 can	75	0	0	19	25	1	33	0
Cherry, canned	1/8 can	85	0	0	21	27	0	13	0
PIES									
Apple, commercially prepared	1 piece	296	2	13	43	32	2	333	0
Apple, prepared from recipe	1 piece	411	4	18	58	N.A.	N.A.	327	0
Banana cream, prepared from mix, no-bake type	1 piece	231	3	11	29	31	1	267	27
Banana cream, prepared from recipe	1 pie	3190	52	151	390	32	8	2846	605
Blueberry, commercially prepared	1 piece	290	2	12	44	33	1	406	0
Blueberry, prepared from recipe	1 piece	360	4	16	49	N.A.	N.A.	272	0
Cherry, commercially prepared	1 piece	325	3	13	50	39	1	308	0
Cherry, prepared from recipe	1 piece	486	5	21	69	N.A.	N.A.	344	0
Chocolate creme, commercially prepared	1 piece	301	3	18	33	31	2	135	5
Chocolate mousse, prepared from mix, no-bake type	1 piece	247	3	13	28	N.A.	N.A.	437	33
Coconut cream, prepared from mix, no-bake type	1 piece	259	3	16	27	28	0	309	22
Coconut creme, commercially prepared	1 piece	191	1	10	24	36	1	163	0
Coconut custard, commercially prepared	1 piece	270	6	13	31	28	2	348	36
CONAGRA, BANQUET Apple Pie, frozen, ready to bake	1 serving	292	3	13	41	36	1	361	9

Description	Serving Size	Cal	Prot (g)	Fat (g)	Carbs (g)	Net Carb(g)	Fiber (g)	Sod (mg)	Chol (mg)
PIES (continued)									
Egg custard, commercially prepared	1 piece	221	6	11	22	19	2	252	35
Fried pies, cherry	1 pie	404	4	20	55	40	3	479	0
Fried pies, fruit	1 pie	404	4	20	55	40	3	479	0
Fried pies, lemon	1 pie	404	4	20	55	40	3	479	0
Lemon meringue, commercially prepared	1 piece	303	2	9	53	46	1	165	51
Lemon meringue, prepared from recipe	1 piece	362	5	15	50	N.A.	N.A.	307	67
Mince, prepared from recipe	1 piece	477	4	17	79	45	4	419	0
NABISCO NILLA Pie Crust, ready to use	1 serving	144	1	7	18	62	0	63	3
Peach	1 piece	261	2	11	38	32	1	316	0
Pecan, commercially prepared	1 piece	452	5	20	65	54	4	479	36
Pecan, prepared from recipe	1 piece	503	6	25	64	N.A.	N.A.	320	106
PEPPERIDGE FARM Apple Turnovers, frozen, ready to bake	1 serving	284	4	4	31	33	2	176	0
Pumpkin, commercially prepared	1 piece	229	4	10	30	25	3	307	22
Pumpkin, prepared from recipe	1 piece	316	7	13	41	N.A.	N.A.	349	65
Strudel, apple	1 piece	195	2	8	29	39	2	191	4
Vanilla cream, prepared from recipe	1 piece	350	6	17	41	32	1	328	78

Description	Serving Size	Cal	Prot (g)	Fat (g)	Carbs (g)	Net Carb(g)	Fiber (g)	Sod (mg)	Chol (mg)
Biscuit with egg and sausage	1 biscuit	581	19	36	41	40	1	1141	302
Biscuit with egg and steak	1 biscuit	410	18	26	21	N.A.	N.A.	888	272
Biscuit, with egg	1 biscuit	373	12	20	32	31	1	891	245
Biscuit, with egg and bacon	1 biscuit	458	17	29	29	28	1	999	353
Biscuit, with egg and ham	1 biscuit	442	20	25	30	30	1	1382	300
Biscuit, with egg, cheese, and bacon	1 biscuit	477	16	29	33	N.A.	N.A.	1260	261
Biscuit, with ham	1 biscuit	386	13	17	44	43	1	1433	25
Biscuit, with sausage	1 biscuit	485	12	30	40	39	1	1071	35
Brownie	1 brownie	243	3	10	39	N.A.	N.A.	153	10
Burrito, with beans	2 pieces	447	14	13	71	N.A.	N.A.	985	4
Burrito, with beans and cheese	2 pieces	378	15	11	55	N.A.	N.A.	1166	28
Burrito, with beans and chili peppers	2 pieces	412	16	14	58	N.A.	N.A.	1044	33
Burrito, with beans and meat	2 pieces	508	22	17	66	N.A.	N.A.	1335	49
Burrito, with beans, cheese, and beef	2 pieces	331	15	13	40	N.A.	N.A.	991	124
Burrito, with beans, cheese, and chili peppers	2 pieces	662	33	21	85	N.A.	N.A.	2060	158
Burrito, with beef	2 pieces	524	27	19	59	N.A.	N.A.	1492	64
Burrito, with beef and chili peppers	2 pieces	426	22	15	49	N.A.	N.A.	1116	54
Burrito, with beef, cheese, and chili peppers	2 pieces	632	41	23	64	N.A.	N.A.	2092	170
Burrito, with fruit (apple or cherry)	1 burrito	484	5	19	73	N.A.	N.A.	443	8
Cheeseburger, large, double patty, with condiments and vegetables	1 sandwich	704	38	40	40	N.A.	N.A.	1148	142
Cheeseburger, large, single meat patty, plain	1 sandwich	609	30	30	47	N.A.	N.A.	1589	96
Cheeseburger, large, single meat patty, with bacon and condiments	1 sandwich	608	32	33	37	N.A.	N.A.	1043	111
Cheeseburger, large, single patty, with condiments and vegetables	1 sandwich	563	28	30	38	N.A.	N.A.	1108	88
Cheeseburger, large, single patty, with ham, condiments and vegetables	1 sandwich	744	39	44	38	N.A.	N.A.	1712	122
Cheeseburger, regular, double patty and bun, plain	1 sandwich	461	22	20	44	N.A.	N.A.	891	80
Cheeseburger, regular, double patty and bun, with condiments and vegetables	1 sandwich	650	30	32	53	N.A.	N.A.	921	93
Cheeseburger, regular, double patty, plain	1 sandwich	457	28	26	22	N.A.	N.A.	636	110
Cheeseburger, regular, double patty, with condiments and vegetables	1 sandwich	417	21	19	35	N.A.	N.A.	1051	60
Cheeseburger, regular, single meat patty, plain	1 sandwich	319	15	14	32	N.A.	N.A.	500	50

Description	Serving Size	Cal	Prot (g)	Fat (g)	Carbs (g)	Net Carb(g)	Fiber (g)	Sod (mg)	Chol (mg)
Cheeseburger, regular, single patty, with condiments	1 sandwich	295	16	13	27	N.A.	N.A.	616	37
Cheeseburger, regular, single patty, with condiments and vegetables	1 sandwich	359	18	18	28	N.A.	N.A.	976	52
Cheeseburger, triple patty, plain	1 sandwich	796	56	46	27	N.A.	N.A.	1213	161
Chicken fillet sandwich, plain	1 sandwich	515	24	27	39	N.A.	N.A.	957	60
Chicken fillet sandwich, with cheese	1 sandwich	632	29	36	42	N.A.	N.A.	1238	78
Chicken, breaded and fried, boneless pieces, plain	1 piece	53	3	3	3	3	0	86	10
Chicken, breaded and fried, boneless pieces, with bbq sauce	6 pieces	330	17	17	25	N.A.	N.A.	829	61
Chicken, breaded and fried, boneless pieces, with honey	6 pieces	329	17	16	27	N.A.	N.A.	537	61
Chicken, breaded and fried, boneless pieces, with mustard sauce	6 pieces	322	17	18	21	N.A.	N.A.	790	61
Chicken, breaded and fried, boneless pieces, with sweet & sour sauce	6 pieces	346	17	16	29	N.A.	N.A.	677	61
Chicken, breaded and fried, dark meat (drumstick or thigh)	2 pieces	431	30	24	16	N.A.	N.A.	755	166
Chicken, breaded and fried, light meat (breast or wing)	2 pieces	494	36	27	20	N.A.	N.A.	975	148
Chili con carne	1 cup	256	25	7	22	N.A.	N.A.	1007	134
Chimichanga, with beef	1 chimichanga	425	20	18	43	N.A.	N.A.	910	9
Chimichanga, with beef and cheese	1 chimichanga	443	20	21	39	N.A.	N.A.	957	51
Chimichanga, with beef and red chili peppers	1 chimichanga	424	18	17	46	N.A.	N.A.	1169	10
Chimichanga, with beef, cheese, and red chili peppers	1 chimichanga	364	15	16	38	N.A.	N.A.	895	50
Clams, breaded and fried	3/4 cup	451	13	25	39	N.A.	N.A.	834	87
Coleslaw	3/4 cup	147	1	10	13	N.A.	N.A.	267	5
Cookies, animal crackers	1 box	299	4	8	50	N.A.	N.A.	273	11
Cookies, chocolate chip	1 box	233	3	11	36	N.A.	N.A.	188	12
Corn on the cob with butter	1 ear	155	4	3	32	N.A.	N.A.	29	6
Corndog	1 sandwich	460	17	18	56	N.A.	N.A.	973	79
Crab cake	1 cake	160	11	10	5	5	0	491	82
Croissant, with egg and cheese	1 croissant	368	13	23	24	N.A.	N.A.	551	216
Croissant, with egg, cheese, and bacon	1 croissant	413	16	26	24	N.A.	N.A.	889	215
Croissant, with egg, cheese, and ham	1 croissant	474	19	31	24	N.A.	N.A.	1081	213
Croissant, with egg, cheese, and sausage	1 croissant	523	20	35	25	N.A.	N.A.	1115	216

Description	Serving Size	Cal	Prot (g)	Fat (g)	Carbs (g)	Net Carb(g)	Fiber (g)	Sod (mg)	Chol (mg)
Danish pastry, cheese	1 pastry	353	6	23	29	N.A.	N.A.	319	20
Danish pastry, cinnamon	1 pastry	349	5	16	47	N.A.	N.A.	326	27
Danish pastry, fruit	1 pastry	335	5	15	45	N.A.	N.A.	333	19
Egg and cheese sandwich	1 sandwich	340	16	17	26	N.A.	N.A.	804	291
Egg, scrambled	2 eggs	199	13	13	2	2	0	211	400
Enchilada, with cheese	1 enchilada	319	10	18	29	N.A.	N.A.	784	44
Enchilada, with cheese and beef	1 enchilada	323	12	17	30	N.A.	N.A.	1319	40
Enchirito, with cheese, beef, and beans	1 enchirito	344	18	15	34	N.A.	N.A.	1251	50
English muffin, with butter	1 muffin	189	5	5	30	N.A.	N.A.	386	13
English muffin, with cheese and sausage	1 muffin	393	15	23	29	28	1	1036	59
English muffin, with egg, cheese, and Canadian bacon	1 sandwich	289	17	11	27	25	2	729	234
English muffin, with egg, cheese, and sausage	1 muffin	487	22	28	31	N.A.	N.A.	1135	274
Fish fillet, battered or breaded, and fried	1 fillet	211	13	11	15	15	0	484	31
Fish sandwich, with tartar sauce	1 sandwich	431	17	21	41	N.A.	N.A.	615	55
Fish sandwich, with tartar sauce and cheese	1 sandwich	523	21	26	48	N.A.	N.A.	939	68
French toast sticks	5 pieces	513	8	27	58	55	3	499	75
French toast with butter	2 slices	356	10	17	36	N.A.	N.A.	513	116
Frijoles with cheese	1 cup	225	11	7	29	N.A.	N.A.	882	37
Ham and cheese sandwich	1 sandwich	352	21	15	33	N.A.	N.A.	771	58
Ham, egg, and cheese sandwich	1 sandwich	347	19	15	31	N.A.	N.A.	1005	246
Hamburger, large, double patty, with condiments and vegetables	1 sandwich	540	34	24	40	N.A.	N.A.	791	122
Hamburger, large, single meat patty, plain	1 sandwich	426	23	20	32	N.A.	N.A.	474	71
Hamburger, large, single meat patty, with condiments and vegetables	1 sandwich	512	26	24	40	N.A.	N.A.	824	87
Hamburger, large, single patty, with condiments	1 sandwich	425	23	19	37	35	2	729	70
Hamburger, large, triple patty, with condiments	1 sandwich	692	50	37	29	N.A.	N.A.	712	142
Hamburger, regular, double patty, plain	1 sandwich	544	30	25	43	N.A.	N.A.	554	99
Hamburger, regular, double patty, with condiments	1 sandwich	576	32	29	39	N.A.	N.A.	742	103
Hamburger, regular, single patty, plain	1 sandwich	275	12	11	31	N.A.	N.A.	387	35
Hamburger, regular, single patty, with condiments	1 sandwich	272	12	8	34	32	2	534	30

Description	Serving Size	Cal	Prot (g)	Fat (g)	Carbs (g)	Net Carb(g)	Fiber (g)	Sod (mg)	Chol (mg)
Hamburger, regular, single patty, with condiments and vegetables	1 sandwich	279	13	12	27	N.A.	N.A.	504	26
Hotdog, plain	1 sandwich	242	10	14	18	N.A.	N.A.	670	44
Hotdog, with chili	1 sandwich	296	14	13	31	N.A.	N.A.	480	51
Hush puppies	5 pieces	257	5	11	35	N.A.	N.A.	965	135
Ice milk, vanilla, soft-serve, with cone	1 cone	164	4	6	24	24	0	92	28
Nachos, with cheese	1 portion	346	9	18	36	N.A.	N.A.	816	18
Nachos, with cheese and jalapeno peppers	1 portion	608	17	32	60	N.A.	N.A.	1736	84
Nachos, with cheese, beans, ground beef, and peppers	1 portion	569	20	29	56	N.A.	N.A.	1800	20
Nachos, with cinnamon and sugar	1 portion	592	7	34	63	N.A.	N.A.	439	39
Onion rings, breaded and fried	1 portion	276	4	14	31	N.A.	N.A.	430	14
Oysters, battered or breaded, and fried	6 pieces	368	13	16	40	N.A.	N.A.	677	108
Pancakes with butter and syrup	2 cakes	520	8	13	91	N.A.	N.A.	1104	58
Pizza with cheese	1 slice	140	8	3	21	N.A.	N.A.	336	9
Pizza with cheese, meat, and vegetables	1 slice	184	13	5	21	N.A.	N.A.	382	21
Pizza with pepperoni	1 slice	181	10	7	20	N.A.	N.A.	267	14
Potato salad	1/3 cup	108	1	5	13	N.A.	N.A.	312	57
Potato, baked and topped with cheese sauce	1 piece	474	15	27	47	N.A.	N.A.	382	18
Potato, baked and topped with cheese sauce and bacon	1 piece	451	18	25	44	N.A.	N.A.	972	30
Potato, baked and topped with cheese sauce and broccoli	1 piece	403	14	20	47	N.A.	N.A.	485	20
Potato, baked and topped with cheese sauce and chili	1 piece	482	23	21	56	N.A.	N.A.	699	32
Potato, baked and topped with sour cream and chives	1 piece	393	7	21	50	N.A.	N.A.	181	24
Potato, French fried in vegetable oil	1 large	578	7	30	67	61	6	335	0
Potato, French fried in vegetable oil	1 medium	458	6	24	53	49	5	265	0
Potato, mashed	1/3 cup	66	2	1	13	N.A.	N.A.	182	2
Potatoes, hashed brown	1/2 cup	151	2	9	16	N.A.	N.A.	290	9
Roast beef sandwich with cheese	1 sandwich	473	32	16	45	N.A.	N.A.	1633	77
Roast beef sandwich, plain	1 sandwich	346	22	12	33	N.A.	N.A.	792	51
Salad, vegetable, tossed, without dressing	1-1/2 cup	33	3	0	7	N.A.	N.A.	54	0
Salad, vegetable, tossed, without dressing, with cheese and egg	1-1/2 cup	102	9	5	5	N.A.	N.A.	119	98
Salad, vegetable, tossed, without dressing, with chicken	1-1/2 cup	105	17	2	4	N.A.	N.A.	209	72

Description	Serving Size	Cal	Prot (g)	Fat (g)	Carbs (g)	Net Carb(g)	Fiber (g)	Sod (mg)	Chol (mg)
Salad, vegetable, tossed, without dressing, with pasta and seafood	1-1/2 cup	379	16	16	32	N.A.	N.A.	1572	50
Salad, vegetable, tossed, without dressing, with shrimp	1-1/2 cup	106	15	2	7	N.A.	N.A.	489	179
Salad, vegetables tossed, without dressing, with turkey, ham and cheese	1-1/2 cup	267	26	15	5	N.A.	N.A.	743	140
Scallops, breaded and fried	6 pieces	386	16	18	38	N.A.	N.A.	919	108
Shrimp, breaded and fried	1 shrimp	454	19	23	40	N.A.	N.A.	1446	200
Steak sandwich	1 sandwich	459	30	13	52	N.A.	N.A.	798	73
Submarine sandwich, with cold cuts	1 submarine	456	22	17	51	N.A.	N.A.	1651	36
Submarine sandwich, with roast beef	1 submarine	410	29	12	44	N.A.	N.A.	845	73
Submarine sandwich, with tuna salad	1 submarine	584	30	26	55	N.A.	N.A.	1293	49
Sundae, caramel	1 sundae	304	7	9	49	49	0	195	25
Sundae, hot fudge	1 sundae	284	6	8	48	48	0	182	21
Sundae, strawberry	1 sundae	268	6	7	45	45	0	92	21
Taco	1 large	568	32	29	41	N.A.	N.A.	1233	87
Taco	1 small	369	21	19	27	N.A.	N.A.	802	56
Taco salad	1-1/2 cup	279	13	14	24	N.A.	N.A.	762	44
Taco salad with chili con carne	1-1/2 cup	290	17	12	27	N.A.	N.A.	885	5
Tostada, with beans and cheese	1 piece	223	10	9	27	N.A.	N.A.	543	30
Tostada, with beans, beef, and cheese	1 piece	333	16	16	30	N.A.	N.A.	871	74
Tostada, with beef and cheese	1 piece	315	19	15	23	N.A.	N.A.	897	41
Tostada, with guacamole	2 pieces	360	12	21	32	N.A.	N.A.	799	39

Description	Serving Size	Cal	Prot (g)	Fat (g)	Carbs (g)	Net Carb(g)	Fiber (g)	Sod (mg)	Chol (mg)
Fat & Lard									
Beef tallow, chicken, duck, goose, mutton tallow, turkey, lard (pork)	1 tbsp	115	0	13	0	0	0	0	14
Beef tallow, chicken, duck, goose, mutton tallow, turkey, lard (pork)	1 cup	1849	0	205	0	0	0	0	223
Margarine									
Margarine, 70% vegetable oil spread, soybean and soybean (hydrogenated)	1 tbsp	87	0	10	0	0	0	98	0
Margarine, 80% fat, stick, includes regular and hydrogenated corn and soybean oils	1 tbsp	99	0	11	0	0	0	92	0
Margarine-butter blend, 60% corn oil margarine and 40% butter	1 tbsp	102	0	11	0	0	0	127	12
Margarine-butter blend, 60% corn oil margarine and 40% butter	1 cup	1630	2	183	1	1	0	2036	200
Margarine-like spread, approx 40% fat	1 tsp	17	0	2	0	0	0	46	0
Margarine-like spread, approx 40% fat	1 cup	800	1	90	1	1	0	2227	0
Margarine-like spread, approx 60% fat, stick	1 tsp	26	0	3	0	0	0	48	0
Margarine-like spread, approx 60% fat, stick	1 cup	1237	1	139	0	0	0	2276	0
Margarine-like spread, approx 60% fat, tub	1 tsp	26	0	3	0	0	0	48	0
Margarine-like spread, approx 60% fat, tub	1 cup	1237	1	139	0	0	0	2276	0
Regular, hard, with salt	1 stick	815	1	91	1	1	0	1069	0
Regular, hard, with salt	1 tsp	34	0	4	0	0	0	44	0
Regular, hard, without salt	1 stick	810	1	91	1	1	0	2	0
Regular, hard, without salt	1 tsp	34	0	4	0	0	0	0	0
Regular, liquid	1 tbsp	102	0	11	0	0	0	111	0
Regular, liquid	1 cup	1637	4	183	0	0	0	1773	0
Soft, with salt	1 tsp	34	0	4	0	0	0	51	0
Soft, with salt	1 cup	1625	2	183	1	1	0	2449	0
Soft, without salt	1 tsp	34	0	4	0	0	0	1	0
Soft, without salt	1 cup	1625	2	182	2	2	0	64	0
Oil									
Coconut	1 tbsp	117	0	14	0	0	0	0	0

Description	Serving Size	Cal	Prot (g)	Fat (g)	Carbs (g)	Net Carb(g)	Fiber (g)	Sod (mg)	Chol (mg)
OIL (continued)									
Coconut	1 cup	1879	0	218	0	0	0	0	0
Fish oil, cod liver	1 tbsp	123	0	14	0	0	0	0	78
Fish oil, cod liver	1 cup	1966	0	218	0	0	0	0	1243
Fish oil, herring	1 tbsp	123	0	14	0	0	0	0	104
Fish oil, herring	1 cup	1966	0	218	0	0	0	0	1670
Fish oil, menhaden	1 tbsp	123	0	14	0	0	0	0	71
Fish oil, menhaden	1 cup	1966	0	218	0	0	0	0	1136
Fish oil, menhaden, fully hydrogenated	1 tbsp	113	0	13	0	0	0	0	63
Fish oil, menhaden, fully hydrogenated	1 cup	1849	0	205	0	0	0	0	1025
Fish oil, salmon	1 tbsp	123	0	14	0	0	0	0	66
Fish oil, salmon	1 cup	1966	0	218	0	0	0	0	1057
Fish oil, sardine	1 tbsp	123	0	14	0	0	0	0	97
Fish oil, sardine	1 cup	1966	0	218	0	0	0	0	1548
Olive, salad or cooking	1 tbsp	119	0	14	0	0	0	0	0
Olive, salad or cooking	1 cup	1909	0	216	0	0	0	0	0
Peanut, salad or cooking	1 tbsp	119	0	14	0	0	0	0	0
Peanut, salad or cooking	1 cup	1909	0	216	0	0	0	0	0
Sesame, salad or cooking	1 tbsp	120	0	14	0	0	0	0	0
Sesame, salad or cooking	1 cup	1927	0	218	0	0	0	0	0
Soybean, salad or cooking	1 tbsp	120	0	14	0	0	0	0	0
Soybean, salad or cooking	1 cup	1927	0	218	0	0	0	0	0
Soybean, salad or cooking, (hydrogenated)	1 tbsp	120	0	14	0	0	0	0	0
Soybean, salad or cooking, (hydrogenated)	1 cup	1927	0	218	0	0	0	0	0
Soybean, salad or cooking, (hydrogenated) and cottonseed	1 tbsp	120	0	14	0	0	0	0	0
Soybean, salad or cooking, (hydrogenated) and cottonseed	1 cup	1927	0	218	0	0	0	0	0
Vegetable safflower, salad or cooking, linoleic, (over 70%)	1 tbsp	120	0	14	0	0	0	0	0
Vegetable safflower, salad or cooking, linoleic, (over 70%)	1 cup	1927	0	218	0	0	0	0	0
Vegetable safflower, salad or cooking, oleic, over 70% (primary safflower oil of commerce)	1 tbsp	120	0	14	0	0	0	0	0
Vegetable safflower, salad or cooking, oleic, over 70% (primary safflower oil of commerce)	1 cup	1927	0	218	0	0	0	0	0

Description	Serving Size	Cal	Prot (g)	Fat (g)	Carbs (g)	Net Carb(g)	Fiber (g)	Sod (mg)	Chol (mg)
Vegetable, almond	1 tbsp	120	0	14	0	0	0	0	0
Vegetable, almond	1 cup	1927	0	218	0	0	0	0	0
Vegetable, apricot kernel	1 tbsp	120	0	14	0	0	0	0	0
Vegetable, apricot kernel	1 cup	1927	0	218	0	0	0	0	0
Vegetable, avocado	1 tbsp	124	0	14	0	0	0	0	0
Vegetable, avocado	1 cup	1927	0	218	0	0	0	0	0
Vegetable, babassu	1 tbsp	120	0	14	0	0	0	0	0
Vegetable, babassu	1 cup	1927	0	218	0	0	0	0	0
Vegetable, canola	1 tbsp	124	0	14	0	0	0	0	0
Vegetable, canola	1 cup	1927	0	218	0	0	0	0	0
Vegetable, cocoa butter	1 tbsp	120	0	14	0	0	0	0	0
Vegetable, cocoa butter	1 cup	1927	0	218	0	0	0	0	0
Vegetable, corn, industrial and retail, all purpose salad or cooking	1 tbsp	120	0	14	0	0	0	0	0
Vegetable, corn, industrial and retail, all purpose salad or cooking	1 cup	1927	0	218	0	0	0	0	0
Vegetable, cottonseed, salad or cooking	1 tbsp	120	0	14	0	0	0	0	0
Vegetable, cottonseed, salad or cooking	1 cup	1927	0	218	0	0	0	0	0
Vegetable, cupu assu	1 tbsp	120	0	14	0	0	0	0	0
Vegetable, cupu assu	1 cup	1927	0	218	0	0	0	0	0
Vegetable, grape seed	1 tbsp	120	0	14	0	0	0	0	0
Vegetable, grape seed	1 cup	1927	0	218	0	0	0	0	0
Vegetable, hazelnut	1 tbsp	120	0	14	0	0	0	0	0
Vegetable, hazelnut	1 cup	1927	0	218	0	0	0	0	0
Vegetable, mustard	1 tbsp	124	0	14	0	0	0	0	0
Vegetable, mustard	1 cup	1927	0	218	0	0	0	0	0
Vegetable, nutmeg butter	1 tbsp	120	0	14	0	0	0	0	0
Vegetable, nutmeg butter	1 cup	1927	0	218	0	0	0	0	0
Vegetable, oat	1 tbsp	120	0	14	0	0	0	0	0
Vegetable, oat	1 cup	1927	0	218	0	0	0	0	0
Vegetable, palm	1 tbsp	120	0	14	0	0	0	0	0
Vegetable, palm	1 cup	1909	0	216	0	0	0	0	0
Vegetable, palm kernel	1 tbsp	117	0	14	0	0	0	0	0
Vegetable, palm kernel	1 cup	1879	0	218	0	0	0	0	0
Vegetable, poppy seed	1 tbsp	120	0	14	0	0	0	0	0
Vegetable, poppy seed	1 cup	1927	0	218	0	0	0	0	0
Vegetable, rice bran	1 tbsp	120	0	14	0	0	0	0	0
Vegetable, rice bran	1 cup	1927	0	218	0	0	0	0	0

Description	Serving Size	Cal	Prot (g)	Fat (g)	Carbs (g)	Net Carb(g)	Fiber (g)	Sod (mg)	Chol (mg)
OILS (continued)									
Vegetable, shea nut	1 tbsp	120	0	14	0	0	0	0	0
Vegetable, shea nut	1 cup	1927	0	218	0	0	0	0	0
Vegetable, soybean lecithin	1 tbsp	104	0	14	0	0	0	0	0
Vegetable, soybean lecithin	1 cup	1663	0	218	0	0	0	0	0
Vegetable, sunflower, high oleic (70% and over)	1 tbsp	124	0	14	0	0	0	0	0
Vegetable, sunflower, high oleic (70% and over)	1 cup	1927	0	218	0	0	0	0	0
Vegetable, sunflower, linoleic, (approx 65%)	1 tbsp	120	0	14	0	0	0	0	0
Vegetable, sunflower, linoleic, (approx 65%)	1 cup	1927	0	218	0	0	0	0	0
Vegetable, sunflower, linoleic, (hydrogenated)	1 tbsp	120	0	14	0	0	0	0	0
Vegetable, sunflower, linoleic, (hydrogenated)	1 cup	1927	0	218	0	0	0	0	0
Vegetable, sunflower, linoleic (less than 60%)	1 tbsp	120	0	14	0	0	0	0	0
Vegetable, sunflower, linoleic (less than 60%)	1 cup	1927	0	218	0	0	0	0	0
Vegetable, tea seed	1 tbsp	120	0	14	0	0	0	0	0
Vegetable, tea seed	1 cup	1927	0	218	0	0	0	0	0
Vegetable, tomato seed	1 tbsp	120	0	14	0	0	0	0	0
Vegetable, tomato seed	1 cup	1927	0	218	0	0	0	0	0
Vegetable, ucuhuba butter	1 tbsp	120	0	14	0	0	0	0	0
Vegetable, ucuhuba butter	1 cup	1927	0	218	0	0	0	0	0
Vegetable, walnut	1 tbsp	120	0	14	0	0	0	0	0
Vegetable, walnut	1 cup	1927	0	218	0	0	0	0	0
Wheat germ	1 tbsp	120	0	14	0	0	0	0	0
Wheat germ	1 cup	1927	0	218	0	0	0	0	0

Salad Dressing

Description	Serving Size	Cal	Prot (g)	Fat (g)	Carbs (g)	Net Carb(g)	Fiber (g)	Sod (mg)	Chol (mg)
Blue + Roquefort cheese, commercial, regular, without salt	1 tbsp	77	1	8	1	1	0	5	3
Blue + Roquefort cheese, commercial, regular, without salt	1 cup	1235	12	128	18	18	0	74	42
Blue or Roquefort cheese dressing, commercial, regular	1 tbsp	77	1	8	1	1	0	167	3
Blue or Roquefort cheese dressing, commercial, regular	1 cup	1235	12	128	18	18	0	2680	42

Description	Serving Size	Cal	Prot (g)	Fat (g)	Carbs (g)	Net Carb(g)	Fiber (g)	Sod (mg)	Chol (mg)
French dressing, commercial, regular	1 tbsp	67	0	6	3	3	0	214	0
French dressing, commercial, regular	1 cup	1075	2	103	44	44	0	3425	0
French dressing, reduced fat	1 tbsp	22	0	1	4	4	0	128	0
French dressing, reduced fat	1 cup	348	1	15	56	56	0	2046	0
French dressing, reduced fat, without salt	1 tbsp	22	0	1	4	3	0	5	0
French dressing, reduced fat, without salt	1 cup	348	1	15	56	56	1	78	0
French, cottonseed, oil, home recipe	1 tbsp	88	0	10	0	0	0	92	0
French, cottonseed, oil, home recipe	1 cup	1388	0	154	7	7	0	1448	0
French, home recipe	1 tbsp	88	0	10	0	0	0	92	0
French, home recipe	1 cup	1388	0	154	7	7	0	1448	0
Home recipe, cooked	1 tbsp	25	1	2	2	2	0	117	9
Home recipe, cooked	1 cup	400	11	24	38	38	0	1872	145
Home recipe, cooked, with margarine	1 tbsp	25	1	2	2	2	0	117	0
Home recipe, cooked, with margarine	1 cup	400	11	24	38	38	0	1872	0
Home recipe, cooked, with soft margarine	1 tbsp	25	1	2	2	2	0	117	0
Home recipe, cooked, with soft margarine	1 cup	400	11	24	38	38	0	1872	0
Home recipe, vinegar and oil	1 tbsp	70	0	8	0	0	0	0	0
Home recipe, vinegar and oil	1 cup	1123	0	125	6	6	0	3	0
Italian dressing, commercial, regular	1 tbsp	69	0	7	1	1	0	116	0
Italian dressing, commercial, regular	1 cup	1097	2	114	24	24	0	1849	0
Italian dressing, commercial, regular, without salt	1 tbsp	69	0	7	1	1	0	4	10
Italian dressing, commercial, regular, without salt	1 cup	1097	2	114	24	24	0	71	157
Italian dressing, reduced fat	1 tbsp	16	0	1	1	1	0	118	1
Italian dressing, reduced fat	1 cup	252	0	24	12	12	0	1889	14
Italian dressing, reduced fat, without salt	1 tbsp	16	0	1	1	1	0	5	1
Italian dressing, reduced fat, without salt	1 cup	252	0	24	12	12	0	72	14
KRAFT FREE Fat Free Italian Dressing	2 tbsp	20	0	0	4	3	0	430	1
KRAFT FREE Fat Free Ranch Dressing	2 tbsp	48	0	0	11	11	0	354	0
KRAFT LIGHT DONE RIGHT! Italian Dressing	2 tbsp	53	0	4	2	2	0	228	0
KRAFT LIGHT DONE RIGHT! Ranch Dressing	2 tbsp	77	0	7	3	3	0	303	8

Description	Serving Size	Cal	Prot (g)	Fat (g)	Carbs (g)	Net Carb(g)	Fiber (g)	Sod (mg)	Chol (mg)
SALAD DRESSING (continued)									
KRAFT Mayo Fat Free Mayonnaise Dressing	1 tbsp	11	0	0	2	2	0	120	2
KRAFT Mayo Light Mayonnaise	1 tbsp	50	0	5	1	1	0	120	5
KRAFT MIRACLE WHIP FREE Nonfat Dressing	1 tbsp	13	0	0	2	2	0	126	1
KRAFT MIRACLE WHIP LIGHT Dressing	1 tbsp	37	0	3	2	2	0	131	4
KRAFT Ranch Dressing	2 tbsp	148	0	16	1	1	0	287	8
KRAFT Zesty Italian Dressing	2 tbsp	109	0	11	2	2	0	505	0
Mayonnaise type, regular, with salt	1 tbsp	57	0	5	4	4	0	105	4
Mayonnaise type, regular, with salt	1 cup	917	2	78	56	56	0	1671	61
Mayonnaise, imitation, milk cream	1 tbsp	15	0	1	2	2	0	76	6
Mayonnaise, imitation, milk cream	1 cup	233	5	12	27	27	0	1210	103
Mayonnaise, imitation, soybean	1 tbsp	35	0	3	2	2	0	75	4
Mayonnaise, imitation, soybean	1 cup	557	1	46	38	38	0	1193	58
Mayonnaise, imitation, soybean without cholesterol	1 tbsp	68	0	7	2	2	0	50	0
Mayonnaise, imitation, soybean without cholesterol	1 cup	1085	0	107	36	36	0	794	0
Mayonnaise, soybean and safflower oil, with salt	1 tbsp	99	0	11	0	0	0	78	8
Mayonnaise, soybean and safflower oil, with salt	1 cup	1577	2	175	6	6	0	1250	130
Mayonnaise, soybean oil, with salt	1 tbsp	99	0	11	0	0	0	78	8
Mayonnaise, soybean oil, with salt	1 cup	1577	2	175	6	6	0	1250	130
Mayonnaise, soybean oil, without salt	1 tbsp	99	0	11	0	0	0	4	8
Mayonnaise, soybean oil, without salt	1 cup	1577	2	175	6	6	0	66	130
Russian dressing	1 tbsp	76	0	8	2	2	0	133	3
Russian dressing	1 cup	1210	4	124	25	25	0	2127	44
Russian dressing, low calorie	1 tbsp	23	0	1	4	4	0	141	1
Russian dressing, low calorie	1 cup	367	1	10	72	71	1	2257	16
Sesame seed dressing, regular	1 tbsp	68	0	7	1	1	0	153	0
Sesame seed dressing, regular	1 cup	1085	8	111	21	19	2	2450	0
Thousand island dressing, reduced fat	1 tbsp	24	0	2	2	2	0	153	2
Thousand island dressing, reduced fat	1 cup	390	2	26	40	37	3	2450	37
Thousand island, commercial, regular	1 tbsp	59	0	6	2	2	0	109	4
Thousand island, commercial, regular	1 cup	943	2	89	38	38	0	1750	65

Description	Serving Size	Cal	Prot (g)	Fat (g)	Carbs (g)	Net Carb(g)	Fiber (g)	Sod (mg)	Chol (mg)
Sandwich Spread									
Sandwich spread, with chopped pickle, regular, unspecified oils	1 tbsp	60	0	5	3	3	0	153	12
Sandwich spread, with chopped pickle, regular, unspecified oils	1 cup	953	2	83	55	54	1	2450	186
Shortening									
Shortening, all	1 tbsp	115	0	13	0	0	0	0	13
Shortening, all	1 cup	1845	0	205	0	0	0	0	205

Description	Serving Size	Cal	Prot (g)	Fat (g)	Carbs (g)	Net Carb(g)	Fiber (g)	Sod (mg)	Chol (mg)
Crustaceans									
CRAB									
Alaska king, imitation, made from surimi	3 oz	87	10	1	9	9	0	715	17
Alaska king, raw	1 leg	144	31	1	0	0	0	1438	72
Alaska king, raw	3 oz	71	16	0	0	0	0	711	36
Alaska king, steamed	1 leg	130	26	1	0	0	0	1436	71
Alaska king, steamed	3 oz	82	16	1	0	0	0	911	45
Blue, canned	1 cup	134	28	1	0	0	0	450	120
Blue, canned	1 oz	28	6	0	0	0	0	94	25
Blue, crab cakes	1 cake	93	12	4	0	0	0	198	90
Blue, raw	3 oz	74	15	1	0	0	0	249	66
Blue, raw	1 crab	18	4	0	0	0	0	62	16
Blue, steamed	1 cup, flaked and pieces	120	24	1	0	0	0	329	118
Blue, steamed	1 cup	138	27	2	0	0	0	377	135
Dungeness, raw	3 oz	73	15	1	1	1	0	251	50
Dungeness, raw	1 crab	140	28	1	1	1	0	481	96
Dungeness, steamed	3 oz	94	19	1	1	1	0	321	65
Dungeness, steamed	1 crab	140	28	1	1	1	0	480	97
Queen, raw	3 oz	77	16	1	0	0	0	458	47
Queen, steamed	3 oz	98	20	1	0	0	0	587	60
CRAYFISH									
Mixed species, farmed, raw	3 oz	61	13	1	0	0	0	53	91
Mixed species, farmed, steamed	3 oz	74	15	1	0	0	0	82	116
Mixed species, wild, raw	3 oz	65	14	1	0	0	0	49	97
Mixed species, wild, steamed	3 oz	70	14	1	0	0	0	80	113
LOBSTER									
Northern, raw	1 lobster	135	28	1	1	1	0	444	143
Northern, raw	3 oz	77	16	1	0	0	0	252	81
Northern, steamed	1 cup	142	30	1	2	2	0	551	104
Northern, steamed	3 oz	83	17	0	1	1	0	323	61
SHRIMP									
Mixed species, breaded and fried	3 oz	206	18	9	10	9	0	292	150
Mixed species, breaded and fried	4 large	73	6	3	3	3	0	103	53
Mixed species, canned	1 cup	154	30	2	1	1	0	216	221
Mixed species, canned	1 oz	34	7	0	0	0	0	48	49

Description	Serving Size	Cal	Prot (g)	Fat (g)	Carbs (g)	Net Carb(g)	Fiber (g)	Sod (mg)	Chol (mg)
CRUSTACEANS(continued)									
Mixed species, imitation, made from surimi	3 oz	86	11	1	8	8	0	599	31
Mixed species, raw	1 medium	6	1	0	0	0	0	9	9
Mixed species, raw	1 small	5	1	0	0	0	0	7	8
Mixed species, steamed	3 oz	84	18	1	0	0	0	190	166
Mixed species, steamed	4 large	22	5	0	0	0	0	49	43
SPINY LOBSTER									
Mixed species, raw	1 lobster	234	43	2	5	5	0	370	146
Mixed species, raw	3 oz	95	18	1	2	2	0	150	60
Mixed species, steamed	1 lobster	233	43	2	5	5	0	370	147
Mixed species, steamed	3 oz	122	22	1	3	3	0	193	77

Fish

ANCHOVY

Description	Serving Size	Cal	Prot (g)	Fat (g)	Carbs (g)	Net Carb(g)	Fiber (g)	Sod (mg)	Chol (mg)
European, canned in oil, drained solids	1 oz, boneless	60	8	2	0	0	0	1040	24
European, canned in oil, drained solids	1 anchovy	8	1	0	0	0	0	147	3
European, raw	3 oz	111	17	3	0	0	0	88	51
BASS									
Fresh water, mixed species, raw	1 fillet	90	15	3	0	0	0	55	54
Fresh water, mixed species, raw	3 oz	97	16	3	0	0	0	60	58
Freshwater, mixed species, dry heat	1 fillet	91	15	3	0	0	0	56	54
Freshwater, mixed species, dry heat	3 oz	124	21	4	0	0	0	77	74
Striped, dry heat	1 fillet	154	28	3	0	0	0	109	128
Striped, dry heat	3 oz	105	19	2	0	0	0	75	88
Striped, raw	1 fillet	154	28	3	0	0	0	110	127
Striped, raw	3 oz	82	15	2	0	0	0	59	68
BLUEFISH									
Dry heat	1 fillet	186	30	6	0	0	0	90	89
Dry heat	3 oz	135	22	4	0	0	0	65	65
Raw	1 fillet	186	30	6	0	0	0	90	89
Raw	3 oz	105	17	3	0	0	0	51	50
BURBOT									
Dry heat	1 fillet	104	22	1	0	0	0	112	69
Dry heat	3 oz	98	21	1	0	0	0	105	65
Raw	1 fillet	104	22	1	0	0	0	113	70
Raw	3 oz	77	16	1	0	0	0	82	51

Description	Serving Size	Cal	Prot (g)	Fat (g)	Carbs (g)	Net Carb(g)	Fiber (g)	Sod (mg)	Chol (mg)
BUTTERFISH									
Dry heat	1 fillet	47	6	0	0	0	0	29	21
Dry heat	3 oz	159	19	0	0	0	0	97	71
Raw	1 fillet	47	6	2	0	0	0	28	21
Raw	3 oz	124	15	6	0	0	0	76	55
CARP									
Dry heat	1 fillet	275	39	11	0	0	0	107	143
Dry heat	3 oz	138	19	5	0	0	0	54	71
Raw	1 fillet	277	39	11	0	0	0	107	144
Raw	3 oz	108	15	4	0	0	0	42	56
CATFISH									
Channel, breaded and fried	1 fillet	199	16	11	7	6	1	244	70
Channel, breaded and fried	3 oz	195	15	10	7	6	1	238	69
Channel, farmed, dry heat	1 fillet	217	27	10	0	0	0	114	92
Channel, farmed, dry heat	3 oz	129	16	6	0	0	0	68	54
Channel, farmed, raw	1 fillet	215	25	11	0	0	0	84	75
Channel, farmed, raw	3 oz	115	13	6	0	0	0	45	40
Channel, wild, dry heat	1 fillet	150	26	4	0	0	0	72	103
Channel, wild, dry heat	3 oz	89	16	2	0	0	0	43	61
Channel, wild, raw	1 fillet	151	26	4	0	0	0	68	92
Channel, wild, raw	3 oz	81	14	2	0	0	0	37	49
CAVIAR									
Black and red, granular	1 tbsp	40	4	3	1	1	0	240	94
Black and red, granular	1 oz	71	7	5	1	1	0	425	167
CISCO									
Raw	1 fillet	77	15	1	0	0	0	43	40
Raw	3 oz	83	16	1	0	0	0	47	43
Smoked	1 oz	50	5	3	0	0	0	136	9
Smoked	3 oz	150	14	8	0	0	0	409	27
COD									
Atlantic, canned, solids and liquid	1 can	328	71	2	0	0	0	680	172
Atlantic, canned, solids and liquid	3 oz	89	19	0	0	0	0	185	47
Atlantic, dried and salted	1 oz	82	18	0	0	0	0	1992	43
Atlantic, dried and salted	1 piece	232	50	1	0	0	0	5622	122
Atlantic, dry heat	1 fillet	189	41	1	0	0	0	140	99
Atlantic, dry heat	3 oz	89	19	0	0	0	0	66	47

Description	Serving Size	Cal	Prot (g)	Fat (g)	Carbs (g)	Net Carb(g)	Fiber (g)	Sod (mg)	Chol (mg)
FISH (continued)									
Atlantic, raw	1 fillet	189	41	1	0	0	0	125	99
Atlantic, raw	3 oz	70	15	0	0	0	0	46	37
Pacific, dry heat	1 fillet	95	21	0	0	0	0	82	42
Pacific, dry heat	3 oz	89	20	0	0	0	0	77	40
Pacific, raw	1 fillet	95	21	0	0	0	0	82	43
Pacific, raw	3 oz	70	15	0	0	0	0	60	31
CROAKER									
Atlantic, breaded and fried	1 fillet	192	16	10	7	6	0	303	73
Atlantic, breaded and fried	3 oz	188	15	10	6	6	0	296	71
Atlantic, raw	1 fillet	82	14	2	0	0	0	44	48
Atlantic, raw	3 oz	88	15	2	0	0	0	48	52
CUSK									
Dry heat	1 fillet	106	23	0	0	0	0	38	50
Dry heat	3 oz	95	21	0	0	0	0	34	45
Raw	1 fillet	106	23	1	0	0	0	38	50
Raw	3 oz	74	16	0	0	0	0	26	35
DOLPHINFISH									
Dry heat	1 fillet	173	38	1	0	0	0	180	149
Dry heat	3 oz	93	20	1	0	0	0	96	80
Raw	1 fillet	173	38	1	0	0	0	180	149
Raw	3 oz	72	16	0	0	0	0	75	62
DRUM									
Freshwater, dry heat	1 fillet	236	35	9	0	0	0	148	126
Freshwater, dry heat	3 oz	130	19	5	0	0	0	82	70
Freshwater, raw	1 fillet	236	35	9	0	0	0	149	127
Freshwater, raw	3 oz	101	15	4	0	0	0	64	54
EEL									
Mixed species, dry heat, boneless	1 oz	67	7	4	0	0	0	18	46
Mixed species, dry heat, with bone	1 oz	52	5	3	0	0	0	14	35
Mixed species, raw	1 fillet	375	38	21	0	0	0	104	257
Mixed species, raw	3 oz	156	16	9	0	0	0	43	107
FISH PORTIONS AND STICK									
Frozen, preheated	1 stick	76	4	3	7	7	0	163	31
FLATFISH (FLOUNDER & SOLE)									
Dry heat	1 fillet	149	31	2	0	0	0	133	86

Description	Serving Size	Cal	Prot (g)	Fat (g)	Carbs (g)	Net Carb(g)	Fiber (g)	Sod (mg)	Chol (mg)
Dry heat	3 oz	99	21	1	0	0	0	89	58
Raw	1 oz, boneless	26	5	0	0	0	0	23	14
Raw	1 fillet	148	31	1	0	0	0	132	78
GEFILTE FISH									
Commercial, sweet recipe	1 piece	35	4	1	3	3	0	220	13
GROUPER									
Mixed species, dry heat	1 fillet	238	50	2	0	0	0	107	95
Mixed species, dry heat	3 oz	100	21	1	0	0	0	45	40
Mixed species, raw	1 fillet	238	50	2	0	0	0	137	96
Mixed species, raw	3 oz	78	16	1	0	0	0	45	31
HADDOCK									
Dry heat	1 fillet	168	36	1	0	0	0	131	111
Dry heat	3 oz	95	21	1	0	0	0	74	63
Raw	1 fillet	168	36	1	0	0	0	131	110
Raw	3 oz	74	16	0	0	0	0	58	48
Smoked	1 oz, boneless	33	7	0	0	0	0	216	22
Smoked	1 cubic inch, boneless	20	4	0	0	0	0	130	13
HALIBUT									
Atlantic and Pacific, dry heat	1/2 fillet	223	42	4	0	0	0	110	65
Atlantic and Pacific, dry heat	3 oz	119	23	2	0	0	0	59	35
Atlantic and Pacific, raw	1/2 fillet	224	42	4	0	0	0	110	65
Atlantic and Pacific, raw	3 oz	94	18	2	0	0	0	46	27
Greenland, dry heat	1/2 fillet	380	29	25	0	0	0	164	94
Greenland, dry heat	3 oz	203	16	13	0	0	0	88	50
Greenland, raw	1/2 fillet	379	29	25	0	0	0	163	94
Greenland, raw	3 oz	158	12	10	0	0	0	68	39
HERRING									
Atlantic, dry heat	1 fillet	290	33	15	0	0	0	164	110
Atlantic, dry heat	3 oz	173	20	9	0	0	0	98	65
Atlantic, kippered	1 oz, boneless	62	7	3	0	0	0	260	23
Atlantic, kippered	1 cubic inch, boneless	37	4	2	0	0	0	156	14
Atlantic, pickled	1 cup	367	20	22	13	13	0	1218	18
Atlantic, pickled	1 oz, boneless	74	4	5	3	3	0	247	4
Atlantic, raw	1 oz, boneless	45	5	2	0	0	0	26	17
Atlantic, raw	1 fillet	291	33	15	0	0	0	166	110

Description	Serving Size	Cal	Prot (g)	Fat (g)	Carbs (g)	Net Carb(g)	Fiber (g)	Sod (mg)	Chol (mg)
FISH (continued)									
Pacific, dry heat	1 fillet	360	30	23	0	0	0	137	143
Pacific, dry heat	3 oz	213	18	14	0	0	0	81	84
Pacific, raw	1 fillet	359	30	23	0	0	0	136	142
Pacific, raw	3 oz	166	14	11	0	0	0	63	65
LING									
Dry heat	1 fillet	168	37	0	0	0	0	261	77
Dry heat	3 oz	94	21	0	0	0	0	147	43
Raw	1 fillet	168	37	1	0	0	0	261	77
Raw	3 oz	74	16	0	0	0	0	115	34
LINGCOD									
Dry heat	1/2 fillet	165	34	2	0	0	0	115	101
Dry heat	3 oz	93	19	1	0	0	0	65	57
Raw	1/2 fillet	164	34	2	0	0	0	114	100
Raw	3 oz	72	15	1	0	0	0	50	44
MACKEREL									
Atlantic, dry heat	1 fillet	231	21	14	0	0	0	73	66
Atlantic, dry heat	3 oz	223	20	13	0	0	0	71	64
Atlantic, raw	1 fillet	230	21	14	0	0	0	101	78
Atlantic, raw	3 oz	174	16	10	0	0	0	77	60
Jack, canned, drained solids	1 cup	296	44	11	0	0	0	720	150
Jack, canned, drained solids	1 oz, boneless	44	7	2	0	0	0	107	22
King, dry heat	1/2 fillet	206	40	3	0	0	0	313	105
King, dry heat	3 oz	114	22	2	0	0	0	173	58
King, raw	1/2 fillet	208	40	3	0	0	0	313	105
King, raw	3 oz	89	17	1	0	0	0	134	45
Pacific and jack, mixed species, dry heat	1 oz, boneless	57	7	2	0	0	0	31	17
Pacific and jack, mixed species, dry heat	1 cubic inch, boneless	34	4	1	0	0	0	19	10
Pacific and jack, mixed species, raw	1 fillet	356	45	15	0	0	0	194	106
Pacific and jack, mixed species, raw	3 oz	134	17	6	0	0	0	73	40
Spanish, dry heat	1 fillet	231	34	8	0	0	0	96	107
Spanish, dry heat	3 oz	134	20	5	0	0	0	56	62
Spanish, raw	1 fillet	260	36	10	0	0	0	110	142
Spanish, raw	3 oz	118	16	4	0	0	0	50	65

Description	Serving Size	Cal	Prot (g)	Fat (g)	Carbs (g)	Net Carb(g)	Fiber (g)	Sod (mg)	Chol (mg)
MILKFISH									
Dry heat	3 oz	162	22	0	0	0	0	78	57
Raw	3 oz	126	17	5	0	0	0	61	44
MONKFISH									
Dry heat	3 oz	82	16	0	0	0	0	20	27
Raw	3 oz	65	12	1	0	0	0	15	21
MULLET									
Striped, dry heat	1 fillet	140	23	3	0	0	0	66	59
Striped, dry heat	3 oz	128	21	3	0	0	0	60	54
Striped, raw	1 oz	33	5	1	0	0	0	18	14
Striped, raw	1 fillet	139	23	3	0	0	0	77	58
PERCH									
Atlantic, dry heat	1 fillet	61	12	1	0	0	0	48	27
Atlantic, dry heat	3 oz	103	20	1	0	0	0	82	46
Atlantic, raw	1 oz, boneless	27	5	0	0	0	0	21	12
Atlantic, raw	1 fillet	60	12	1	0	0	0	48	27
Mixed species, dry heat	1 fillet	54	11	0	0	0	0	36	53
Mixed species, dry heat	3 oz	99	21	1	0	0	0	67	98
Mixed species, raw	1 fillet	55	12	0	0	0	0	37	54
Mixed species, raw	3 oz	77	16	1	0	0	0	53	77
PIKE									
Northern, dry heat	1/2 fillet	175	38	1	0	0	0	76	78
Northern, dry heat	3 oz	96	21	1	0	0	0	42	43
Northern, raw	1/2 fillet	174	38	1	0	0	0	77	77
Northern, raw	3 oz	75	16	0	0	0	0	33	33
Walleye, dry heat	1 fillet	148	30	2	0	0	0	81	136
Walleye, dry heat	3 oz	101	21	1	0	0	0	55	94
Walleye, raw	1 fillet	148	30	2	0	0	0	81	137
Walleye, raw	3 oz	79	16	1	0	0	0	43	73
POLLOCK									
Atlantic, dry heat	1/2 fillet	178	38	1	0	0	0	166	137
Atlantic, dry heat	3 oz	100	21	1	0	0	0	94	77
Atlantic, raw	1/2 fillet	178	38	1	0	0	0	166	137
Atlantic, raw	3 oz	78	17	1	0	0	0	73	60
Walleye, dry heat	1 fillet	68	14	1	0	0	0	70	58
Walleye, dry heat	3 oz	96	20	1	0	0	0	99	82

Description	Serving Size	Cal	Prot (g)	Fat (g)	Carbs (g)	Net Carb(g)	Fiber (g)	Sod (mg)	Chol (mg)
FISH (continued)									
Walleye, raw	1 fillet	62	13	1	0	0	0	76	55
Walleye, raw	3 oz	69	15	1	0	0	0	84	60
POMPANO									
Florida, dry heat	1 fillet	186	21	8	0	0	0	67	56
Florida, dry heat	3 oz	179	20	8	0	0	0	65	54
Florida, raw	1 oz, boneless	46	5	2	0	0	0	18	14
Florida, raw	1 fillet	184	21	8	0	0	0	73	56
POUT									
Ocean, dry heat	1/2 fillet	140	29	1	0	0	0	107	92
Ocean, dry heat	3 oz	87	18	1	0	0	0	66	57
Ocean, raw	1/2 fillet	139	29	1	0	0	0	107	92
Ocean, raw	3 oz	67	14	1	0	0	0	52	44
ROCKFISH									
Pacific, mixed species, dry heat	1 fillet	180	36	2	0	0	0	115	66
Pacific, mixed species, dry heat	3 oz	103	20	1	0	0	0	65	37
Pacific, mixed species, raw	1 fillet	180	36	2	0	0	0	115	67
Pacific, mixed species, raw	3 oz	80	16	1	0	0	0	51	30
ROE									
Mixed species, dry heat	1 oz	58	8	2	1	1	0	33	136
Mixed species, dry heat	3 oz	173	24	6	2	2	0	99	407
Mixed species, raw	1 tbsp	20	3	1	0	0	0	13	52
Mixed species, raw	1 oz	40	6	2	0	0	0	26	106
ROUGHY									
Orange, dry heat	3 oz	76	16	1	0	0	0	69	22
Orange, raw	3 oz	59	12	0	0	0	0	54	17
SABLEFISH									
Dry heat	1/2 fillet	378	26	26	0	0	0	109	95
Dry heat	3 oz	213	15	14	0	0	0	61	54
Raw	1/2 fillet	376	26	26	0	0	0	108	95
Raw	3 oz	166	11	11	0	0	0	48	42
Smoked	1 oz	73	5	5	0	0	0	209	18
Smoked	3 oz	218	15	15	0	0	0	626	54
SALMON									
Atlantic, farmed, dry heat	1/2 fillet	367	39	20	0	0	0	109	112
Atlantic, farmed, dry heat	3 oz	175	19	10	0	0	0	52	54

Description	Serving Size	Cal	Prot (g)	Fat (g)	Carbs (g)	Net Carb(g)	Fiber (g)	Sod (mg)	Chol (mg)
Atlantic, farmed, raw	1/2 fillet	362	39	20	0	0	0	117	117
Atlantic, farmed, raw	3 oz	156	17	8	0	0	0	50	50
Atlantic, wild, dry heat	1/2 fillet	280	39	11	0	0	0	86	109
Atlantic, wild, dry heat	3 oz	155	22	6	0	0	0	48	60
Atlantic, wild, raw	1/2 fillet	281	39	11	0	0	0	87	109
Atlantic, wild, raw	3 oz	121	17	5	0	0	0	37	47
Chinook, dry heat	1/2 fillet	356	40	18	0	0	0	92	131
Chinook, dry heat	3 oz	196	22	10	0	0	0	51	72
Chinook, raw	1/2 fillet	356	40	18	0	0	0	93	131
Chinook, raw	3 oz	153	17	8	0	0	0	40	56
Chinook, smoked	1 cup, cooked	159	25	5	0	0	0	1066	31
Chinook, smoked	1 oz, boneless	33	5	1	0	0	0	222	7
Chinook, smoked, (lox), regular	1 oz	33	5	1	0	0	0	567	7
Chinook, smoked, (lox), regular	3 oz	99	16	3	0	0	0	1700	20
Chum, canned, without salt, drained solids with bone	1 can	520	79	18	0	0	0	277	144
Chum, canned, without salt, drained solids with bone	3 oz	120	18	4	0	0	0	64	33
Chum, drained solids with bone	1 can	520	79	18	0	0	0	1797	144
Chum, drained solids with bone	3 oz	120	18	4	0	0	0	414	33
Chum, dry heat	1/2 fillet	237	40	6	0	0	0	99	146
Chum, dry heat	3 oz	131	22	4	0	0	0	54	81
Chum, raw	1/2 fillet	238	40	6	0	0	0	99	147
Chum, raw	3 oz	102	17	3	0	0	0	43	63
Coho, farmed, dry heat	1 fillet	255	35	11	0	0	0	74	90
Coho, farmed, dry heat	3 oz	151	21	6	0	0	0	44	54
Coho, farmed, raw	1 fillet	254	34	11	0	0	0	75	81
Coho, farmed, raw	3 oz	136	18	6	0	0	0	40	43
Coho, wild, dry heat	1/2 fillet	247	42	7	0	0	0	103	98
Coho, wild, dry heat	3 oz	118	20	3	0	0	0	49	47
Coho, wild, raw	1/2 fillet	289	43	11	0	0	0	91	89
Coho, wild, raw	3 oz	124	18	5	0	0	0	39	38
Coho, wild, steamed	1/2 fillet	285	42	11	0	0	0	82	88
Coho, wild, steamed	3 oz	156	23	6	0	0	0	45	48
Pink, canned, solids with bone and liquid	1 can	631	90	24	0	0	0	2513	249
Pink, canned, solids with bone and liquid	3 oz	118	17	5	0	0	0	471	47

Description	Serving Size	Cal	Prot (g)	Fat (g)	Carbs (g)	Net Carb(g)	Fiber (g)	Sod (mg)	Chol (mg)
FISH (continued)									
Pink, canned, without salt, solids with bone and liquid	1 can	631	90	25	0	0	0	341	250
Pink, canned, without salt, solids with bone and liquid	3 oz	118	17	5	0	0	0	64	47
Pink, dry heat	1/2 fillet	185	32	5	0	0	0	107	83
Pink, dry heat	3 oz	127	22	3	0	0	0	73	57
Pink, raw	1/2 fillet	184	32	5	0	0	0	107	83
Pink, raw	3 oz	99	17	2	0	0	0	57	44
Sockeye, canned, drained solids with bone	1 can	565	76	25	0	0	0	1985	162
Sockeye, canned, drained solids with bone	3 oz	130	17	6	0	0	0	457	37
Sockeye, canned, without salt, drained solids with bone	1 can	565	76	25	0	0	0	277	162
Sockeye, canned, without salt, drained solids with bone	3 oz	130	17	6	0	0	0	64	37
Sockeye, dry heat	1/2 fillet	335	42	15	0	0	0	102	135
Sockeye, dry heat	3 oz	184	23	8	0	0	0	56	74
Sockeye, raw	1 oz, boneless	48	6	2	0	0	0	13	18
Sockeye, raw	1/2 fillet	333	42	15	0	0	0	93	123
SARDINE									
Atlantic, canned in oil, drained solids with bone	1 cup	310	37	16	0	0	0	752	212
Atlantic, canned in oil, drained solids with bone	1 oz	59	7	3	0	0	0	143	40
Pacific, canned in tomato sauce, drained solids with bone	1 cup	158	15	10	0	0	0	368	54
Pacific, canned in tomato sauce, drained solids with bone	1 can	659	60	41	0	0	0	1532	226
SCUP									
Dry heat	1 fillet	68	12	0	0	0	0	27	34
Dry heat	3 oz	115	21	0	0	0	0	46	57
Raw	1 cup	174	31	4	0	0	0	70	86
Raw	1 oz, boneless	30	5	1	0	0	0	12	15
SEA BASS									
Mixed species, dry heat	1 fillet	125	24	2	0	0	0	88	54
Mixed species, dry heat	3 oz	105	20	2	0	0	0	74	45
Mixed species, raw	1 fillet	125	24	2	0	0	0	88	53
Mixed species, raw	3 oz	82	16	1	0	0	0	58	35

Description	Serving Size	Cal	Prot (g)	Fat (g)	Carbs (g)	Net Carb(g)	Fiber (g)	Sod (mg)	Chol (mg)
SEATROUT									
Mixed species, dry heat	1 fillet	247	40	6	0	0	0	138	197
Mixed species, dry heat	3 oz	113	18	3	0	0	0	63	90
Mixed species, raw	1 fillet	248	40	6	0	0	0	138	198
Mixed species, raw	3 oz	88	14	2	0	0	0	49	71
SHAD									
American, dry heat	1 fillet	363	31	0	0	0	0	94	138
American, dry heat	3 oz	214	18	0	0	0	0	55	82
American, raw	1 fillet	362	31	22	0	0	0	94	138
American, raw	3 oz	167	14	10	0	0	0	43	64
Mixed species, batter-dipped and fried	3 oz	194	16	11	5	5	0	104	50
SHEEPSHEAD									
Dry heat	1 fillet	234	48	2	0	0	0	136	119
Dry heat	3 oz	107	22	1	0	0	0	62	54
Raw	1 fillet	257	48	4	0	0	0	169	119
Raw	3 oz	92	17	2	0	0	0	60	43
SMELT									
Rainbow, dry heat	3 oz	105	19	2	0	0	0	65	77
Rainbow, raw	3 oz	82	15	2	0	0	0	51	60
SNAPPER									
Mixed species, dry heat	1 fillet	218	45	2	0	0	0	97	80
Mixed species, dry heat	3 oz	109	22	1	0	0	0	48	40
Mixed species, raw	1 fillet	218	45	2	0	0	0	140	81
Mixed species, raw	3 oz	85	17	1	0	0	0	54	31
SPOT									
Dry heat	1 fillet	79	12	2	0	0	0	19	39
Dry heat	3 oz	134	20	4	0	0	0	31	65
Raw	1 fillet	79	12	2	0	0	0	19	38
Raw	3 oz	105	16	3	0	0	0	25	51
STURGEON									
Mixed species, dry heat	1 cup, cooked	184	28	6	0	0	0	94	105
Mixed species, dry heat	1 oz, boneless	38	6	1	0	0	0	20	22
Mixed species, raw	3 oz	89	14	3	0	0	0	46	51
Mixed species, smoked	1 oz	49	9	1	0	0	0	210	23
Mixed species, smoked	3 oz	147	27	3	0	0	0	628	68

Description	Serving Size	Cal	Prot (g)	Fat (g)	Carbs (g)	Net Carb(g)	Fiber (g)	Sod (mg)	Chol (mg)
FISH (continued)									
SUCKER									
White, dry heat	1 fillet	148	27	3	0	0	0	63	66
White, dry heat	3 oz	101	18	2	0	0	0	43	45
White, raw	1 fillet	146	27	3	0	0	0	64	65
White, raw	3 oz	78	14	2	0	0	0	34	35
SUNFISH									
Pumpkin seed, dry heat	1 fillet	42	9	0	0	0	0	38	32
Pumpkin seed, dry heat	3 oz	97	21	1	0	0	0	88	73
Pumpkin seed, raw	1 fillet	43	9	0	0	0	0	38	32
Pumpkin seed, raw	3 oz	76	16	0	0	0	0	68	57
SURIMI									
Raw	1 oz	28	4	0	2	2	0	41	9
Raw	3 oz	84	13	1	6	6	0	122	26
SWORDFISH									
Dry heat	3 oz	132	22	4	0	0	0	98	43
Raw	3 oz	103	17	3	0	0	0	77	33
TILEFISH									
Dry heat	1/2 fillet	221	37	5	0	0	0	89	96
Dry heat	3 oz	125	21	3	0	0	0	50	54
Raw	1/2 fillet	185	34	3	0	0	0	102	97
Raw	3 oz	82	15	1	0	0	0	45	43
TROUT									
Mixed species, dry heat	1 fillet	118	17	5	0	0	0	42	46
Mixed species, dry heat	3 oz	162	23	6	0	0	0	57	63
Mixed species, raw	1 fillet	117	16	5	0	0	0	41	46
Mixed species, raw	3 oz	126	18	5	0	0	0	44	49
Rainbow, farmed, dry heat	1 fillet	120	17	5	0	0	0	30	48
Rainbow, farmed, dry heat	3 oz	144	21	6	0	0	0	36	58
Rainbow, farmed, raw	1 fillet	109	16	4	0	0	0	28	47
Rainbow, farmed, raw	3 oz	117	18	4	0	0	0	30	50
Rainbow, wild, dry heat	1 fillet	215	33	7	0	0	0	80	99
Rainbow, wild, dry heat	3 oz	128	19	4	0	0	0	48	59
Rainbow, wild, raw	1 fillet	189	33	5	0	0	0	49	94
Rainbow, wild, raw	3 oz	101	17	3	0	0	0	26	50

Description	Serving Size	Cal	Prot (g)	Fat (g)	Carbs (g)	Net Carb(g)	Fiber (g)	Sod (mg)	Chol (mg)
TUNA									
Fresh, bluefin, dry heat	3 oz	156	25	5	0	0	0	43	42
Fresh, bluefin, raw	3 oz	122	20	4	0	0	0	33	32
Fresh, skipjack, raw	1/2 fillet	204	44	2	0	0	0	73	93
Fresh, skipjack, raw	3 oz	88	19	1	0	0	0	31	40
Fresh, yellowfin, raw	1 oz, boneless	31	7	0	0	0	0	10	13
Fresh, yellowfin, raw	1 cubic inch, boneless	17	4	0	0	0	0	6	7
Light, canned in oil, drained solids	1 cup, solid or chunks	289	43	11	0	0	0	517	26
Light, canned in oil, drained solids	1 oz	56	8	2	0	0	0	100	5
Light, canned in oil, without salt, drained solids	1 can	339	50	13	0	0	0	86	31
Light, canned in oil, without salt, drained solids	3 oz	168	25	6	0	0	0	43	15
Light, canned in water, drained solids	1 cup, solid or chunks	179	39	1	0	0	0	521	46
Light, canned in water, drained solids	1 oz	33	7	0	0	0	0	96	9
Light, canned in water, without salt, drained solids	1 can	191	42	1	0	0	0	83	50
Light, canned in water, without salt, drained solids	3 oz	99	22	1	0	0	0	43	26
Skipjack, fresh, dry heat	1/2 fillet	203	43	2	0	0	0	72	92
Skipjack, fresh, dry heat	3 oz	112	24	1	0	0	0	40	51
Tuna salad	1 cup	383	33	18	19	19	0	824	27
Tuna salad	3 oz	159	14	7	8	8	0	342	11
White, canned in oil, drained solids	1 can	331	47	13	0	0	0	705	55
White, canned in oil, drained solids	3 oz	158	23	6	0	0	0	337	26
White, canned in oil, without salt, drained solids	1 can	331	47	13	0	0	0	89	55
White, canned in oil, without salt, drained solids	3 oz	158	23	6	0	0	0	43	26
White, canned in water, drained solids	1 can	220	41	5	0	0	0	648	72
White, canned in water, drained solids	3 oz	109	20	2	0	0	0	320	36
White, canned in water, without salt, drained solids	1 can	220	41	5	0	0	0	86	72
White, canned in water, without salt, drained solids	3 oz	109	20	2	0	0	0	43	36
Yellowfin, fresh, dry heat	3 oz	118	25	1	0	0	0	40	49

Description	Serving Size	Cal	Prot (g)	Fat (g)	Carbs (g)	Net Carb(g)	Fiber (g)	Sod (mg)	Chol (mg)
FISH (continued)									
TURBOT									
European, dry heat	1/2 fillet	194	33	0	0	0	0	305	99
European, dry heat	3 oz	104	17	0	0	0	0	163	53
European, raw	1/2 fillet	194	33	5	0	0	0	306	98
European, raw	3 oz	81	14	2	0	0	0	128	41
WHITEFISH									
Mixed species, dry heat	1 fillet	265	38	10	0	0	0	100	119
Mixed species, dry heat	3 oz	146	21	6	0	0	0	55	65
Mixed species, raw	1 fillet	265	38	10	0	0	0	101	119
Mixed species, raw	3 oz	114	16	4	0	0	0	43	51
Mixed species, smoked	1 cup, cooked	147	32	1	0	0	0	1386	45
Mixed species, smoked	1 oz, boneless	31	7	0	0	0	0	289	9
WHITING									
Mixed species, dry heat	1 fillet	84	17	1	0	0	0	95	60
Mixed species, dry heat	3 oz	99	20	1	0	0	0	112	71
Mixed species, raw	1 fillet	83	17	1	0	0	0	66	62
Mixed species, raw	3 oz	77	16	1	0	0	0	61	57
WOLFFISH									
Atlantic, dry heat	1/2 fillet	146	27	3	0	0	0	130	70
Atlantic, dry heat	3 oz	105	19	2	0	0	0	93	50
Atlantic, raw	1/2 fillet	147	27	3	0	0	0	130	70
Atlantic, raw	3 oz	82	15	2	0	0	0	72	39
YELLOWTAIL									
Mixed species, dry heat	1/2 fillet	273	43	0	0	0	0	73	104
Mixed species, dry heat	3 oz	159	25	0	0	0	0	43	60
Mixed species, raw	1/2 fillet	273	43	9	0	0	0	73	103
Mixed species, raw	3 oz	124	20	4	0	0	0	33	47

Mollusks

Description	Serving Size	Cal	Prot (g)	Fat (g)	Carbs (g)	Net Carb(g)	Fiber (g)	Sod (mg)	Chol (mg)
ABALONE									
Mixed species, fried	3 oz	161	17	5	9	9	0	502	80
Mixed species, raw	3 oz	89	15	0	5	5	0	256	72
CLAM									
Mixed species, breaded and fried	3 oz	172	12	9	9	9	0	309	52
Mixed species, breaded and fried	20 small	380	27	19	19	19	0	684	115

Description	Serving Size	Cal	Prot (g)	Fat (g)	Carbs (g)	Net Carb(g)	Fiber (g)	Sod (mg)	Chol (mg)
Mixed species, canned, drained solids	1 cup	237	41	1	8	8	0	179	107
Mixed species, canned, drained solids	3 oz	126	22	1	4	4	0	95	57
Mixed species, canned, liquid	1 cup	5	1	0	0	0	0	516	7
Mixed species, canned, liquid	3 oz	2	0	0	0	0	0	183	3
Mixed species, raw	1 cup	168	29	1	6	6	0	127	77
Mixed species, raw	1 large	15	3	0	1	1	0	11	7
Mixed species, steamed	3 oz	126	22	1	4	4	0	95	57
Mixed species, steamed	20 small	281	49	2	10	10	0	213	127
CUTTLEFISH									
Mixed species, raw	3 oz	67	14	0	1	1	0	316	95
Mixed species, steamed	3 oz	134	28	1	1	1	0	632	190
MUSSEL									
Blue, raw	1 cup	129	18	2	6	6	0	429	42
Blue, raw	1 oz	24	3	0	1	1	0	81	8
Blue, steamed	3 oz	146	20	3	6	6	0	314	48
OCTOPUS									
Common, raw	3 oz	70	13	1	2	2	0	196	41
Common, steamed	3 oz	139	25	1	4	4	0	391	82
OYSTER									
Eastern, breaded and fried	3 oz	167	7	10	10	10	0	354	69
Eastern, breaded and fried	6 medium	173	8	10	10	10	0	367	71
Eastern, canned	1 cup	112	11	3	6	6	0	181	89
Eastern, canned	1 cup	171	18	4	10	10	0	278	136
Eastern, farmed, dry heat	3 oz	67	6	1	6	6	0	139	32
Eastern, farmed, dry heat	6 medium	47	4	1	4	4	0	96	22
Eastern, farmed, raw	3 oz	50	4	1	5	5	0	151	21
Eastern, farmed, raw	6 medium	50	4	1	5	5	0	150	21
Eastern, wild, dry heat	3 oz	61	7	1	4	4	0	207	42
Eastern, wild, dry heat	6 medium	42	5	1	3	3	0	144	29
Eastern, wild, raw	1 cup	169	17	5	10	10	0	523	131
Eastern, wild, raw	6 medium	57	6	2	3	3	0	177	45
Eastern, wild, steamed	3 oz	116	12	3	7	7	0	359	89
Eastern, wild, steamed	6 medium	58	6	2	3	3	0	177	44
Pacific, raw	1 medium	41	5	1	2	2	0	53	25
Pacific, raw	3 oz	69	8	1	4	4	0	90	43
Pacific, steamed	1 medium	41	5	1	2	2	0	53	25

Description	Serving Size	Cal	Prot (g)	Fat (g)	Carbs (g)	Net Carb(g)	Fiber (g)	Sod (mg)	Chol (mg)
MOLLUSKS (continued)									
Pacific, steamed	3 oz	139	16	3	8	8	0	180	85
SCALLOP									
Mixed species, breaded and fried	2 large	67	6	3	3	3	0	144	19
Mixed species, imitation, made from surimi	3 oz	84	11	0	9	9	0	676	19
Mixed species, raw	3 oz	75	14	0	2	2	0	137	28
SQUID									
Mixed species, fried	3 oz	149	15	6	7	7	0	260	221
Mixed species, raw	1 oz, boneless	26	4	0	1	1	0	12	66
Mixed species, raw	3 oz	78	13	1	3	3	0	37	198
WHELK									
Raw	3 oz	116	20	0	7	7	0	175	55
Steamed	3 oz	234	41	0	13	13	0	350	111

Description	Serving Size	Cal	Prot (g)	Fat (g)	Carbs (g)	Net Carb(g)	Fiber (g)	Sod (mg)	Chol (mg)
Abiyuch									
Raw	1/2 cup	79	2	0	20	14	6	23	0
Acerola									
West Indian cherry, raw	1 fruit, w/o refuse	2	0	0	0	0	0	0	0
Apples									
Applesauce, canned, sweetened, with salt	1 cup	194	0	0	51	48	3	71	0
Applesauce, canned, sweetened, without salt	1 cup	194	0	0	51	48	3	8	0
Applesauce, canned, unsweetened, with added ascorbic acid	1 cup	105	0	0	28	25	3	5	0
Applesauce, canned, unsweetened, without added ascorbic acid	1 cup	105	0	0	28	25	3	5	0
Canned, sweetened, sliced, drained, heated	1 cup, sliced	137	0	0	34	30	4	6	0
Canned, sweetened, sliced, drained, unheated	1 cup, sliced	137	0	0	34	31	3	6	0
Crabapples, raw	1 cup, sliced	84	0	0	22	NA	NA	1	0
Dehydrated (low moisture), sulfured, stewed	1 cup	143	1	0	38	33	5	50	0
Dehydrated (low moisture), sulfured, uncooked	1 cup	208	1	0	56	49	7	74	0
Dried, sulfured, stewed, with added sugar	1 cup	232	1	0	58	53	5	53	0
Dried, sulfured, stewed, without added sugar	1 cup	145	1	0	39	34	5	51	0
Dried, sulfured, uncooked	1 ring	16	0	0	4	4	1	6	0
Frozen, unsweetened, heated	1 cup, sliced	97	1	0	25	21	4	6	0
Frozen, unsweetened, unheated	1 cup, sliced	83	0	0	21	18	3	5	0
Raw, with skin	1 cup, quartered or chopped	74	0	0	19	16	3	0	0
Raw, with skin	1 cup, sliced	65	0	0	17	14	3	0	0
Raw, without skin	1 cup, sliced	63	0	0	16	14	2	0	0
Raw, without skin	1 medium	73	0	0	19	17	2	0	0
Apricots									
Canned, extra heavy syrup pack, without skin, solids and liquids	1 cup, whole, without pits	236	1	0	61	57	4	32	0

Description	Serving Size	Cal	Prot (g)	Fat (g)	Carbs (g)	Net Carb(g)	Fiber (g)	Sod (mg)	Chol (mg)
APRICOTS (continued)									
Canned, extra light syrup pack, with skin, solids and liquids	1 cup	121	1	0	31	27	4	5	0
Canned, heavy syrup pack, with skin, solids and liquids	1 cup	214	1	0	55	51	4	10	0
Canned, heavy syrup pack, without skin, solids and liquids	1 cup, whole, without pits	214	1	0	55	51	4	28	0
Canned, juice pack, with skin, solids and liquids	1 cup	117	2	0	30	26	4	10	0
Canned, light syrup pack, with skin, solids and liquids	1 cup	159	1	0	42	38	4	10	0
Canned, water pack, with skin, solids and liquids	1 cup	66	2	0	16	12	4	7	0
Canned, water pack, without skin, solids and liquids	1 cup, whole, without pits	50	2	0	12	10	2	25	0
Dehydrated (low-moisture), sulfured, stewed	1 cup	314	5	0	81	N.A.	NA	12	0
Dehydrated (low-moisture), sulfured, uncooked	1 cup	381	6	1	99	NA	NA	15	0
Dried, sulfured, stewed, with added sugar	1 cup	305	3	0	79	68	11	8	0
Dried, sulfured, stewed, without added sugar	1 cup	213	3	0	55	47	8	8	0
Dried, sulfured, uncooked	1 cup	309	5	0	80	69	12	13	0
Frozen, sweetened	1 cup	237	2	0	61	55	5	10	0
Raw	1 cup	74	2	0	17	14	4	2	0

Avocados

Description	Serving Size	Cal	Prot (g)	Fat (g)	Carbs (g)	Net Carb(g)	Fiber (g)	Sod (mg)	Chol (mg)
Raw, all commercial varieties	1 cup, cubes	242	3	21	11	4	8	15	0
Raw, California	1 cup, pureed	407	5	36	16	5	11	28	0
Raw, Florida	1 cup, pureed	258	4	19	20	8	12	12	0

Bananas

Description	Serving Size	Cal	Prot (g)	Fat (g)	Carbs (g)	Net Carb(g)	Fiber (g)	Sod (mg)	Chol (mg)
Dehydrated, or banana powder	1 tbsp	21	0	0	5	5	0	0	0
Raw	1 cup, mashed	207	2	1	53	47	5	2	0
Raw	1 cup, sliced	138	2	0	35	32	4	2	0

Blackberries

Description	Serving Size	Cal	Prot (g)	Fat (g)	Carbs (g)	Net Carb(g)	Fiber (g)	Sod (mg)	Chol (mg)
Canned, heavy syrup, solids and liquids	1 cup	236	3	0	59	50	9	8	0
Frozen, unsweetened	1 cup	97	2	0	24	16	8	2	0
Raw	1 cup	75	1	0	18	11	8	0	0

Description	Serving Size	Cal	Prot (g)	Fat (g)	Carbs (g)	Net Carb(g)	Fiber (g)	Sod (mg)	Chol (mg)
Blueberries									
Frozen, sweetened	1 cup	186	1	0	50	46	5	2	0
Frozen, unsweetened	1 cup	79	1	1	19	15	4	2	0
Raw	1 cup	81	1	0	20	17	4	9	0
Boysenberries									
Canned, heavy syrup	1 cup	225	3	0	57	50	7	8	0
Frozen, unsweetened	1 cup	66	1	0	16	11	5	1	0
Breadfruit									
Breadfruit, raw	1 cup	227	2	0	60	49	11	4	0
Carambola									
Carambola, (star fruit), raw	1 cup, cubes	45	1	0	11	7	4	3	0
Carissa									
Carissa, (natal-plum), raw	1 fruit, w/o skin and seeds	12	0	0	3	NA	NA	1	0
Cherimoya									
Cherimoya, raw	1 fruit, w/o skin and seeds	514	7	0	131	118	13	0	0
Cherries									
Sour, red, canned, extra heavy syrup pack, solids and liquids	1 cup	298	2	0	76	74	2	18	0
Sour, red, canned, heavy syrup pack, solids and liquids	1 cup	233	2	0	60	57	3	18	0
Sour, red, canned, light syrup pack, solids and liquids	1 cup	189	2	0	49	47	2	18	0
Sour, red, canned, water pack, solids and liquids	1 cup	88	2	0	22	19	3	17	0
Sour, red, frozen, unsweetened	1 cup, unthawed	71	1	1	17	15	2	2	0
Sour, red, raw	1 cup, without pits	78	2	0	19	16	2	5	0
Sour, red, raw	1 cup, with pits	52	1	0	13	11	2	3	0
Sweet, canned, extra heavy syrup pack, solids and liquids	1 cup	266	2	0	68	65	4	8	0
Sweet, canned, heavy syrup pack, solids and liquids	1 cup	210	2	0	54	50	4	8	0

Description	Serving Size	Cal	Prot (g)	Fat (g)	Carbs (g)	Net Carb(g)	Fiber (g)	Sod (mg)	Chol (mg)
CHERRIES (continued)									
Sweet, canned, juice pack, solids and liquids	1 cup	135	2	0	35	31	4	8	0
Sweet, canned, light syrup pack, solids and liquids	1 cup	169	2	0	44	40	4	8	0
Sweet, canned, water pack, solids and liquids	1 cup	114	2	0	29	25	4	2	0
Sweet, frozen, sweetened	1 cup, thawed	231	3	0	58	52	5	3	0
Sweet, raw	1 cup, with pits	84	1	1	19	17	3	0	0
Sweet, raw	1 cup, w/o pits	104	2	1	24	21	3	0	0

Cranberries

Description	Serving Size	Cal	Prot (g)	Fat (g)	Carbs (g)	Net Carb(g)	Fiber (g)	Sod (mg)	Chol (mg)
Cranberry sauce, canned, sweetened	1 slice	86	0	0	22	22	1	17	0
Cranberry-orange relish, canned	1 cup	490	1	0	127	127	0	88	0
Raw	1 cup, chop.	54	0	0	14	9	5	1	0

Currants

Description	Serving Size	Cal	Prot (g)	Fat (g)	Carbs (g)	Net Carb(g)	Fiber (g)	Sod (mg)	Chol (mg)
European black, raw	1 cup	71	2	0	17	NA	NA	2	0
Red and white, raw	1 cup	63	2	0	15	11	5	1	0
Zante, dried	1 cup	408	6	0	107	97	10	12	0

Dates

Description	Serving Size	Cal	Prot (g)	Fat (g)	Carbs (g)	Net Carb(g)	Fiber (g)	Sod (mg)	Chol (mg)
Deglet noor	1 date	23	0	0	6	5	1	0	0

Durian

Description	Serving Size	Cal	Prot (g)	Fat (g)	Carbs (g)	Net Carb(g)	Fiber (g)	Sod (mg)	Chol (mg)
Raw or frozen	1 fruit	885	9	2	163	140	23	6	0

Elderberries

Description	Serving Size	Cal	Prot (g)	Fat (g)	Carbs (g)	Net Carb(g)	Fiber (g)	Sod (mg)	Chol (mg)
Raw	1 cup	106	1	1	27	17	10	9	0

Feijoa

Description	Serving Size	Cal	Prot (g)	Fat (g)	Carbs (g)	Net Carb(g)	Fiber (g)	Sod (mg)	Chol (mg)
Raw	1 fruit, w/o refuse	25	1	0	5	NA	NA	2	0

Figs

Description	Serving Size	Cal	Prot (g)	Fat (g)	Carbs (g)	Net Carb(g)	Fiber (g)	Sod (mg)	Chol (mg)
Canned, extra heavy syrup pack, solids and liquids	1 cup	279	1	0	73	NA	NA	3	0
Canned, heavy syrup pack, solids and liquids	1 cup	228	1	0	59	54	6	3	0
Canned, light syrup pack, solids and liquids	1 cup	174	1	0	45	41	5	3	0
Canned, water pack, solids and liquids	1 cup	131	1	0	35	29	5	2	0
Dried, stewed	1 cup	280	3	1	71	58	13	13	0

Description	Serving Size	Cal	Prot (g)	Fat (g)	Carbs (g)	Net Carb(g)	Fiber (g)	Sod (mg)	Chol (mg)
Dried, uncooked	1 fig	48	1	0	12	10	2	2	0
Raw	1 large	47	0	0	12	10	2	1	0

Gooseberries

Description	Serving Size	Cal	Prot (g)	Fat (g)	Carbs (g)	Net Carb(g)	Fiber (g)	Sod (mg)	Chol (mg)
Canned, light syrup pack, solids and liquids	1 cup	184	2	0	47	41	6	5	0
Raw	1 cup	66	1	1	15	9	6	2	0

Grapefruit

Description	Serving Size	Cal	Prot (g)	Fat (g)	Carbs (g)	Net Carb(g)	Fiber (g)	Sod (mg)	Chol (mg)
Raw, pink and red and white, all areas	1/2 large	53	1	0	13	12	2	0	0
Raw, pink and red, all areas	1/2 fruit	37	1	0	9	NA	NA	0	0
Raw, pink and red, California and Arizona	1/2 fruit	46	1	0	12	NA	NA	1	0
Raw, pink and red, Florida	1/2 fruit	37	1	0	9	8	1	0	0
Raw, white, all areas	1/2 fruit	39	1	0	10	9	1	0	0
Raw, white, California	1/2 fruit	44	1	0	11	NA	NA	0	0
Raw, white, Florida	1/2 fruit	38	1	0	10	NA	NA	0	0
Sections, canned, juice pack, solids and liquids	1 cup	92	2	0	23	22	1	17	0
Sections, canned, light syrup pack, solids and liquids	1 cup	152	1	0	39	38	1	5	0
Sections, canned, water pack, solids and liquids	1 cup	88	1	0	22	21	1	5	0

Grapes

Description	Serving Size	Cal	Prot (g)	Fat (g)	Carbs (g)	Net Carb(g)	Fiber (g)	Sod (mg)	Chol (mg)
Canned, Thompson seedless, heavy syrup pack, solids and liquids	1 cup	187	1	0	50	49	1	13	0
Canned, Thompson seedless, water pack, solids and liquids	1 cup	98	1	0	25	23	2	15	0
Raw, American type (slip skin)	1 cup	62	1	0	16	15	1	2	0
Raw, American type (slip skin)	1 grape	2	0	0	0	0	0	0	0
Raw, red or green (European type varieties, such as, Thompson seedless)	1 cup, seedless	114	1	1	28	27	2	3	0

Guavas

Description	Serving Size	Cal	Prot (g)	Fat (g)	Carbs (g)	Net Carb(g)	Fiber (g)	Sod (mg)	Chol (mg)
Common, raw	1 fruit, w/o refuse	46	1	0	11	6	5	3	0
Guava sauce, cooked	1 cup	86	1	0	23	14	9	10	0
Strawberry, raw	1 fruit, w/o refuse	4	0	0	1	1	0	2	0

Description	Serving Size	Cal	Prot (g)	Fat (g)	Carbs (g)	Net Carb(g)	Fiber (g)	Sod (mg)	Chol (mg)
Jackfruit									
Canned, syrup pack	1 cup	164	1	1	43	41	2	20	0
Raw	1 cup, sliced	155	2	0	40	37	3	5	0
Java-plum									
Raw	3 pieces	5	0	0	1	NA	NA	1	0
Kiwi									
Fresh, raw	1 cup	108	2	1	26	20	6	9	0
Fresh, raw	1 fruit, w/o skin	56	1	0	14	10	3	5	0
Kumquats									
Raw	1 fruit, w/o refuse	12	0	0	3	2	1	1	0
Lemons									
Lemon peel, raw	1 tbsp	3	0	0	1	0	1	0	0
Raw, without peel	1 fruit	17	1	0	5	4	2	1	0
Limes									
Raw	1 fruit	20	0	0	7	5	2	1	0
Litchis									
Dried	1 fruit	7	0	0	2	2	0	0	0
Raw	1 fruit, w/o refuse	6	0	0	2	1	0	0	0
Loganberries									
Frozen	1 cup, unthawed	81	2	0	19	12	7	1	0
Longings									
Raw	1 fruit, w/o refuse	2	0	0	0	0	0	0	0
Loquats									
Raw	1 large	9	0	0	2	2	0	0	0
Mangosteen									
Canned, syrup pack	1 cup	143	1	0	35	32	4	14	0
Melon									
Cantaloupe, raw	1 cup, balls	62	2	0	15	13	1	16	0

Description	Serving Size	Cal	Prot (g)	Fat (g)	Carbs (g)	Net Carb(g)	Fiber (g)	Sod (mg)	Chol (mg)
Casaba, raw	1 cup, cubes	44	2	0	11	9	1	20	0
Honeydew, raw	1 cup, balls	62	1	0	16	15	1	18	0
Melon balls, frozen	1 cup, unthawed	57	1	0	14	13	1	54	0

Mixed Fruit

Description	Serving Size	Cal	Prot (g)	Fat (g)	Carbs (g)	Net Carb(g)	Fiber (g)	Sod (mg)	Chol (mg)
Fruit cocktail (peach and pineapple and pear and grape and cherry), canned, extra heavy syrup, solids and liquids	1 cup	229	1	0	60	57	3	16	0
Fruit cocktail (peach and pineapple and pear and grape and cherry), canned, extra light syrup, solids and liquids	1/2 cup	55	0	0	14	13	1	5	0
Fruit cocktail (peach and pineapple and pear and grape and cherry), canned, heavy syrup, solids and liquids	1 cup	181	1	0	47	44	2	15	0
Fruit cocktail (peach and pineapple and pear and grape and cherry), canned, juice pack, solids and liquids	1 cup	109	1	0	28	26	2	9	0
Fruit cocktail (peach and pineapple and pear and grape and cherry), canned, light syrup, solids and liquids	1 cup	138	1	0	36	34	2	15	0
Fruit cocktail (peach and pineapple and pear and grape and cherry), canned, water pack, solids and liquids	1 cup	76	1	0	20	18	2	9	0
Fruit salad (peach and pear and apricot and pineapple and cherry), canned, extra heavy syrup, solids and liquids	1 cup	228	1	0	59	56	3	13	0
Fruit salad (peach and pear and apricot and pineapple and cherry), canned, heavy syrup, solids and liquids	1 cup	186	1	0	49	46	3	15	0
Fruit salad (peach and pear and apricot and pineapple and cherry), canned, juice pack, solids and liquids	1 cup	125	1	0	32	30	2	12	0
Fruit salad (peach and pear and apricot and pineapple and cherry), canned, light syrup, solids and liquids	1 cup	146	1	0	38	36	3	15	0
Fruit salad (peach and pear and apricot and pineapple and cherry), canned, water pack, solids and liquids	1 cup	74	1	0	19	17	2	7	0
Fruit salad (pineapple and papaya and banana and guava), tropical, canned, heavy syrup, solids and liquids	1 cup	221	1	0	57	54	3	5	0
Fruit, mixed (peach and cherry-sweet and -sour and raspberry and grape and boysenberry), frozen, sweetened	1 cup, thawed	245	4	0	61	56	5	8	0

Description	Serving Size	Cal	Prot (g)	Fat (g)	Carbs (g)	Net Carb(g)	Fiber (g)	Sod (mg)	Chol (mg)
MIXED FRUIT (continued)									
Fruit, mixed (peach and pear and pineapple), canned, heavy syrup, solids and liquids	1 cup	184	1	0	48	45	3	10	0
Fruit, mixed (prune and apricot and pear), dried	1 package	712	7	1	188	165	23	53	0

Mongo

Raw	1 fruit, w/o refuse	135	1	0	35	31	4	4	0

Mulberries

Raw	10 fruit	6	0	0	1	1	0	2	0

Nectarines

Raw	1 fruit	67	1	1	16	14	2	0	0

Oheloberries

Raw	10 fruit	3	0	0	1	NA	NA	0	0

Olives

Ripe, canned (jumbo-super colossal)	1 jumbo	7	0	1	0	0	0	75	0
Ripe, canned (small-extra large)	1 large	5	0	0	0	0	0	38	0

Oranges

Peel, raw	1 tbsp	6	0	0	2	1	1	0	0
Raw, all commercial varieties	1 large	86	2	0	22	17	4	0	0
Raw, California, Valencias	1 fruit	59	1	0	14	11	3	0	0
Raw, Florida	1 fruit	65	1	0	16	13	3	0	0
Raw, navels	1 fruit	64	1	0	16	13	3	1	0
Raw, with peel	1 fruit, w/o seeds	64	2	0	25	17	7	3	0

Papayas

Raw	1 cup, cubes	55	1	0	14	11	3	4	0

Passion-fruit

Purple, raw	1 fruit, w/o refuse	17	0	0	4	2	2	5	0

Peaches

Canned, extra heavy syrup pack, solids and liquids	1 cup, halves or slices	252	1	0	68	66	3	21	0

Description	Serving Size	Cal	Prot (g)	Fat (g)	Carbs (g)	Net Carb(g)	Fiber (g)	Sod (mg)	Chol (mg)
Canned, extra light syrup, solids and liquids	1 cup, halves or slices	104	1	0	27	25	2	12	0
Canned, heavy syrup pack, solids and liquids	1 cup	194	1	0	52	49	3	16	0
Canned, juice pack, solids and liquids	1 cup	110	2	0	29	26	3	10	0
Canned, light syrup pack, solids and liquids	1 cup, halves or slices	136	1	0	37	33	3	13	0
Canned, water pack, solids and liquids	1 cup, halves or slices	59	1	0	15	12	3	7	0
Dehydrated (low-moisture), sulfured, stewed	1 cup	322	5	1	83	NA	NA	10	0
Dehydrated (low-moisture), sulfured, uncooked	1 cup	377	6	1	96	NA	NA	12	0
Dried, sulfured, stewed, with added sugar	1 cup	278	3	1	72	65	6	5	0
Dried, sulfured, stewed, without added sugar	1 cup	199	3	1	51	44	7	5	0
Dried, sulfured, uncooked	1 half	31	0	0	8	7	1	1	0
Frozen, sliced, sweetened	10 slices	146	1	0	37	34	3	9	0
Raw	1 large	68	1	0	17	14	3	0	0
Spiced, canned, heavy syrup pack, solids and liquids	1 cup, whole	182	1	0	49	45	3	10	0

Pears

Description	Serving Size	Cal	Prot (g)	Fat (g)	Carbs (g)	Net Carb(g)	Fiber (g)	Sod (mg)	Chol (mg)
Asian, raw	1 fruit	51	1	0	13	9	4	0	0
Canned, extra light syrup pack, solids and liquids	1 cup	116	1	0	30	26	4	5	0
Canned, heavy syrup pack, solids and liquids	1 cup	197	1	0	51	47	4	13	0
Canned, juice pack, solids and liquids	1 cup	124	1	0	32	28	4	10	0
Canned, light syrup pack, solids and liquids	1 cup	143	0	0	38	34	4	13	0
Canned, water pack, solids and liquids	1 cup	71	0	0	19	15	4	5	0
Dried, sulfured, stewed, with added sugar	1 cup	392	2	0	104	88	16	8	0
Dried, sulfured, stewed, without added sugar	1 cup	324	2	0	86	70	16	8	0
Dried, sulfured, uncooked	1 half	47	0	0	13	11	1	1	0
Pears, canned, extra heavy syrup pack, solids and liquids	1 half	77	0	0	20	19	1	4	0
Raw	1 pear	123	1	0	32	27	5	0	0

Description	Serving Size	Cal	Prot (g)	Fat (g)	Carbs (g)	Net Carb(g)	Fiber (g)	Sod (mg)	Chol (mg)
Persimmons									
Japanese, dried	1 fruit, w/o refuse	93	0	0	25	20	5	1	0
Japanese, raw	1 fruit	118	1	0	31	25	6	2	0
Native, raw	1 fruit, w/o refuse	32	0	0	8	NA	NA	0	0
Pineapple									
Canned, extra heavy syrup pack, solids and liquids	1 cup, crush., sliced, or chunks	216	1	0	56	54	2	3	0
Canned, heavy syrup pack, solids and liquids	1 cup, crush., sliced, or chunks	198	1	0	51	49	2	3	0
Canned, juice pack, solids and liquids	1 cup, crush., sliced, or chunks	149	1	0	39	37	2	2	0
Canned, light syrup pack, solids and liquids	1 cup, crush., sliced, or chunks	131	1	0	34	32	2	3	0
Canned, water pack, solids and liquids	1 cup, crush., sliced, or chunks	79	1	0	20	18	2	2	0
Frozen, chunks, sweetened	1 cup, chunks	208	1	0	54	52	3	5	0
Raw, all varieties	1 fruit	231	2	1	58	53	6	5	0
Pitanga									
Raw	1 fruit, w/o refuse	2	0	0	1	NA	NA	0	0
Plantains									
Cooked	1 cup, sliced	179	1	0	48	44	4	8	0
Raw	1 medium	218	2	0	57	53	4	7	0
Plums									
Canned, purple, extra heavy syrup pack, solids and liquids	1 cup	264	1	0	69	66	3	50	0
Canned, purple, heavy syrup pack, solids and liquids	1 plum	41	0	0	11	10	0	9	0
Canned, purple, juice pack, solids and liquids	1 plum	27	0	0	7	7	0	0	0

Description	Serving Size	Cal	Prot (g)	Fat (g)	Carbs (g)	Net Carb(g)	Fiber (g)	Sod (mg)	Chol (mg)
Canned, purple, light syrup pack, solids and liquids	1 plum	29	0	0	7	7	0	9	0
Canned, purple, water pack, solids and liquids	1 plum	19	0	0	5	5	0	0	0
Dried (prunes), stewed, with added sugar	1 cup	308	3	1	82	72	9	5	0
Dried (prunes), stewed, without added sugar	1 cup	265	3	1	70	53	16	5	0
Dried (prunes), uncooked	1 prune	20	0	0	5	5	1	0	0
Raw	1 fruit	36	1	0	9	8	1	0	0

Pomegranates

Raw	1 fruit	105	1	0	26	26	1	5	0

Prickly Pears

Raw	1 fruit, w/o refuse	42	1	0	10	6	4	5	0

Prunes

Canned, heavy syrup pack, solids and liquids	1 cup	246	2	0	65	56	9	7	0
Dehydrated (low-moisture), stewed	1 cup	316	3	1	83	NA	NA	6	0
Dehydrated (low-moisture), uncooked	1 cup	447	5	1	118	NA	NA	7	0

Pummelo

Raw	1 fruit, w/o refuse	231	5	4	59	52	6	6	0

Quinces

Raw	1 fruit, w/o refuse	52	0	0	14	12	2	4	0

Raisins

Golden seedless	1 cup	498	6	1	131	125	7	20	0
Seeded	1 cup	488	4	1	129	118	11	46	0
Seedless	1 cup	495	5	0	131	124	7	20	0

Rambutan

Canned, syrup pack	1 cup	123	1	0	31	30	1	17	0

Raspberries

Canned, red, heavy syrup pack, solids and liquids	1 cup	233	2	0	60	51	8	8	0

Description	Serving Size	Cal	Prot (g)	Fat (g)	Carbs (g)	Net Carb(g)	Fiber (g)	Sod (mg)	Chol (mg)
RASPBERRIES (continued)									
Frozen, red, sweetened	1 cup, unthawed	258	2	0	65	54	11	3	0
Raw	1 cup	60	1	0	14	6	8	0	0

Rhubarb

Frozen, cooked, with sugar	1 cup	278	1	0	75	70	5	2	0
Frozen, uncooked	1 cup, diced	29	1	0	7	5	2	3	0
Raw	1 stalk	11	0	0	2	1	1	2	0

Roselle

Raw	1 cup	28	1	0	6	NA	NA	3	0

Rowal

Raw	1/2 cup	127	3	1	27	20	7	5	0

Sapodilla

Raw	1 sapodilla	141	1	1	34	25	9	20	0

Sapotes

Raw	1 fruit, w/o refuse	302	5	0	76	70	6	23	0

Soursop

Raw	1 fruit	413	6	1	105	85	21	88	0

Strawberries

Canned, heavy syrup pack, solids and liquids	1 cup	234	1	0	60	55	4	10	0
Frozen, sweetened, sliced	1 cup, thawed	245	1	0	66	61	5	8	0
Frozen, sweetened, whole	1 cup, thawed	199	1	0	54	49	5	3	0
Frozen, unsweetened	1 cup, thawed	77	1	0	20	16	5	4	0
Raw	1 cup	46	1	0	11	7	3	2	0

Tamarinds

Raw	1 cup	287	3	1	75	69	6	34	0

Tangerines

Canned, juice pack	1 cup	92	2	0	24	22	2	12	0
Canned, light syrup pack	1 cup	154	1	0	41	39	2	15	0
Raw	1 large	43	1	0	11	9	2	1	0

Watermelon

Raw	1 cup, balls	49	1	0	11	10	1	3	0

Description	Serving Size	Cal	Prot (g)	Fat (g)	Carbs (g)	Net Carb(g)	Fiber (g)	Sod (mg)	Chol (mg)
Game Meat									
ANTELOPE									
Raw	1 oz	32	6	0	0	0	0	14	27
Roasted	3 oz	128	25	2	0	0	0	46	107
BEAR									
Raw	1 oz	46	6	0	0	0	0	0	0
Simmered	3 oz	220	28	10	0	0	0	60	83
BEAVER									
Raw	1 oz	41	7	0	0	0	0	14	0
Roasted	3 oz	180	30	5	0	0	0	50	99
BEEFALO									
Composite of cuts, raw	1 oz	41	7	1	0	0	0	22	12
Composite of cuts, roasted	3 oz	160	26	5	0	0	0	70	49
BISON									
Lean only, raw	1 oz	31	6	0	0	0	0	15	18
Lean only, roasted	3 oz	122	24	2	0	0	0	48	70
Ribeye, lean only, trimmed to 0" fat, raw	1 oz	33	6	1	0	0	0	14	18
Shoulder clod, lean only, trimmed to 0" fat, raw	1 oz	31	6	1	0	0	0	17	19
Top round, lean only, 0" fat, raw	1 oz	31	6	0	0	0	0	14	19
Top sirloin, lean only, trimmed to 0" fat, raw	1 oz	32	6	1	0	0	0	14	20
BOAR									
Wild, raw	1 oz	35	6	1	0	0	0	14	0
Wild, roasted	3 oz	136	24	3	0	0	0	51	65
BUFFALO									
Water, raw	1 oz	28	6	0	0	0	0	15	13
Water, roasted	3 oz	111	23	1	0	0	0	48	52
CARIBOU									
Raw	1 oz	36	6	1	0	0	0	16	24
Roasted	3 oz	142	25	3	0	0	0	51	93
DEER									
Raw	1 oz	34	7	1	0	0	0	14	24
Roasted	3 oz	134	26	2	0	0	0	46	95

Description	Serving Size	Cal	Prot (g)	Fat (g)	Carbs (g)	Net Carb(g)	Fiber (g)	Sod (mg)	Chol (mg)
GAME MEAT (continued)									
ELK									
Raw	1 oz	31	7	0	0	0	0	16	16
Roasted	3 oz	124	26	1	0	0	0	52	62
GOAT									
Raw	1 oz	31	6	1	0	0	0	23	16
Roasted	3 oz	122	23	2	0	0	0	73	64
HORSE									
Raw	1 oz	38	6	1	0	0	0	15	15
Roasted	3 oz	149	24	4	0	0	0	47	58
MOOSE									
Raw	1 oz	29	6	0	0	0	0	18	17
Roasted	3 oz	114	25	1	0	0	0	59	66
MUSKRAT									
Raw	1 oz	46	6	0	0	0	0	23	0
Roasted	3 oz	199	26	0	0	0	0	81	103
OPOSSUM									
Roasted	3 oz	188	26	7	0	0	0	49	110
RABBIT									
Domesticated, composite of cuts, raw	1 oz	39	6	1	0	0	0	12	16
Domesticated, composite of cuts, roasted	3 oz	167	25	5	0	0	0	40	70
Domesticated, composite of cuts, stewed	3 oz	175	26	5	0	0	0	31	73
Wild, raw	1 oz	32	6	1	0	0	0	14	23
Wild, stewed	3 oz	147	28	2	0	0	0	38	105
RACCOON									
Roasted	3 oz	217	25	10	0	0	0	67	82
SQUIRREL									
Raw	1 oz	34	6	1	0	0	0	29	24
Roasted	3 oz	147	26	3	0	0	0	101	103

Lamb

AUSTRALIAN

Description	Serving Size	Cal	Prot (g)	Fat (g)	Carbs (g)	Net Carb(g)	Fiber (g)	Sod (mg)	Chol (mg)
Composite of trimmed retail cuts, lean and fat, trimmed to 1/8" fat, cooked	3 oz	218	21	13	0	0	0	65	74
Composite of trimmed retail cuts, lean and fat, trimmed to 1/8" fat, raw	1 oz	65	5	4	0	0	0	21	19

Description	Serving Size	Cal	Prot (g)	Fat (g)	Carbs (g)	Net Carb(g)	Fiber (g)	Sod (mg)	Chol (mg)
Composite of trimmed retail cuts, lean only, trimmed to 1/8" fat, cooked	3 oz	171	23	7	0	0	0	68	74
Composite of trimmed retail cuts, lean only, trimmed to 1/8" fat, raw	1 oz	40	6	2	0	0	0	24	18
Foreshank, lean and fat, trimmed to 1/8" fat, braised	3 oz	201	21	11	0	0	0	79	77
Foreshank, lean and fat, trimmed to 1/8" fat, raw	1 oz	55	5	3	0	0	0	27	19
Foreshank, lean only, trimmed to 1/8" fat, braised	3 oz	140	23	4	0	0	0	85	78
Foreshank, lean only, trimmed to 1/8" fat, raw	1 oz	35	6	1	0	0	0	30	19
Leg, center slice, bone-in, lean and fat, trimmed to 1/8" fat, broiled	3 oz	183	22	9	0	0	0	55	72
Leg, center slice, bone-in, lean and fat, trimmed to 1/8" fat, raw	1 oz	55	5	3	0	0	0	17	18
Leg, center slice, bone-in, lean only, trimmed to 1/8" fat, broiled	3 oz	156	23	6	0	0	0	56	72
Leg, center slice, bone-in, lean only, trimmed to 1/8" fat, raw	1 oz	41	6	1	0	0	0	18	18
Leg, shank half, lean and fat, trimmed to 1/8" fat, raw	1 oz	57	5	4	0	0	0	21	19
Leg, shank half, lean and fat, trimmed to 1/8" fat, roasted	3 oz	196	21	11	0	0	0	57	71
Leg, shank half, lean only, trimmed to 1/8" fat, raw	1 oz	38	6	1	0	0	0	23	18
Leg, shank half, lean only, trimmed to 1/8" fat, roasted	3 oz	155	23	5	0	0	0	59	71
Leg, sirloin chops, boneless, lean and fat, trimmed to 1/8" fat, broiled	3 oz	200	22	11	0	0	0	54	72
Leg, sirloin chops, boneless, lean and fat, trimmed to 1/8" fat, raw	1 oz	59	5	4	0	0	0	17	19
Leg, sirloin chops, boneless, lean only, trimmed to 1/8" fat, broiled	3 oz	160	23	6	0	0	0	56	72
Leg, sirloin chops, boneless, lean only, trimmed to 1/8" fat, raw	1 oz	37	6	1	0	0	0	18	18
Leg, sirloin half, boneless, lean and fat, trimmed to 1/8" fat, raw	1 oz	72	5	5	0	0	0	20	19
Leg, sirloin half, boneless, lean and fat, trimmed to 1/8" fat, roasted	3 oz	239	21	15	0	0	0	66	87
Leg, sirloin half, boneless, lean only, trimmed to 1/8" fat, raw	1 oz	39	6	1	0	0	0	23	18
Leg, sirloin half, boneless, lean only, trimmed to 1/8" fat, roasted	3 oz	183	24	8	0	0	0	71	89

Description	Serving Size	Cal	Prot (g)	Fat (g)	Carbs (g)	Net Carb(g)	Fiber (g)	Sod (mg)	Chol (mg)
LAMB (continued)									
Leg, whole (shank and sirloin), lean and fat, trimmed to 1/8" fat, raw	1 oz	61	5	4	0	0	0	21	19
Leg, whole (shank and sirloin), lean and fat, trimmed to 1/8" fat, roasted	3 oz	207	21	12	0	0	0	60	75
Leg, whole (shank and sirloin), lean only, trimmed to 1/8" fat, raw	1 oz	38	6	1	0	0	0	23	18
Leg, whole (shank and sirloin), lean only, trimmed to 1/8" fat, roasted	3 oz	162	23	6	0	0	0	61	76
Loin, lean and fat, trimmed to 1/8" fat, broiled	3 oz	186	22	9	0	0	0	66	70
Loin, lean and fat, trimmed to 1/8" fat, raw	1 oz	58	5	3	0	0	0	20	19
Loin, lean and fat, trimmed to 1/8" fat, raw	3 oz	173	16	10	0	0	0	60	56
Loin, lean only, trimmed to 1/8" fat, broiled	3 oz	163	23	6	0	0	0	68	69
Loin, lean only, trimmed to 1/8" fat, raw	1 oz	41	6	2	0	0	0	21	18
Loin, lean only, trimmed to 1/8" fat, raw	3 oz	124	18	5	0	0	0	64	54
Rib lean and fat, trimmed to 1/8" fat, raw	1 oz	82	5	6	0	0	0	19	19
Rib lean and fat, trimmed to 1/8" fat, roasted	3 oz	235	19	16	0	0	0	65	68
Rib lean only, trimmed to 1/8" fat, raw	1 oz	45	6	2	0	0	0	23	19
Rib lean only, trimmed to 1/8" fat, roasted	3 oz	179	21	9	0	0	0	70	68
Separable fat, cooked	3 oz	543	8	54	0	0	0	43	71
Separable fat, raw	1 oz	184	2	19	0	0	0	9	22
Shoulder, arm, lean and fat, trimmed to 1/8" fat, braised	3 oz	264	25	16	0	0	0	62	90
Shoulder, arm, lean and fat, trimmed to 1/8" fat, raw	1 oz	69	5	5	0	0	0	20	18
Shoulder, arm, lean and fat, trimmed to 1/8" fat, raw	3 oz	207	15	15	0	0	0	61	55
Shoulder, arm, lean only, trimmed to 1/8" fat, braised	3 oz	202	29	8	0	0	0	66	94
Shoulder, arm, lean only, trimmed to 1/8" fat, raw	1 oz	39	6	1	0	0	0	24	18
Shoulder, arm, lean only, trimmed to 1/8" fat, raw	3 oz	116	17	4	0	0	0	71	53
Shoulder, blade, lean and fat, trimmed to 1/8" fat, broiled	3 oz	247	18	17	0	0	0	75	71
Shoulder, blade, lean and fat, trimmed to 1/8" fat, raw	1 oz	74	5	6	0	0	0	22	19

Description	Serving Size	Cal	Prot (g)	Fat (g)	Carbs (g)	Net Carb(g)	Fiber (g)	Sod (mg)	Chol (mg)
Shoulder, blade, lean only, trimmed to 1/8" fat, raw	1 oz	46	5	2	0	0	0	26	18
Shoulder, whole (arm and blade), lean and fat, trimmed to 1/8" fat, cooked	3 oz	252	20	17	0	0	0	72	76
Shoulder, whole (arm and blade), lean and fat, trimmed to 1/8" fat, raw	1 oz	73	5	5	0	0	0	22	19
Shoulder, whole (arm and blade), lean only, trimmed to 1/8" fat, cooked	3 oz	198	22	10	0	0	0	77	77
Shoulder, whole (arm and blade), lean only, trimmed to 1/8" fat, raw	1 oz	44	5	2	0	0	0	25	18
Shoulder,blade, lean only, trimmed to 1/8" fat, broiled	3 oz	196	20	11	0	0	0	80	72

DOMESTIC

Description	Serving Size	Cal	Prot (g)	Fat (g)	Carbs (g)	Net Carb(g)	Fiber (g)	Sod (mg)	Chol (mg)
Composite of trimmed retail cuts, lean and fat, trimmed to 1/4" fat, choice, cooked	3 oz	250	21	16	0	0	0	61	82
Composite of trimmed retail cuts, lean and fat, trimmed to 1/4" fat, choice, raw	1 oz	76	5	6	0	0	0	16	20
Composite of trimmed retail cuts, lean and fat, trimmed to 1/8" fat, choice, cooked	3 oz	230	22	14	0	0	0	61	82
Composite of trimmed retail cuts, lean and fat, trimmed to 1/8" fat, choice, raw	1 oz	69	5	5	0	0	0	17	20
Composite of trimmed retail cuts, lean only, trimmed to 1/4" fat, choice, cooked	3 oz	175	24	7	0	0	0	65	78
Composite of trimmed retail cuts, lean only, trimmed to 1/4" fat, choice, raw	1 oz	38	6	1	0	0	0	19	18
Composite of trimmed retail cuts, separable fat, trimmed to 1/4" fat, choice, cooked	3 oz	498	10	48	0	0	0	49	97
Composite of trimmed retail cuts, separable fat, trimmed to 1/4" fat, choice, raw	1 oz	189	2	19	0	0	0	9	26
Cubed for stew or kabob (leg and shoulder), lean only, trimmed to 1/4" fat, braised	3 oz	190	29	6	0	0	0	60	92
Cubed for stew or kabob (leg and shoulder), lean only, trimmed to 1/4" fat, broiled	3 oz	158	24	5	0	0	0	65	77

Description	Serving Size	Cal	Prot (g)	Fat (g)	Carbs (g)	Net Carb(g)	Fiber (g)	Sod (mg)	Chol (mg)
LAMB (continued)									
Cubed for stew or kabob (leg and shoulder), lean only, trimmed to 1/4" fat, raw	1 oz	38	6	1	0	0	0	18	18
Foreshank, lean and fat, trimmed to 1/4" fat, choice, braised	3 oz	207	24	10	0	0	0	61	90
Foreshank, lean and fat, trimmed to 1/4" fat, choice, raw	1 oz	57	5	4	0	0	0	20	20
Foreshank, lean and fat, trimmed to 1/8" fat, braised	3 oz	207	24	10	0	0	0	61	90
Foreshank, lean and fat, trimmed to 1/8" fat, choice, raw	1 oz	57	5	4	0	0	0	20	20
Foreshank, lean only, trimmed to 1/4" fat, choice, braised	3 oz	159	26	4	0	0	0	63	88
Foreshank, lean only, trimmed to 1/4" fat, choice, raw	1 oz	34	6	1	0	0	0	22	20
Ground, boiled	3 oz	241	21	15	0	0	0	69	82
Ground, raw	1 oz	80	5	6	0	0	0	17	21
Ground, raw	4 oz	319	19	24	0	0	0	67	82
Leg, shank half, lean and fat, trimmed to 1/4" fat, choice, raw	1 oz	57	5	4	0	0	0	16	19
Leg, shank half, lean and fat, trimmed to 1/4" fat, choice, roasted	3 oz	191	22	10	0	0	0	55	77
Leg, shank half, lean and fat, trimmed to 1/8" fat, choice, raw	1 oz	52	5	3	0	0	0	16	19
Leg, shank half, lean and fat, trimmed to 1/8" fat, choice, roasted	3 oz	184	23	9	0	0	0	55	77
Leg, shank half, lean only, trimmed to 1/4" fat, choice, raw	1 oz	35	6	1	0	0	0	17	18
Leg, shank half, lean only, trimmed to 1/4" fat, choice, roasted	3 oz	153	24	5	0	0	0	56	74
Leg, sirloin half, lean and fat, trimmed to 1/4" fat, choice, raw	1 oz	77	5	6	0	0	0	16	20
Leg, sirloin half, lean and fat, trimmed to 1/4" fat, choice, roasted	3 oz	248	21	16	0	0	0	58	82
Leg, sirloin half, lean and fat, trimmed to 1/8" fat, choice, raw	1 oz	74	5	5	0	0	0	16	20
Leg, sirloin half, lean and fat, trimmed to 1/8" fat, choice, roasted	3 oz	241	21	15	0	0	0	58	82
Leg, sirloin half, lean only, trimmed to 1/4" fat, choice, raw	1 oz	38	6	1	0	0	0	18	19
Leg, sirloin half, lean only, trimmed to 1/4" fat, choice, roasted	3 oz	173	24	7	0	0	0	60	78

Description	Serving Size	Cal	Prot (g)	Fat (g)	Carbs (g)	Net Carb(g)	Fiber (g)	Sod (mg)	Chol (mg)
Leg, whole (shank and sirloin), lean and fat, trimmed to 1/4" fat, choice, raw	1 oz	65	5	4	0	0	0	16	20
Leg, whole (shank and sirloin), lean and fat, trimmed to 1/4" fat, choice, roasted	3 oz	219	22	13	0	0	0	56	79
Leg, whole (shank and sirloin), lean and fat, trimmed to 1/8" fat, choice, raw	1 oz	59	5	4	0	0	0	16	19
Leg, whole (shank and sirloin), lean and fat, trimmed to 1/8" fat, choice, roasted	3 oz	206	22	11	0	0	0	57	78
Leg, whole (shank and sirloin), lean only, trimmed to 1/4" fat, choice, raw	1 oz	36	6	1	0	0	0	18	18
Leg, whole (shank and sirloin), lean only, trimmed to 1/4" fat, choice, roasted	3 oz	162	24	6	0	0	0	58	76
Loin, lean and fat, trimmed to 1/4" fat, choice, broiled	3 oz	269	21	18	0	0	0	65	85
Loin, lean and fat, trimmed to 1/4" fat, choice, broiled	1 chop, exclud. refuse	202	16	14	0	0	0	49	64
Loin, lean and fat, trimmed to 1/4" fat, choice, raw	1 oz	88	5	7	0	0	0	16	21
Loin, lean and fat, trimmed to 1/4" fat, choice, raw	1 chop, exclud. refuse	295	16	24	0	0	0	53	70
Loin, lean and fat, trimmed to 1/4" fat, choice, roasted	3 oz	263	19	19	0	0	0	54	81
Loin, lean and fat, trimmed to 1/8" fat, choice, broiled	3 oz	252	22	16	0	0	0	66	84
Loin, lean and fat, trimmed to 1/8" fat, choice, raw	1 oz	79	5	6	0	0	0	17	20
Loin, lean and fat, trimmed to 1/8" fat, choice, roasted	3 oz	247	20	17	0	0	0	54	79
Loin, lean only, trimmed to 1/4" fat, choice, broiled	3 oz	184	25	7	0	0	0	71	81
Loin, lean only, trimmed to 1/4" fat, choice, broiled	1 chop, exclud. refuse	99	14	4	0	0	0	39	44
Loin, lean only, trimmed to 1/4" fat, choice, raw	1 oz	41	6	1	0	0	0	19	19
Loin, lean only, trimmed to 1/4" fat, choice, raw	1 chop, exclud. refuse	93	14	3	0	0	0	44	43

Description	Serving Size	Cal	Prot (g)	Fat (g)	Carbs (g)	Net Carb(g)	Fiber (g)	Sod (mg)	Chol (mg)
LAMB (continued)									
Loin, lean only, trimmed to 1/4" fat, choice, roasted	3 oz	172	23	7	0	0	0	56	74
Rib lean and fat, trimmed to 1/4" fat, choice, broiled	3 oz	307	19	23	0	0	0	65	84
Rib lean and fat, trimmed to 1/4" fat, choice, raw	1 oz	105	4	9	0	0	0	16	22
Rib lean and fat, trimmed to 1/4" fat, choice, roasted	3 oz	305	18	23	0	0	0	62	82
Rib lean and fat, trimmed to 1/8" fat, choice, broiled	3 oz	289	20	21	0	0	0	65	83
Rib lean and fat, trimmed to 1/8" fat, choice, raw	1 oz	97	4	8	0	0	0	16	21
Rib lean and fat, trimmed to 1/8" fat, choice, roasted	3 oz	290	19	21	0	0	0	63	82
Rib lean only, trimmed to 1/4" fat, choice, broiled	3 oz	200	24	9	0	0	0	72	77
Rib lean only, trimmed to 1/4" fat, choice, raw	1 oz	48	6	2	0	0	0	20	19
Rib lean only, trimmed to 1/4" fat, choice, roasted	3 oz	197	22	10	0	0	0	69	75
Shoulder, arm, lean and fat, trimmed to 1/4" fat, choice, braised	3 oz	294	26	18	0	0	0	61	102
Shoulder, arm, lean and fat, trimmed to 1/4" fat, choice, braised	1 chop, exclud. refuse	242	21	15	0	0	0	50	84
Shoulder, arm, lean and fat, trimmed to 1/4" fat, choice, broiled	3 oz	239	21	15	0	0	0	65	82
Shoulder, arm, lean and fat, trimmed to 1/4" fat, choice, broiled	1 chop, exclud. refuse	261	23	17	0	0	0	72	89
Shoulder, arm, lean and fat, trimmed to 1/4" fat, choice, raw	1 oz	74	5	5	0	0	0	17	20
Shoulder, arm, lean and fat, trimmed to 1/4" fat, choice, raw	1 chop, exclud. refuse	346	22	26	0	0	0	80	94
Shoulder, arm, lean and fat, trimmed to 1/4" fat, choice, roasted	3 oz	237	19	16	0	0	0	55	78
Shoulder, arm, lean and fat, trimmed to 1/8" fat, broiled	3 oz	229	21	14	0	0	0	66	82
Shoulder, arm, lean and fat, trimmed to 1/8" fat, choice, braised	3 oz	286	26	17	0	0	0	61	102
Shoulder, arm, lean and fat, trimmed to 1/8" fat, choice, raw	1 oz	69	5	5	0	0	0	17	20

Description	Serving Size	Cal	Prot (g)	Fat (g)	Carbs (g)	Net Carb(g)	Fiber (g)	Sod (mg)	Chol (mg)
Shoulder, arm, lean and fat, trimmed to 1/8" fat, choice, roasted	3 oz	227	19	15	0	0	0	55	77
Shoulder, arm, lean only, trimmed to 1/4" fat, choice, braised	3 oz	237	30	10	0	0	0	65	103
Shoulder, arm, lean only, trimmed to 1/4" fat, choice, braised	1 chop, exclud. refuse	153	20	7	0	0	0	42	67
Shoulder, arm, lean only, trimmed to 1/4" fat, choice, broiled	3 oz	170	24	7	0	0	0	70	78
Shoulder, arm, lean only, trimmed to 1/4" fat, choice, broiled	1 chop, exclud. refuse	148	21	6	0	0	0	61	68
Shoulder, arm, lean only, trimmed to 1/4" fat, choice, raw	1 oz	37	6	1	0	0	0	20	18
Shoulder, arm, lean only, trimmed to 1/4" fat, choice, raw	1 chop, exclud. refuse	133	20	4	0	0	0	70	65
Shoulder, arm, lean only, trimmed to 1/4" fat, choice, roasted	3 oz	163	22	7	0	0	0	57	73
Shoulder, blade, lean and fat, trimmed to 1/4" fat, choice, braised	3 oz	293	24	19	0	0	0	64	99
Shoulder, blade, lean and fat, trimmed to 1/4" fat, choice, broiled	3 oz	236	20	15	0	0	0	70	81
Shoulder, blade, lean and fat, trimmed to 1/4" fat, choice, raw	1 oz	73	5	5	0	0	0	18	20
Shoulder, blade, lean and fat, trimmed to 1/4" fat, choice, roasted	3 oz	239	19	16	0	0	0	56	78
Shoulder, blade, lean and fat, trimmed to 1/8" fat, choice, braised	3 oz	288	25	18	0	0	0	64	99
Shoulder, blade, lean and fat, trimmed to 1/8" fat, choice, broiled	3 oz	227	20	14	0	0	0	71	81
Shoulder, blade, lean and fat, trimmed to 1/8" fat, choice, raw	1 oz	69	5	5	0	0	0	18	20
Shoulder, blade, lean and fat, trimmed to 1/8" fat, choice, roasted	3 oz	230	19	15	0	0	0	57	78
Shoulder, blade, lean only, trimmed to 1/4" fat, choice, braised	3 oz	245	27	12	0	0	0	67	99
Shoulder, blade, lean only, trimmed to 1/4" fat, choice, broiled	3 oz	179	22	8	0	0	0	75	77
Shoulder, blade, lean only, trimmed to 1/4" fat, choice, raw	1 oz	43	5	2	0	0	0	20	19
Shoulder, blade, lean only, trimmed to 1/4" fat, choice, roasted	3 oz	178	21	9	0	0	0	58	74

Description	Serving Size	Cal	Prot (g)	Fat (g)	Carbs (g)	Net Carb(g)	Fiber (g)	Sod (mg)	Chol (mg)
LAMB (continued)									
Shoulder, whole (arm and blade), lean and fat, trimmed to 1/4" fat, choice, braised	3 oz	292	24	19	0	0	0	64	99
Shoulder, whole (arm and blade), lean and fat, trimmed to 1/4" fat, choice, broiled	3 oz	236	21	15	0	0	0	66	82
Shoulder, whole (arm and blade), lean and fat, trimmed to 1/4" fat, choice, raw	1 oz	75	5	6	0	0	0	17	20
Shoulder, whole (arm and blade), lean and fat, trimmed to 1/4" fat, choice, roasted	3 oz	235	19	15	0	0	0	56	78
Shoulder, whole (arm and blade), lean and fat, trimmed to 1/8" fat, choice, braised	3 oz	287	25	18	0	0	0	63	99
Shoulder, whole (arm and blade), lean and fat, trimmed to 1/8" fat, choice, broiled	3 oz	228	20	14	0	0	0	70	81
Shoulder, whole (arm and blade), lean and fat, trimmed to 1/8" fat, choice, raw	1 oz	69	5	5	0	0	0	18	20
Shoulder, whole (arm and blade), lean and fat, trimmed to 1/8" fat, choice, roasted	3 oz	229	19	15	0	0	0	56	77
Shoulder, whole (arm and blade), lean only, trimmed to 1/4" fat, choice, braised	3 oz	241	28	12	0	0	0	67	99
Shoulder, whole (arm and blade), lean only, trimmed to 1/4" fat, choice, broiled	3 oz	179	23	8	0	0	0	71	79
Shoulder, whole (arm and blade), lean only, trimmed to 1/4" fat, choice, raw	1 oz	41	6	2	0	0	0	20	19
Shoulder, whole (arm and blade), lean only, trimmed to 1/4" fat, choice, roasted	3 oz	173	21	8	0	0	0	58	74
NEW ZEALAND									
Composite of trimmed retail cuts, lean and fat, cooked	3 oz	259	21	18	0	0	0	39	93
Composite of trimmed retail cuts, lean and fat, raw	1 oz	79	5	6	0	0	0	11	22
Composite of trimmed retail cuts, lean and fat, trimmed to 1/8" fat, cooked	3 oz	230	21	14	0	0	0	39	90
Composite of trimmed retail cuts, lean and fat, trimmed to 1/8" fat, raw	1 oz	66	5	5	0	0	0	12	22

Description	Serving Size	Cal	Prot (g)	Fat (g)	Carbs (g)	Net Carb(g)	Fiber (g)	Sod (mg)	Chol (mg)
Composite of trimmed retail cuts, lean only, cooked	3 oz	175	25	7	0	0	0	43	93
Composite of trimmed retail cuts, lean only, raw	1 oz	36	6	1	0	0	0	13	21
Composite of trimmed retail cuts, separable fat, cooked	3 oz	498	8	49	0	0	0	30	93
Composite of trimmed retail cuts, separable fat, raw	1 oz	181	2	18	0	0	0	6	25
Foreshank, lean and fat, braised	3 oz	219	23	12	0	0	0	40	87
Foreshank, lean and fat, raw	1 oz	63	5	4	0	0	0	13	20
Foreshank, lean and fat, trimmed to 1/8" fat, braised	3 oz	219	23	12	0	0	0	40	87
Foreshank, lean and fat, trimmed to 1/8" fat, raw	1 oz	63	5	4	0	0	0	13	20
Foreshank, lean only, braised	3 oz	158	26	5	0	0	0	42	86
Foreshank, lean only, raw	1 oz	33	6	1	0	0	0	14	19
Leg, whole (shank and sirloin), lean and fat, raw	1 oz	61	5	4	0	0	0	11	22
Leg, whole (shank and sirloin), lean and fat, roasted	3 oz	209	21	12	0	0	0	37	86
Leg, whole (shank and sirloin), lean and fat, trimmed to 1/8" fat, raw	1 oz	57	5	4	0	0	0	12	21
Leg, whole (shank and sirloin), lean and fat, trimmed to 1/8" fat, roasted	3 oz	199	22	11	0	0	0	37	86
Leg, whole (shank and sirloin), lean only, raw	1 oz	35	6	1	0	0	0	12	21
Leg, whole (shank and sirloin), lean only, roasted	3 oz	154	24	5	0	0	0	38	85
Loin, lean and fat, broiled	3 oz	268	20	19	0	0	0	42	95
Loin, lean and fat, broiled	1 chop, exclud. refuse	135	10	10	0	0	0	21	48
Loin, lean and fat, raw	1 oz	86	5	7	0	0	0	10	24
Loin, lean and fat, raw	1 chop, exclud. refuse	197	11	16	0	0	0	24	54
Loin, lean and fat, trimmed to 1/8" fat, broiled	3 oz	252	21	17	0	0	0	43	96
Loin, lean and fat, trimmed to 1/8" fat, broiled	1 chop, exclud. refuse	124	10	8	0	0	0	21	47
Loin, lean and fat, trimmed to 1/8" fat, raw	1 oz	77	5	6	0	0	0	11	23

Description	Serving Size	Cal	Prot (g)	Fat (g)	Carbs (g)	Net Carb(g)	Fiber (g)	Sod (mg)	Chol (mg)
LAMB (continued)									
Loin, lean and fat, trimmed to 1/8" fat, raw	1 chop, exclud. refuse	172	11	13	0	0	0	25	52
Loin, lean only, broiled	3 oz	169	25	6	0	0	0	47	97
Loin, lean only, broiled	1 chop, exclud. refuse	60	9	2	0	0	0	17	34
Loin, lean only, raw	1 oz	37	6	1	0	0	0	13	23
Loin, lean only, raw	1 chop, exclud. refuse	55	9	2	0	0	0	19	34
Rib lean and fat, raw	1 oz	98	4	8	0	0	0	11	23
Rib lean and fat, roasted	3 oz	289	16	23	0	0	0	37	85
Rib lean and fat, trimmed to 1/8" fat, raw	1 oz	88	4	7	0	0	0	12	23
Rib lean and fat, trimmed to 1/8" fat, roasted	3 oz	269	17	20	0	0	0	37	84
Rib lean only, raw	1 oz	40	6	1	0	0	0	15	22
Rib lean only, roasted	3 oz	167	21	8	0	0	0	41	80
Shoulder, whole (arm and blade), lean and fat, braised	3 oz	303	24	21	0	0	0	43	105
Shoulder, whole (arm and blade), lean and fat, raw	1 oz	77	5	6	0	0	0	12	21
Shoulder, whole (arm and blade), lean and fat, trimmed to 1/8" fat, braised	3 oz	291	25	19	0	0	0	44	105
Shoulder, whole (arm and blade), lean and fat, trimmed to 1/8" fat, raw	1 oz	71	5	5	0	0	0	12	21
Shoulder, whole (arm and blade), lean only, braised	3 oz	242	29	12	0	0	0	48	108
Shoulder, whole (arm and blade), lean only, raw	1 oz	38	6	1	0	0	0	13	20
VARIETY MEATS & BY-PRODUCTS									
Brain, braised	3 oz	123	11	5	0	0	0	114	1737
Brain, pan-fried	3 oz	232	14	10	0	0	0	133	2128
Brain, raw	1 oz	35	3	1	0	0	0	32	383
Brain, raw	4 oz	138	12	5	0	0	0	127	1533
Heart, braised	3 oz	157	21	5	2	2	0	54	212
Heart, raw	1 oz	35	5	1	0	0	0	25	38
Heart, raw	4 oz	138	19	5	0	0	0	101	153
Kidneys, braised	3 oz	116	20	2	1	1	0	128	480
Kidneys, raw	1 oz	27	4	1	0	0	0	44	96
Kidneys, raw	4 oz	110	18	2	1	1	0	177	382

Description	Serving Size	Cal	Prot (g)	Fat (g)	Carbs (g)	Net Carb(g)	Fiber (g)	Sod (mg)	Chol (mg)
Liver, braised	3 oz	187	26	6	2	2	0	48	426
Liver, pan-fried	3 oz	202	22	8	3	3	0	105	419
Liver, raw	1 oz	39	6	1	1	1	0	20	105
Liver, raw	4 oz	158	23	4	2	2	0	79	421
Lungs, braised	3 oz	96	17	2	0	0	0	71	241
Lungs, raw	1 oz	27	5	1	0	0	0	45	0
Lungs, raw	4 oz	108	19	2	0	0	0	178	0
Mechanically separated, raw	1 oz	78	4	6	0	0	0	17	60
Pancreas, braised	3 oz	199	19	11	0	0	0	44	340
Pancreas, raw	1 oz	43	4	2	0	0	0	21	74
Pancreas, raw	4 oz	172	17	10	0	0	0	85	295
Spleen, braised	3 oz	133	22	3	0	0	0	49	327
Spleen, raw	1 oz	29	5	1	0	0	0	24	71
Spleen, raw	4 oz	115	20	2	0	0	0	95	284
Tongue, braised	3 oz	234	18	16	0	0	0	57	161
Tongue, raw	1 oz	63	4	5	0	0	0	22	44
Tongue, raw	4 oz	252	18	18	0	0	0	88	177

Veal

VARIETY MEATS & BY-PRODUCTS

Description	Serving Size	Cal	Prot (g)	Fat (g)	Carbs (g)	Net Carb(g)	Fiber (g)	Sod (mg)	Chol (mg)
Brain, pan-fried	3 oz	181	12	9	0	0	0	150	1802
Brain, raw	1 oz	33	3	1	0	0	0	36	451
Brain, raw	4 oz	134	12	5	0	0	0	144	1803
Heart, braised	3 oz	158	25	4	0	0	0	49	150
Heart, raw	1 oz	31	5	1	0	0	0	22	29
Heart, raw	4 oz	125	19	3	0	0	0	87	118
Kidneys, braised	3 oz	139	22	3	0	0	0	94	672
Kidneys, raw	1 oz	28	4	1	0	0	0	50	103
Kidneys, raw	4 oz	112	18	3	1	1	0	202	413
Liver, braised	3 oz	140	18	4	2	2	0	45	477
Liver, pan-fried	3 oz	208	25	7	3	3	0	112	281
Liver, raw	1 oz	38	5	1	1	1	0	18	88
Liver, raw	4 oz	152	20	4	5	5	0	70	350
Lungs, braised	3 oz	88	16	2	0	0	0	48	224
Lungs, raw	1 oz	26	5	0	0	0	0	31	65
Lungs, raw	4 oz	102	18	2	0	0	0	122	260
Pancreas, braised	3 oz	218	25	11	0	0	0	58	0
Pancreas, raw	1 oz	52	4	3	0	0	0	19	49

Description	Serving Size	Cal	Prot (g)	Fat (g)	Carbs (g)	Net Carb(g)	Fiber (g)	Sod (mg)	Chol (mg)
VEAL (continued)									
Pancreas, raw	4 oz	206	17	13	0	0	0	76	196
Spleen, braised	3 oz	110	20	2	0	0	0	49	380
Spleen, raw	1 oz	28	5	0	0	0	0	27	96
Spleen, raw	4 oz	111	21	2	0	0	0	110	386
Thymus, braised	3 oz	148	27	3	0	0	0	56	399
Thymus, raw	1 oz	28	5	1	0	0	0	24	76
Thymus, raw	4 oz	112	20	2	0	0	0	94	304
Tongue, braised	3 oz	172	22	8	0	0	0	54	202
Tongue, raw	1 oz	37	5	1	1	1	0	23	18
Tongue, raw	4 oz	149	19	6	2	2	0	93	70
Veal, variety meats and by-products, brain, braised	3 oz	116	10	5	0	0	0	133	2635
Breast, plate half, boneless, lean and fat, braised	3 oz	240	22	15	0	0	0	54	95
Breast, point half, boneless, lean and fat, braised	3 oz	211	24	11	0	0	0	56	97
Breast, separable fat, cooked	1 oz	148	3	14	0	0	0	14	27
Breast, whole, boneless, lean and fat, braised	3 oz	226	23	13	0	0	0	55	96
Breast, whole, boneless, lean and fat, raw	1 oz	59	5	4	0	0	0	20	20
Breast, whole, boneless, lean only, braised	3 oz	185	26	8	0	0	0	58	99
Composite of trimmed retail cuts, lean and fat, cooked	3 oz	196	26	8	0	0	0	74	97
Composite of trimmed retail cuts, lean and fat, raw	1 oz	41	5	2	0	0	0	23	23
Composite of trimmed retail cuts, lean only, cooked	3 oz	167	27	4	0	0	0	76	100
Composite of trimmed retail cuts, lean only, raw	1 oz	32	6	1	0	0	0	24	24
Composite of trimmed retail cuts, separable fat, cooked	3 oz	546	8	54	0	0	0	48	62
Composite of trimmed retail cuts, separable fat, raw	1 oz	181	2	18	0	0	0	7	21
Cubed for stew (leg and shoulder), lean only, braised	3 oz	160	30	3	0	0	0	79	123
Cubed for stew (leg and shoulder), lean only, raw	1 oz	31	6	1	0	0	0	24	24
Ground, broiled	3 oz	146	21	5	0	0	0	71	88

Description	Serving Size	Cal	Prot (g)	Fat (g)	Carbs (g)	Net Carb(g)	Fiber (g)	Sod (mg)	Chol (mg)
Ground, raw	1 oz	41	5	2	0	0	0	23	23
Ground, raw	4 oz	163	22	7	0	0	0	93	93
Leg (top round), lean and fat, braised	3 oz	179	31	5	0	0	0	57	114
Leg (top round), lean and fat, pan-fried, breaded	3 oz	194	23	7	8	8	0	386	95
Leg (top round), lean and fat, pan-fried, not breaded	3 oz	179	27	6	0	0	0	65	89
Leg (top round), lean and fat, raw	1 oz	33	6	1	0	0	0	18	22
Leg (top round), lean and fat, roasted	3 oz	136	24	3	0	0	0	58	88
Leg (top round), lean only, braised	3 oz	173	31	4	0	0	0	57	115
Leg (top round), lean only, pan-fried, breaded	3 oz	175	24	4	8	8	0	387	96
Leg (top round), lean only, pan-fried, not breaded	3 oz	156	28	3	0	0	0	65	91
Leg (top round), lean only, raw	1 oz	30	6	0	0	0	0	18	22
Leg (top round), lean only, roasted	3 oz	128	24	2	0	0	0	58	88
Loin, lean and fat, braised	3 oz	241	26	12	0	0	0	68	100
Loin, lean and fat, braised	1 chop, exclud. refuse	227	24	12	0	0	0	64	94
Loin, lean and fat, raw	1 oz	46	5	2	0	0	0	24	22
Loin, lean and fat, raw	1 chop, exclud. refuse	204	24	10	0	0	0	106	99
Loin, lean and fat, roasted	3 oz	184	21	9	0	0	0	79	88
Loin, lean only, braised	3 oz	192	29	6	0	0	0	71	106
Loin, lean only, braised	1 chop, exclud. refuse	156	23	5	0	0	0	58	86
Loin, lean only, raw	1 oz	33	6	1	0	0	0	26	23
Loin, lean only, raw	1 chop, exclud. refuse	131	23	3	0	0	0	103	90
Loin, lean only, roasted	3 oz	149	22	5	0	0	0	82	90
Rib, lean and fat, braised	3 oz	213	28	9	0	0	0	81	118
Rib, lean and fat, raw	1 oz	46	5	2	0	0	0	25	23
Rib, lean and fat, roasted	3 oz	194	20	10	0	0	0	78	94
Rib, lean only, braised	3 oz	185	29	5	0	0	0	84	122
Rib, lean only, raw	1 oz	34	6	1	0	0	0	27	24
Rib, lean only, roasted	3 oz	150	22	5	0	0	0	82	98
Shank (fore and hind), lean and fat, braised	3 oz	162	27	4	0	0	0	79	105
Shank (fore and hind), lean and fat, raw	1 oz	32	5	1	0	0	0	24	21

Description	Serving Size	Cal	Prot (g)	Fat (g)	Carbs (g)	Net Carb(g)	Fiber (g)	Sod (mg)	Chol (mg)
VEAL (continued)									
Shank (fore and hind), lean only, braised	3 oz	150	27	3	0	0	0	80	107
Shank (fore and hind), lean only, raw	1 oz	31	5	1	0	0	0	24	21
Shoulder, arm, lean and fat, braised	3 oz	201	29	7	0	0	0	74	126
Shoulder, arm, lean and fat, raw	1 oz	37	5	1	0	0	0	24	23
Shoulder, arm, lean and fat, roasted	3 oz	156	22	6	0	0	0	77	92
Shoulder, arm, lean only, braised	3 oz	171	30	3	0	0	0	77	132
Shoulder, arm, lean only, raw	1 oz	30	6	0	0	0	0	24	24
Shoulder, arm, lean only, roasted	3 oz	139	22	4	0	0	0	77	93
Shoulder, blade, lean and fat, braised	3 oz	191	27	7	0	0	0	83	130
Shoulder, blade, lean and fat, raw	1 oz	37	5	1	0	0	0	27	26
Shoulder, blade, lean and fat, roasted	3 oz	158	21	6	0	0	0	85	99
Shoulder, blade, lean only, braised	3 oz	168	28	4	0	0	0	86	134
Shoulder, blade, lean only, raw	1 oz	32	6	1	0	0	0	27	26
Shoulder, blade, lean only, roasted	3 oz	145	22	5	0	0	0	87	101
Shoulder, whole (arm and blade), lean and fat, braised	3 oz	194	27	7	0	0	0	81	107
Shoulder, whole (arm and blade), lean and fat, raw	1 oz	37	5	1	0	0	0	26	25
Shoulder, whole (arm and blade), lean and fat, roasted	3 oz	156	22	6	0	0	0	82	96
Shoulder, whole (arm and blade), lean only, braised	3 oz	169	29	4	0	0	0	82	111
Shoulder, whole (arm and blade), lean only, raw	1 oz	32	6	1	0	0	0	26	24
Shoulder, whole (arm and blade), lean only, roasted	3 oz	145	22	5	0	0	0	82	97
Sirloin, lean and fat, braised	3 oz	214	27	10	0	0	0	67	92
Sirloin, lean and fat, raw	1 oz	43	5	2	0	0	0	22	22
Sirloin, lean and fat, roasted	3 oz	172	21	8	0	0	0	71	87
Sirloin, lean only, braised	3 oz	173	29	4	0	0	0	69	96
Sirloin, lean only, raw	1 oz	31	6	1	0	0	0	23	22
Sirloin, lean only, roasted	3 oz	143	22	4	0	0	0	72	88

Description	Serving Size	Cal	Prot (g)	Fat (g)	Carbs (g)	Net Carb(g)	Fiber (g)	Sod (mg)	Chol (mg)
Beans									
ADZUKI									
Boiled	1 cup	294	17	0	57	40	17	18	0
Canned, sweetened	1 cup	702	11	0	163	NA	NA	645	0
Raw	1 cup	648	39	0	124	99	25	10	0
Yokan	1 slice	36	0	0	9	NA	NA	12	0
BAKED									
Canned, plain or vegetarian	1 cup	236	12	1	52	39	13	1008	0
Canned, with beef	1 cup	322	17	9	45	NA	NA	1264	59
Canned, with franks	1 cup	368	17	16	40	22	18	1114	16
Canned, with pork	1 cup	268	13	4	51	37	14	1047	18
Canned, with pork and sweet sauce	1 cup	281	13	3	53	40	13	850	18
Canned, with pork and tomato sauce	1 cup	248	13	2	49	37	12	1113	18
Home prepared	1 cup	382	14	12	54	40	14	1068	13
BLACK									
Black, mature seeds, raw	1 cup	662	42	2	121	92	29	10	0
Boiled	1 cup	227	15	1	41	26	15	2	0
BLACK TURTLE SOUP									
Boiled	1 cup	241	15	0	45	35	10	6	0
Canned	1 cup	218	14	1	40	23	17	922	0
Raw	1 cup	624	39	1	116	71	46	17	0
BROADBEANS									
Boiled	1 cup	187	13	1	33	24	9	9	0
Canned	1 cup	182	14	0	32	22	9	1160	0
Raw	1 cup	512	39	2	87	50	38	20	0
CRANBERRY									
Boiled	1 cup	241	17	1	43	26	18	2	0
Canned	1 cup	216	14	1	39	23	16	863	0
Raw	1 cup	653	45	2	117	69	48	12	0
FRENCH									
Boiled	1 cup	228	12	1	43	26	17	11	0
Raw	1 cup	631	35	3	118	72	46	33	0
GREAT NORTHERN									
Boiled	1 cup	209	15	1	37	25	12	4	0
Canned	1 cup	299	19	1	55	42	13	10	0

Description	Serving Size	Cal	Prot (g)	Fat (g)	Carbs (g)	Net Carb(g)	Fiber (g)	Sod (mg)	Chol (mg)
BEANS (continued)									
Raw	1 cup	620	40	2	114	77	37	26	0
HYACINTH									
Boiled	1 cup	227	16	1	40	NA	NA	14	0
Raw	1 cup	722	50	1	128	NA	NA	44	0
KIDNEY									
Boiled	1 cup	225	15	1	40	29	11	4	0
California red, boiled	1 cup	219	16	0	40	23	16	7	0
California red, raw	1 cup	607	45	0	110	64	46	20	0
Canned	1 cup	207	13	1	38	29	9	888	0
Raw	1 cup	613	43	1	110	65	46	44	0
Red, boiled	1 cup	225	15	1	40	27	13	4	0
Red, canned	1 cup	218	13	1	40	24	16	873	0
Red, raw	1 cup	620	41	2	113	85	28	22	0
Royal red, boiled	1 cup	218	17	0	39	22	16	9	0
Royal red, raw	1 cup	605	47	1	107	62	46	24	0
LIMA BEANS									
Baby, boiled	1 cup	229	15	1	42	28	14	5	0
Baby, raw	1 cup	677	42	1	127	85	42	26	0
Large, boiled	1 cup	216	15	1	39	26	13	4	0
Large, canned	1 cup	190	12	0	36	24	12	810	0
Large, raw	1 cup	602	38	1	113	79	34	32	0
MOTHBEANS									
Boiled	1 cup	207	14	1	37	NA	NA	18	0
Raw	1 cup	672	45	2	121	NA	NA	59	0
MUNG BEANS									
Boiled	1 cup	212	14	1	39	23	15	4	0
Raw	1 cup	718	49	2	130	96	34	31	0
MUNGO BEANS									
Boiled	1 cup	189	14	1	33	21	12	13	0
Raw	1 cup	706	52	3	122	84	38	79	0
NAVY									
Boiled	1 cup	258	16	1	48	36	12	2	0
Canned	1 cup	296	20	1	54	40	13	1174	0
Raw	1 cup	697	46	2	126	75	51	29	0

Description	Serving Size	Cal	Prot (g)	Fat (g)	Carbs (g)	Net Carb(g)	Fiber (g)	Sod (mg)	Chol (mg)
PINK									
Boiled	1 cup	252	15	1	47	38	9	3	0
Raw	1 cup	720	44	2	135	108	27	17	0
PINTO									
Boiled	1 cup	234	14	1	44	29	15	3	0
Canned	1 cup	206	12	1	37	26	11	706	0
Raw	1 cup	656	40	2	122	75	47	19	0
SMALL WHITE									
Boiled	1 cup	254	16	1	46	28	19	4	0
Raw	1 cup	722	45	2	134	80	54	26	0
WHITE									
Boiled	1 cup	249	17	0	45	34	11	11	0
Canned	1 cup	307	19	1	57	45	13	13	0
Raw	1 cup	673	47	1	122	91	31	32	0
WINGED									
Boiled	1 cup	253	18	8	26	NA	NA	22	0
Raw	1 cup	744	54	23	76	NA	NA	69	0
YARDLONG BEANS									
Boiled	1 cup	202	14	1	36	30	6	9	0
Raw	1 cup	579	41	2	103	85	18	28	0
YELLOW									
Boiled	1 cup	255	16	1	45	26	18	9	0
Raw	1 cup	676	43	4	119	70	49	24	0

Peas

Description	Serving Size	Cal	Prot (g)	Fat (g)	Carbs (g)	Net Carb(g)	Fiber (g)	Sod (mg)	Chol (mg)
CHICKPEAS (GARBANZO BEANS)									
Boiled	1 cup	269	15	3	45	32	12	11	0
Canned	1 cup	286	12	2	54	44	11	718	0
Raw	1 cup	728	39	9	121	87	35	48	0
COWPEAS									
Boiled	1 cup	200	14	1	35	29	6	32	0
Boiled (blackeyes, crowder, southern)	1 cup	200	13	1	36	25	11	7	0
Canned, plain (blackeyes, crowder, southern)	1 cup	185	11	1	33	25	8	718	0
Canned, with pork (blackeyes, crowder, southern)	1 cup	199	7	4	40	32	8	840	17
Raw	1 cup	573	40	3	100	82	18	97	0

Description	Serving Size	Cal	Prot (g)	Fat (g)	Carbs (g)	Net Carb(g)	Fiber (g)	Sod (mg)	Chol (mg)
PEAS (continued)									
Raw (blackeyes, crowder, southern)	1 cup	561	39	2	100	83	18	27	0
PIGEON PEAS									
Boiled	1 cup	203	11	0	39	28	11	8	0
Raw	1 cup	703	44	2	129	98	31	35	0
SPLIT PEAS									
Peas, split, mature seeds, cooked, boiled, without salt	1 cup	231	16	1	41	25	16	4	0
Peas, split, mature seeds, raw	1 cup	672	48	2	119	69	50	30	0

Soybean Products

Description	Serving Size	Cal	Prot (g)	Fat (g)	Carbs (g)	Net Carb(g)	Fiber (g)	Sod (mg)	Chol (mg)
SOY FLOUR									
Soy flour, defatted	1 cup	329	47	1	38	21	18	20	0
Soy flour, defatted, crude protein basis (N x 6 1/4)	1 cup	327	51	1	34	16	18	20	0
Soy flour, full-fat, raw	1 cup	366	29	16	30	22	8	11	0
Soy flour, full-fat, raw, crude protein basis (N x 6 1/4)	1 cup	369	32	16	27	19	8	11	0
Soy flour, full-fat, roasted	1 cup	375	30	17	29	20	8	10	0
Soy flour, full-fat, roasted, crude protein basis (N x 6 1/4)	1 cup	373	32	17	26	26	0	10	0
Soy flour, low-fat	1 cup	327	41	5	33	24	9	16	0
Soy flour, low-fat, crude protein basis (N x 6 1/4)	1 cup	325	45	5	30	21	9	16	0
SOY MEAL									
Soy meal, defatted, raw	1 cup	414	55	2	49	NA	NA	4	0
Soy meal, defatted, raw, crude protein basis (N x 6 1/4)	1 cup	411	60	2	44	NA	NA	4	0
SOY MILK									
Fluid	1 cup	81	7	3	4	1	3	29	0
SOY PROTEIN CONCENTRATE									
Crude protein basis (N x 6 1/4), produced by acid wash	1 oz	93	18	0	7	6	2	255	0
Produced by acid wash	1 oz	94	16	0	9	7	2	255	0
Produced by alcohol extraction	1 oz	94	16	0	9	7	2	1	0
SOY PROTEIN ISOLATE									
Potassium type	1 oz	96	23	1	2	0	2	14	0
Potassium type, crude protein basis	1 oz	91	25	0	1	0	1	14	0

Description	Serving Size	Cal	Prot (g)	Fat (g)	Carbs (g)	Net Carb(g)	Fiber (g)	Sod (mg)	Chol (mg)
PROTEIN TECHNOLOGIES INTERNATIONAL, ProPlus	1 oz	108	24	1	0	NA	NA	11	0
PROTEIN TECHNOLOGIES INTERNATIONAL, SUPRO	1 oz	110	25	1	0	NA	NA	337	0
Regular	1 oz	96	23	1	2	0	2	285	0
SOY SAUCE									
Made from hydrolyzed vegetable protein	1 tbsp	7	0	0	1	1	0	1024	0
Made from soy (tamari)	1 tbsp	11	2	0	1	1	0	1005	0
Made from soy and wheat (shoyu)	1 cup	135	13	0	22	20	2	14573	0
Made from soy and wheat (shoyu), low sodium	1 cup	135	13	0	22	20	2	8499	0
SOYBEANS									
Boiled	1 cup	298	29	14	17	7	10	2	0
Dry roasted	1 cup	774	68	35	56	42	14	3	0
Raw	1 cup	774	68	34	56	39	17	4	0
Roasted, no salt	1 cup	810	61	41	58	27	30	7	0
Roasted, salted	1 cup	810	61	41	58	27	30	280	0
TEMPEH									
Cooked		0	0	0	0	NA	NA	0	0
Raw	1 cup	320	31	15	16	NA	NA	15	0
TOFU									
Dried-frozen (koyadofu)	1 piece	82	8	5	2	1	1	1	0
Dried-frozen (koyadofu), prepared with calcium sulfate	1 piece	82	8	5	2	2	0	1	0
Extra firm, prepared with nigari	1/5 block	87	9	5	2	1	0	9	0
Firm, prepared with calcium sulfate and magnesium chloride (nigari)	1/2 cup	97	10	5	4	3	1	10	0
Firm, prepared with calcium sulfate and magnesium chloride (nigari)	1/4 block	62	7	3	2	2	0	6	0
Fried	1 oz	77	5	5	3	2	1	5	0
Fried	1 piece	35	2	2	1	1	1	2	0
Fried, prepared with calcium sulfate	1 piece	35	2	2	1	1	1	2	0
Hard, prepared with nigari	1/4 block	178	15	11	5	5	1	2	0
MORI-NU, Tofu, silken, extra firm	1 slice	46	6	1	2	2	0	53	0
MORI-NU, Tofu, silken, firm	1 slice	52	6	2	2	2	0	30	0
MORI-NU, Tofu, silken, lite extra firm	1 slice	32	6	1	1	1	0	82	0
MORI-NU, Tofu, silken, soft	1 slice	46	4	2	2	2	0	4	0

Description	Serving Size	Cal	Prot (g)	Fat (g)	Carbs (g)	Net Carb(g)	Fiber (g)	Sod (mg)	Chol (mg)
SOYBEAN PRODUCTS (continued)									
MOR-NU, Tofu, silken, lite firm	1 slice	31	5	1	1	1	0	71	0
Okara	1 cup	94	4	2	15	NA	NA	11	0
Raw, firm, prepared with calcium sulfate	1/2 cup	183	20	10	5	2	3	18	0
Raw, firm, prepared with calcium sulfate	1/4 block	117	13	7	3	2	2	11	0
Raw, regular, prepared with calcium sulfate	1/2 cup	94	10	6	2	2	0	9	0
Raw, regular, prepared with calcium sulfate	1/4 block	88	9	5	2	2	0	8	0
Salted and fermented (fuyu)	1 block	13	1	1	1	NA	NA	316	0
Salted and fermented (fuyu), prepared with calcium sulfate	1 block	13	1	1	1	NA	NA	316	0
Soft, prepared with calcium sulfate and magnesium chloride (nigari)	1 cup	151	16	9	4	4	0	20	0
Soft, prepared with calcium sulfate and magnesium chloride (nigari)	1 cubic inch	11	1	1	0	0	0	1	0
Natto	1 cup	371	31	18	25	16	9	12	0
OTHER LEGUMES									
Carob flour	1 cup	229	5	1	92	51	41	36	0
Carob flour	1 tbsp	18	0	0	7	4	3	3	0
Chickpea flour (besan)	1 cup	339	21	5	53	43	10	59	0
Falafel, home-prepared	1 patty	57	2	3	5	NA	NA	50	0
Hummus, commercial	1 cup	415	20	23	36	21	15	948	0
Hummus, commercial	1 tbsp	23	1	1	2	1	1	53	0
Hummus, home prepared	1 cup	421	12	20	50	37	13	600	0
Hummus, home prepared	1 tbsp	26	1	1	3	2	1	37	0
Lentils, mature seeds, cooked, boiled, with salt	1 cup	230	18	1	40	24	16	471	0
Lentils, mature seeds, cooked, boiled, without salt	1 cup	230	18	1	40	24	16	4	0
Lentils, mature seeds, cooked, boiled, without salt	1 tbsp	14	1	0	2	2	1	0	0
Lentils, mature seeds, raw	1 cup	649	54	1	110	51	59	19	0
Lentils, mature seeds, raw	1 tbsp	41	3	0	7	3	4	1	0
Lentils, pink, raw	1 cup	664	48	4	114	93	21	13	0
Lupins, mature seeds, cooked, boiled, with salt	1 cup	198	26	4	16	12	5	398	0
Lupins, mature seeds, cooked, boiled, without salt	1 cup	198	26	4	16	12	5	7	0
Lupins, mature seeds, raw	1 cup	668	65	14	73	NA	NA	27	0
Meat extender	1 cup	275	34	2	34	18	15	9	0

Description	Serving Size	Cal	Prot (g)	Fat (g)	Carbs (g)	Net Carb(g)	Fiber (g)	Sod (mg)	Chol (mg)
Meat extender	1 oz	89	11	1	11	6	5	3	0
Meatless bacon	1 cup	446	15	39	9	5	4	2110	0
Meatless bacon	1 oz, cooked	50	2	4	1	1	0	234	0
Meatless sausage	1 link	64	5	4	2	2	1	222	0
Meatless sausage	1 patty	97	7	6	4	3	1	337	0
Miso	1 cup	567	32	16	77	62	15	10029	0

Description	Serving Size	Cal	Prot (g)	Fat (g)	Carbs (g)	Net Carb(g)	Fiber (g)	Sod (mg)	Chol (mg)
Nuts									
ACORNS									
Acorn flour, full fat	1 oz	142	2	8	15	NA	NA	0	0
Dried	1 oz	144	2	9	15	NA	NA	0	0
Raw	1 oz	110	2	6	12	NA	NA	0	0
ALMONDS									
Almond butter, plain, with salt added	1 tbsp	101	2	9	3	3	1	72	0
Almond butter, plain, without salt added	1 tbsp	101	2	9	3	3	1	2	0
Almond paste	1 oz	130	3	8	14	12	1	3	0
Blanched	1 tbsp	53	2	4	2	1	1	3	0
Dry roasted, with salt added	1 oz	169	6	14	5	2	3	96	0
Dry roasted, without salt added	1 oz	169	6	14	5	2	3	0	0
Honey roasted, unblanched	1 oz	168	5	13	8	4	4	37	0
Oil roasted, with salt added	1 oz	172	6	15	5	2	3	96	0
Oil roasted, without salt added	1 oz	172	6	15	5	2	3	0	0
Plain	1 cup, ground or sliced	549	20	46	19	8	11	1	0
BEECHNUTS									
Dried	1 oz	163	2	14	9	NA	NA	11	0
BRAZILNUTS									
Dried, unblanched	1 oz	186	4	18	4	2	2	1	0
BUTTERNUTS									
Nuts, butternuts, dried	1 oz	174	7	15	3	2	1	0	0
CASHEWS									
Cashew butter, plain, with salt added	1 oz	166	5	13	8	7	1	174	0
Cashew butter, plain, without salt added	1 oz	166	5	13	8	7	1	4	0
Dry roasted, with salt added	1 oz	163	4	13	9	8	1	181	0
Dry roasted, without salt added	1 tbsp	49	1	4	3	3	0	1	0
Oil roasted, with salt added	1 oz	163	5	13	8	7	1	177	0
Oil roasted, without salt added	1 oz	163	5	13	8	7	1	5	0
CHESTNUTS									
Chinese, boiled and steamed	1 oz	43	1	0	10	NA	NA	1	0
Chinese, dried	1 oz	103	2	0	23	NA	NA	1	0
Chinese, raw	1 oz	64	1	0	14	NA	NA	1	0
Chinese, roasted	1 oz	68	1	0	15	NA	NA	1	0

Description	Serving Size	Cal	Prot (g)	Fat (g)	Carbs (g)	Net Carb(g)	Fiber (g)	Sod (mg)	Chol (mg)
NUTS (continued)									
European, boiled and steamed	1 oz	37	1	0	8	NA	NA	8	0
European, dried, peeled	1 oz	105	1	1	22	NA	NA	10	0
European, dried, unpeeled	1 oz	106	2	1	22	19	3	10	0
European, raw, peeled	1 oz	56	0	0	13	NA	NA	1	0
European, raw, unpeeled	1 oz	60	1	1	13	11	2	1	0
European, roasted	1 oz	69	1	1	15	14	1	1	0
Japanese, boiled and steamed	1 oz	16	0	0	4	NA	NA	1	0
Japanese, dried	1 oz	102	1	0	23	NA	NA	10	0
Japanese, raw	1 oz	44	1	0	10	NA	NA	4	0
Japanese, roasted	1 oz	57	1	0	13	NA	NA	5	0
COCONUTS									
Coconut cream, canned (liquid expressed from grated meat)	1 tbsp	36	1	3	2	1	0	10	0
Coconut cream, raw (liquid expressed from grated meat)	1 tbsp	50	1	5	1	1	0	1	0
Coconut milk, canned (liquid expressed from grated meat and water)	1 tbsp	30	0	3	0	NA	NA	2	0
Coconut milk, frozen (liquid expressed from grated meat and water)	1 tbsp	30	0	3	1	NA	NA	2	0
Coconut milk, raw (liquid expressed from grated meat and water)	1 tbsp	35	0	3	1	1	0	2	0
Coconut water (liquid from coconuts)	1 tbsp	3	0	0	1	0	0	16	0
Dried (desiccated), creamed	1 oz	194	2	18	6	NA	NA	10	0
Dried (desiccated), not sweetened	1 oz	187	2	17	7	2	5	10	0
Dried (desiccated), sweetened, flaked, canned	4 oz	505	4	34	47	42	5	23	0
Dried (desiccated), sweetened, flaked, packaged	1 oz	134	1	9	13	12	1	73	0
Dried (desiccated), sweetened, shredded	1 cup	466	3	31	44	40	4	244	0
Dried (desiccated), toasted	1 oz	168	2	13	13	NA	NA	10	0
Raw	1 medium	1405	13	125	60	25	36	79	0
GINKGO									
Canned	1 oz	31	1	0	6	4	3	87	0
Dried	1 oz	99	3	1	21	NA	NA	4	0
Raw	1 oz	52	1	0	11	NA	NA	2	0
HAZELNUTS									
Dry roasted, without salt added	1 oz	183	4	17	5	2	3	0	0

Description	Serving Size	Cal	Prot (g)	Fat (g)	Carbs (g)	Net Carb(g)	Fiber (g)	Sod (mg)	Chol (mg)
Raw	1 cup, chop.	722	17	67	19	8	11	0	0
Blanched	1 oz	178	4	17	5	2	3	0	0
HICKORYNUTS									
Dried	1 oz	186	4	17	5	3	2	0	0
MACADAMIA NUTS									
Dry roasted, with salt added	1 oz	203	2	21	4	1	2	75	0
Dry roasted, without salt added	1 oz	204	2	21	4	2	2	1	0
Raw	1 oz	204	2	21	4	1	2	1	0
MIXED NUTS									
Dry roasted, with peanuts, with salt added	1 oz	168	5	14	7	5	3	190	0
Dry roasted, with peanuts, without salt added	1 oz	168	5	14	7	5	3	3	0
Oil roasted, with peanuts, with salt added	1 oz	175	5	15	6	4	3	185	0
Oil roasted, with peanuts, without salt added	1 tbsp	55	1	5	2	1	1	1	0
Oil roasted, without peanuts, without salt added	1 oz	174	4	15	6	5	2	3	0
Without peanuts, oil roasted, with salt added	1 oz	174	4	15	6	5	2	198	0
PEANUTS									
All types, cooked, boiled, with salt	1 cup	200	9	13	13	8	6	473	0
All types, cooked, boiled, with salt	1 cup, shelled	572	24	38	38	22	16	1352	0
All types, dry-roasted, with salt	1 oz	166	7	13	6	4	2	230	0
All types, dry-roasted, with salt	1 peanut	6	0	0	0	0	0	8	0
All types, dry-roasted, without salt	1 cup	854	35	69	31	20	12	9	0
All types, dry-roasted, without salt	1 oz	166	7	13	6	4	2	2	0
All types, oil-roasted, with salt	1 cup, chop.	837	38	68	27	14	13	624	0
All types, oil-roasted, with salt	1 cup, halves and whole	837	38	68	27	14	13	624	0
All types, oil-roasted, without salt	1 cup, chop.	773	35	62	25	16	9	8	0
All types, oil-roasted, without salt	1 oz, shelled	165	7	13	5	3	2	2	0
All types, raw	1 cup	828	38	68	24	11	12	26	0
All types, raw	1 oz	161	7	13	5	2	2	5	0
Peanut butter, chunk style, with salt	1 cup	1520	62	122	56	39	17	1254	0
Peanut butter, chunk style, with salt	2 tbsp	188	8	15	7	5	2	156	0
Peanut butter, chunk style, without salt	1 cup	1520	62	122	56	39	17	44	0
Peanut butter, chunk style, without salt	2 tbsp	188	8	15	7	5	2	5	0

Description	Serving Size	Cal	Prot (g)	Fat (g)	Carbs (g)	Net Carb(g)	Fiber (g)	Sod (mg)	Chol (mg)
NUTS (continued)									
Peanut butter, smooth style, with salt	1 cup	1530	65	125	50	35	15	1205	0
Peanut butter, smooth style, with salt	2 tbsp	190	8	15	6	4	2	149	0
Peanut butter, smooth style, without salt	1 cup	1530	65	125	50	35	15	44	0
Peanut butter, smooth style, without salt	2 tbsp	190	8	15	6	4	2	5	0
Peanut flour, defatted	1 cup	196	31	0	21	11	9	108	0
Peanut flour, defatted	1 oz	93	15	0	10	5	4	51	0
Peanut flour, low fat	1 cup	257	20	12	19	9	9	1	0
Peanut flour, low fat	1 oz	121	10	6	9	4	4	0	0
Spanish, oil-roasted, with salt	1 cup	851	41	69	26	13	13	637	0
Spanish, oil-roasted, with salt	1 oz	164	8	13	5	2	3	123	0
Spanish, oil-roasted, without salt	1 cup	851	41	69	26	13	13	9	0
Spanish, oil-roasted, without salt	1 oz	164	8	13	5	2	3	2	0
Spanish, raw	1 cup	832	38	69	23	9	14	32	0
Spanish, raw	1 oz	162	7	13	4	2	3	6	0
Valencia, oil-roasted, with salt	1 cup	848	39	70	23	11	13	1112	0
Valencia, oil-roasted, with salt	1 oz	167	8	14	5	2	3	219	0
Valencia, oil-roasted, without salt	1 cup	848	39	70	23	11	13	9	0
Valencia, oil-roasted, without salt	1 oz	167	8	14	5	2	3	2	0
Valencia, raw	1 cup	832	37	66	31	18	13	1	0
Valencia, raw	1 oz	162	7	13	6	3	2	0	0
Virginia, oil-roasted, with salt	1 cup	827	37	66	28	16	13	619	0
Virginia, oil-roasted, with salt	1 oz	164	7	13	6	3	3	123	0
Virginia, oil-roasted, without salt	1 cup	827	37	66	28	16	13	9	0
Virginia, oil-roasted, without salt	1 oz	164	7	13	6	3	3	2	0
Virginia, raw	1 cup	822	37	68	24	12	12	15	0
Virginia, raw	1 oz	160	7	13	5	2	2	3	0
PECANS									
Dry roasted, with salt added	1 oz	201	3	20	4	1	3	109	0
Dry roasted, without salt added	1 oz	201	3	20	4	1	3	0	0
Oil roasted, with salt added	1 oz	203	3	20	4	1	3	111	0
Oil roasted, without salt added	1 oz	203	3	20	4	1	3	0	0
Raw	1 cup	746	10	74	15	5	10	0	0
PINE NUTS									
Dried	1 tbsp	49	2	4	1	1	0	0	0
Dried	10 nuts	6	0	1	0	0	0	1	0

Description	Serving Size	Cal	Prot (g)	Fat (g)	Carbs (g)	Net Carb(g)	Fiber (g)	Sod (mg)	Chol (mg)
PISTACHIO NUTS									
Dry roasted, with salt added	1 oz	161	6	12	8	5	3	115	0
Dry roasted, without salt added	1 oz	162	6	12	8	5	3	3	0
Raw	1 oz	158	6	12	8	5	3	0	0
WALNUTS									
Black, dried	1 tbsp	47	2	4	1	1	0	0	0
English	1 cup, chop.	785	18	75	16	8	8	2	0

Seds

Description	Serving Size	Cal	Prot (g)	Fat (g)	Carbs (g)	Net Carb(g)	Fiber (g)	Sod (mg)	Chol (mg)
BREADFRUIT SEEDS									
Boiled	1 oz	48	2	1	9	8	1	7	0
Dried	1 oz	104	2	0	23	18	4	15	0
Raw	1 oz	54	2	1	8	7	1	7	0
Raw	1 oz	62	2	0	13	NA	NA	9	0
Roasted	1 oz	59	2	1	11	10	2	8	0
CHIA SEEDS									
Dried	1 oz	134	5	7	14	NA	NA	11	0
COTTONSEEDS									
Cottonseed flour, low fat (glandless)	1 oz	94	14	0	10	NA	NA	10	0
Cottonseed flour, partially defatted (glandless)	1 tbsp	18	2	0	2	2	0	2	0
Cottonseed meal, partially defatted (glandless)	1 oz	104	14	1	11	NA	NA	10	0
Kernels, roasted (glandless)	1 tbsp	51	3	3	2	2	1	3	0
FLAXSEED									
Raw	1 tbsp	59	2	4	4	1	3	4	0
LOTUS SEEDS									
Dried	1 oz	94	4	1	18	NA	NA	1	0
Raw	1 oz	25	1	0	5	NA	NA	0	0
PUMPKIN & SQUASH SEEDS									
Kernels, dried	1 oz, hulled	153	7	12	5	4	1	5	0
Kernels, roasted, with salt added	1 oz	148	9	11	4	3	1	163	0
Kernels, roasted, without salt	1 oz	148	9	11	4	3	1	5	0
Whole, roasted, with salt added	1 oz	126	5	5	15	NA	NA	163	0
Whole, roasted, without salt	1 oz	126	5	5	15	NA	NA	5	0
SAFFLOWER SEEDS									
Kernels, dried	1 oz	147	5	10	10	NA	NA	1	0

Description	Serving Size	Cal	Prot (g)	Fat (g)	Carbs (g)	Net Carb(g)	Fiber (g)	Sod (mg)	Chol (mg)
SEEDS (continued)									
Safflower meal, partially defatted	1 oz	97	10	1	14	NA	NA	1	0
SESAME SEEDS									
Kernels, dried (decorticated)	1 tbsp	47	2	4	1	0	1	3	0
Kernels, toasted, with salt added (decorticated)	1 oz	161	5	13	7	3	5	167	0
Kernels, toasted, without salt added (decorticated)	1 oz	161	5	13	7	3	5	11	0
Sesame butter, paste	1 tbsp	95	3	8	4	3	2	2	0
Sesame butter, tahini, from raw and stone ground kernels	1 oz	162	5	13	7	5	3	21	0
Sesame butter, tahini, from roasted and toasted kernels	1 oz	169	5	15	6	3	3	33	0
Sesame butter, tahini, from unroasted kernels	1 oz	172	5	15	5	2	3	0	0
Sesame butter, tahini, type of kernels unspecified	1 tbsp	89	3	8	3	3	1	5	0
Sesame flour, high-fat	1 oz	149	9	10	8	NA	NA	12	0
Sesame flour, low-fat	1 oz	94	14	0	10	NA	NA	11	0
Sesame flour, partially defatted	1 oz	108	11	3	10	NA	NA	12	0
Sesame meal, partially defatted	1 oz	161	5	13	7	NA	NA	11	0
Whole, dried	1 tbsp	52	2	4	2	1	1	1	0
Whole, roasted and toasted	1 oz	160	5	13	7	3	4	3	0
SUNFLOWER SEEDS									
Kernels, dried	1 cup, w/hulls	262	10	22	9	4	5	1	0
Kernels, dry roasted, with salt added	1 oz	165	5	13	7	4	3	221	0
Kernels, dry roasted, without salt	1 oz	165	5	13	7	4	3	1	0
Kernels, oil roasted, with salt added	1 oz	174	6	16	4	2	2	171	0
Kernels, oil roasted, without salt	1 oz	174	6	16	4	2	2	1	0
Kernels, toasted, with salt added	1 oz	175	5	15	6	3	3	174	0
Kernels, toasted, without salt	1 oz	175	5	15	6	3	3	1	0
Sunflower seed butter, with salt added	1 oz	164	6	13	8	NA	NA	147	0
Sunflower seed butter, without salt	1 oz	164	6	13	8	NA	NA	1	0
Sunflower seed flour, partially defatted	1 tbsp	13	2	0	1	1	0	0	0
WATERMELON SEEDS									
Kernels, dried	1 oz	158	8	13	4	NA	NA	28	0

Description	Serving Size	Cal	Prot (g)	Fat (g)	Carbs (g)	Net Carb(g)	Fiber (g)	Sod (mg)	Chol (mg)
Blade									
Chops or roasts, bone-in, lean and fat, raw	1 chop, exclud. refuse	314	17	24	0	0	0	59	79
Chops or roasts, bone-in, lean only, raw	1 chop, exclud. refuse	129	16	6	0	0	0	55	52
Chops, bone-in, lean and fat, braised	3 oz	275	19	19	0	0	0	47	72
Chops, bone-in, lean and fat, braised	1 chop, exclud. refuse	268	18	19	0	0	0	46	71
Chops, bone-in, lean and fat, broiled	3 oz	272	19	19	0	0	0	60	73
Chops, bone-in, lean and fat, broiled	1 chop, exclud. refuse	256	18	18	0	0	0	56	69
Chops, bone-in, lean and fat, pan-fried	3 oz	291	18	21	0	0	0	57	72
Chops, bone-in, lean and fat, pan-fried	1 chop, exclud. refuse	284	18	21	0	0	0	56	71
Chops, bone-in, lean only, braised	3 oz	191	21	10	0	0	0	53	71
Chops, bone-in, lean only, braised	1 chop, exclud. refuse	142	16	7	0	0	0	39	52
Chops, bone-in, lean only, broiled	3 oz	199	22	10	0	0	0	68	71
Chops, bone-in, lean only, broiled	1 chop, exclud. refuse	147	16	8	0	0	0	50	53
Chops, bone-in, lean only, pan-fried	3 oz	205	21	11	0	0	0	66	70
Chops, bone-in, lean only, pan-fried	1 chop, exclud. refuse	152	16	8	0	0	0	49	52
Roasts, bone-in, lean and fat, roasted	3 oz	275	20	19	0	0	0	26	79
Roasts, bone-in, lean only, roasted	3 oz	210	23	11	0	0	0	25	79
Center Loin									
Chops or roasts, bone-in, lean and fat, raw	1 chop, exclud. refuse	224	23	13	0	0	0	67	75
Chops or roasts, bone-in, lean only, raw	1 chop, exclud. refuse	137	22	4	0	0	0	65	62
Chops, bone-in, lean and fat, braised	3 oz	210	24	11	0	0	0	50	73
Chops, bone-in, lean and fat, braised	1 chop, exclud. refuse	205	23	11	0	0	0	49	71
Chops, bone-in, lean and fat, broiled	3 oz	204	24	10	0	0	0	49	70
Chops, bone-in, lean and fat, broiled	1 chop, exclud. refuse	197	24	10	0	0	0	48	67
Chops, bone-in, lean and fat, pan-fried	3 oz	235	25	13	0	0	0	68	78

Description	Serving Size	Cal	Prot (g)	Fat (g)	Carbs (g)	Net Carb(g)	Fiber (g)	Sod (mg)	Chol (mg)
CENTER LOIN (continued)									
Chops, bone-in, lean and fat, pan-fried	1 chop, exclud. refuse	216	23	12	0	0	0	62	72
Chops, bone-in, lean only, braised	3 oz	172	25	6	0	0	0	53	72
Chops, bone-in, lean only, braised	1 chop, exclud. refuse	149	22	5	0	0	0	46	63
Chops, bone-in, lean only, broiled	3 oz	172	26	6	0	0	0	51	70
Chops, bone-in, lean only, broiled	1 chop, exclud. refuse	149	22	5	0	0	0	44	61
Chops, bone-in, lean only, pan-fried	3 oz	197	27	8	0	0	0	73	78
Chops, bone-in, lean only, pan-fried	1 chop, exclud. refuse	160	22	7	0	0	0	59	63
Roasts, bone-in, lean and fat, roasted	3 oz	199	22	10	0	0	0	54	68
Roasts, bone-in, lean only, roasted	3 oz	169	23	7	0	0	0	56	67

Center Rib

Description	Serving Size	Cal	Prot (g)	Fat (g)	Carbs (g)	Net Carb(g)	Fiber (g)	Sod (mg)	Chol (mg)
Chops or roasts, bone-in, lean and fat, raw	1 chop, exclud. refuse	205	20	12	0	0	0	41	59
Chops or roasts, bone-in, lean only, raw	1 chop, exclud. refuse	128	19	5	0	0	0	39	47
Chops or roasts, boneless, lean and fat, raw	1 chop, exclud. refuse	213	20	13	0	0	0	42	61
Chops or roasts, boneless, lean only, raw	1 chop, exclud. refuse	134	19	5	0	0	0	40	48
Chops, bone-in, lean and fat, braised	3 oz	213	23	12	0	0	0	34	62
Chops, bone-in, lean and fat, braised	1 chop, exclud. refuse	188	20	10	0	0	0	30	55
Chops, bone-in, lean and fat, broiled	3 oz	224	24	12	0	0	0	53	70
Chops, bone-in, lean and fat, broiled	1 chop, exclud. refuse	195	21	10	0	0	0	46	61
Chops, bone-in, lean and fat, pan-fried	3 oz	225	22	13	0	0	0	43	62
Chops, bone-in, lean and fat, pan-fried	1 chop, exclud. refuse	193	19	11	0	0	0	37	53
Chops, bone-in, lean only, braised	3 oz	175	24	8	0	0	0	35	60
Chops, bone-in, lean only, braised	1 chop, exclud. refuse	138	19	6	0	0	0	27	48
Chops, bone-in, lean only, broiled	3 oz	186	26	7	0	0	0	55	69
Chops, bone-in, lean only, broiled	1 chop, exclud. refuse	147	21	6	0	0	0	44	54
Chops, bone-in, lean only, pan-fried	3 oz	185	24	9	0	0	0	44	60

Description	Serving Size	Cal	Prot (g)	Fat (g)	Carbs (g)	Net Carb(g)	Fiber (g)	Sod (mg)	Chol (mg)
Chops, bone-in, lean only, pan-fried	1 chop, exclud. refuse	140	18	7	0	0	0	33	45
Chops, boneless, lean and fat, braised	3 oz	217	22	12	0	0	0	34	62
Chops, boneless, lean and fat, braised	1 chop, exclud. refuse	207	21	12	0	0	0	32	59
Chops, boneless, lean and fat, broiled	3 oz	221	23	12	0	0	0	53	70
Chops, boneless, lean and fat, broiled	1 chop, exclud. refuse	208	22	11	0	0	0	50	66
Chops, boneless, lean and fat, pan-fried	3 oz	190	24	9	0	0	0	44	60
Chops, boneless, lean and fat, pan-fried	1 chop, exclud. refuse	168	21	8	0	0	0	39	53
Chops, boneless, lean only, braised	3 oz	179	24	8	0	0	0	35	60
Chops, boneless, lean only, braised	1 chop, exclud. refuse	152	20	7	0	0	0	30	51
Chops, boneless, lean only, broiled	3 oz	184	25	7	0	0	0	55	69
Chops, boneless, lean only, broiled	1 chop, exclud. refuse	153	21	6	0	0	0	46	58
Chops, boneless, lean only, pan-fried	3 oz	190	24	9	0	0	0	44	60
Chops, boneless, lean only, pan-fried	1 chop, exclud. refuse	148	18	7	0	0	0	34	46
Roasts, bone-in, lean and fat, roasted	3 oz	217	23	12	0	0	0	39	62
Roasts, bone-in, lean only, roasted	3 oz	190	24	9	0	0	0	40	60
Roasts, boneless, lean and fat, roasted	3 oz	214	23	11	0	0	0	41	69
Roasts, boneless, lean only, roasted	3 oz	182	24	8	0	0	0	43	71

Country-style Ribs

Description	Serving Size	Cal	Prot (g)	Fat (g)	Carbs (g)	Net Carb(g)	Fiber (g)	Sod (mg)	Chol (mg)
Lean and fat, braised	3 oz	252	20	16	0	0	0	50	74
Lean and fat, raw	1 oz	68	5	5	0	0	0	16	20
Lean and fat, roasted	3 oz	279	20	19	0	0	0	44	78
Lean only, braised	3 oz	199	22	10	0	0	0	54	73
Lean only, raw	1 oz	45	5	2	0	0	0	19	18
Lean only, roasted	3 oz	210	23	11	0	0	0	25	79

Cured

BACON

Description	Serving Size	Cal	Prot (g)	Fat (g)	Carbs (g)	Net Carb(g)	Fiber (g)	Sod (mg)	Chol (mg)
Broiled, pan-fried or roasted	3 med, slices, cooked	109	6	9	0	0	0	303	16
Raw	1 thick slice	211	3	21	0	0	0	277	25
Raw	3 med. slices	378	6	37	0	0	0	496	46

Description	Serving Size	Cal	Prot (g)	Fat (g)	Carbs (g)	Net Carb(g)	Fiber (g)	Sod (mg)	Chol (mg)
CURED (continued)									
BREAKFAST STRIPS									
Cooked	3 slices, cooked	156	10	12	0	0	0	714	36
Raw or unheated	3 slices	264	8	24	0	0	0	671	47
CANADIAN-STYLE BACON									
Grilled	2 slices	86	11	4	1	1	0	719	27
Unheated	2 slices	89	12	3	1	1	0	799	28
HAM									
Boneless, extra lean (approximately 5% fat), roasted	1 cup	203	29	7	2	2	0	1684	74
Boneless, extra lean (approximately 5% fat), roasted	3 oz	123	18	4	1	1	0	1023	45
Boneless, extra lean and regular, roasted	1 cup	231	31	10	1	1	0	1939	80
Boneless, extra lean and regular, roasted	3 oz	140	19	6	0	0	0	1177	48
Boneless, extra lean and regular, unheated	1 cup	227	26	11	3	3	0	1789	74
Boneless, extra lean and regular, unheated	1 slice	46	5	2	1	1	0	362	15
Boneless, regular (approximately 11% fat), roasted	1 cup	249	32	13	0	0	0	2100	83
Boneless, regular (approximately 11% fat), roasted	3 oz	151	19	8	0	0	0	1275	50
Center slice, country-style, lean only, raw	1 oz	55	8	2	0	0	0	764	20
Center slice, country-style, lean only, raw	4 oz	220	31	9	0	0	0	3045	79
Center slice, lean and fat, unheated	1 oz	58	6	3	0	0	0	393	15
Center slice, lean and fat, unheated	4 oz	229	23	14	0	0	0	1566	61
Extra lean (approximately 4% fat), canned, roasted	1 cup	190	30	6	1	1	0	1589	42
Extra lean (approximately 4% fat), canned, roasted	3 oz	116	18	4	0	0	0	965	26
Extra lean (approximately 4% fat), canned, unheated	1 cup	168	26	6	0	0	0	1757	53
Extra lean (approximately 4% fat), canned, unheated	1 oz	34	5	1	0	0	0	356	11
Extra lean and regular, canned, roasted	1 cup	234	29	11	1	1	0	1495	57
Extra lean and regular, canned, roasted	3 oz	142	18	7	0	0	0	908	35

Description	Serving Size	Cal	Prot (g)	Fat (g)	Carbs (g)	Net Carb(g)	Fiber (g)	Sod (mg)	Chol (mg)
Extra lean and regular, canned, unheated	1 cup	202	25	9	0	0	0	1786	53
Extra lean and regular, canned, unheated	1 oz	41	5	2	0	0	0	362	11
Patties, grilled	1 patty, cooked	203	8	17	1	1	0	632	43
Patties, unheated	1 oz	89	4	7	0	0	0	308	20
Patties, unheated	1 patty	205	8	17	1	1	0	709	46
Regular (approximately 13% fat), canned, roasted	1 cup	316	29	19	1	1	0	1317	87
Regular (approximately 13% fat), canned, roasted	3 oz	192	17	12	0	0	0	800	53
Regular (approximately 13% fat), canned, unheated	1 cup	266	24	17	0	0	0	1736	55
Regular (approximately 13% fat), canned, unheated	1 oz	54	5	3	0	0	0	352	11
Steak, boneless, extra lean, unheated	1 oz	35	6	1	0	0	0	360	13
Steak, boneless, extra lean, unheated	1 slice	69	11	2	0	0	0	720	26
Whole, lean and fat, roasted	1 cup	340	30	22	0	0	0	1662	87
Whole, lean and fat, roasted	3 oz	207	18	13	0	0	0	1009	53
Whole, lean and fat, unheated	1 cup	344	26	24	0	0	0	1798	78
Whole, lean and fat, unheated	1 oz	70	5	5	0	0	0	364	16
Whole, lean only, roasted	1 cup	220	35	7	0	0	0	1858	77
Whole, lean only, roasted	3 oz	133	21	4	0	0	0	1128	47
Whole, lean only, unheated	1 cup	206	31	7	0	0	0	2122	73
Whole, lean only, unheated	1 oz	42	6	1	0	0	0	430	15
SHOULDER									
Arm picnic, lean and fat, roasted	1 cup	392	29	28	0	0	0	1501	81
Arm picnic, lean and fat, roasted	3 oz	238	17	17	0	0	0	911	49
Arm picnic, lean only, roasted	1 cup	238	35	9	0	0	0	1723	67
Arm picnic, lean only, roasted	3 oz	145	21	5	0	0	0	1046	41
Blade roll, lean and fat, roasted	3 oz	244	15	19	0	0	0	827	57
Blade roll, lean and fat, unheated	1 oz	76	5	6	0	0	0	354	15
Blade roll, lean and fat, unheated	4 oz	304	19	23	0	0	0	1413	60
Feet, pickled	1 oz	58	4	4	0	0	0	262	26
Salt pork, raw	1 oz	212	1	22	0	0	0	404	24
Separable fat (from ham and arm picnic), roasted	1 oz	168	2	17	0	0	0	177	24

Description	Serving Size	Cal	Prot (g)	Fat (g)	Carbs (g)	Net Carb(g)	Fiber (g)	Sod (mg)	Chol (mg)
CURED (continued)									
Separable fat (from ham and arm picnic), roasted	3 oz	502	6	50	0	0	0	530	73
Separable fat (from ham and arm picnic), unheated	1 oz	164	2	17	0	0	0	143	19
Separable fat (from ham and arm picnic), unheated	3 oz	492	5	50	0	0	0	429	58

Ground

Description	Serving Size	Cal	Prot (g)	Fat (g)	Carbs (g)	Net Carb(g)	Fiber (g)	Sod (mg)	Chol (mg)
Cooked	3 oz	252	22	16	0	0	0	62	80
Raw	1 oz	75	5	5	0	0	0	16	20
Raw	4 oz	297	19	22	0	0	0	63	81

HORMEL

Description	Serving Size	Cal	Prot (g)	Fat (g)	Carbs (g)	Net Carb(g)	Fiber (g)	Sod (mg)	Chol (mg)
ALWAYS TENDER, Boneless Pork Loin, Fresh Pork	1 oz	41	5	2	0	0	0	100	14
ALWAYS TENDER, Boneless Pork Loin, Fresh Pork	1 serving	162	21	8	1	1	0	401	55
ALWAYS TENDER, Center Cut Chops, Fresh Pork	1 oz	47	5	3	0	0	0	107	15
ALWAYS TENDER, Center Cut Chops, Fresh Pork	1 serving	187	21	10	1	1	0	423	58
ALWAYS TENDER, Pork Loin Filets, Lemon Garlic-Flavored	1 oz	33	5	1	1	1	0	165	12
ALWAYS TENDER, Pork Loin Filets, Lemon Garlic-Flavored	1 serving	132	20	4	2	2	0	661	47
ALWAYS TENDER, Pork Tenderloin, Peppercorn-Flavored	4 oz	123	19	4	2	2	0	665	53
ALWAYS TENDER, Pork Tenderloin, Teriyaki-Flavored	4 oz	133	20	3	5	5	0	463	52
Canadian Style Bacon	1 serving	68	9	3	1	1	0	569	27
Cure 81 Ham	1 serving	89	15	3	0	0	0	872	43

Leg (ham)

Description	Serving Size	Cal	Prot (g)	Fat (g)	Carbs (g)	Net Carb(g)	Fiber (g)	Sod (mg)	Chol (mg)
Rump half, lean and fat, raw	1 oz	63	5	4	0	0	0	17	19
Rump half, lean and fat, roasted	1 cup, diced	340	39	18	0	0	0	84	130
Rump half, lean and fat, roasted	3 oz	214	25	11	0	0	0	53	82
Rump half, lean only, raw	1 oz	39	6	1	0	0	0	20	17
Rump half, lean only, roasted	1 cup, diced	278	42	10	0	0	0	88	130
Rump half, lean only, roasted	3 oz	175	26	6	0	0	0	55	82
Shank half, lean and fat, raw	1 oz	75	5	5	0	0	0	16	19
Shank half, lean and fat, roasted	1 cup, diced	390	34	25	0	0	0	80	124

Description	Serving Size	Cal	Prot (g)	Fat (g)	Carbs (g)	Net Carb(g)	Fiber (g)	Sod (mg)	Chol (mg)
Shank half, lean and fat, roasted	3 oz	246	22	16	0	0	0	50	78
Shank half, lean only, raw	1 oz	39	6	1	0	0	0	19	17
Shank half, lean only, roasted	1 cup, diced	290	38	13	0	0	0	86	124
Shank half, lean only, roasted	3 oz	183	24	8	0	0	0	54	78
Whole, lean and fat, raw	1 oz	69	5	5	0	0	0	13	21
Whole, lean and fat, roasted	1 cup, diced	369	36	22	0	0	0	81	127
Whole, lean and fat, roasted	3 oz	232	23	14	0	0	0	51	80
Whole, lean only, raw	1 oz	39	6	1	0	0	0	16	19
Whole, lean only, roasted	1 cup, diced	285	40	12	0	0	0	86	127
Whole, lean only, roasted	3 oz	179	25	7	0	0	0	54	80

Shoulder

ARM PICNIC

Description	Serving Size	Cal	Prot (g)	Fat (g)	Carbs (g)	Net Carb(g)	Fiber (g)	Sod (mg)	Chol (mg)
Lean and fat, braised	1 cup, diced	444	38	29	0	0	0	119	147
Lean and fat, braised	3 oz	280	24	18	0	0	0	75	93
Lean and fat, raw	1 oz	72	5	5	0	0	0	19	20
Lean and fat, roasted	1 cup, diced	428	32	29	0	0	0	95	127
Lean and fat, roasted	3 oz	269	20	19	0	0	0	60	80
Lean only, braised	3 oz	211	27	9	0	0	0	87	97
Lean only, raw	1 oz	40	6	2	0	0	0	23	18
Lean only, roasted	3 oz	194	23	10	0	0	0	68	81

BLADE

Description	Serving Size	Cal	Prot (g)	Fat (g)	Carbs (g)	Net Carb(g)	Fiber (g)	Sod (mg)	Chol (mg)
Boston (roasts), lean and fat, roasted	3 oz	229	20	14	0	0	0	57	73
Boston (roasts), lean only, roasted	3 oz	197	21	11	0	0	0	75	72
Boston (steaks), lean and fat, braised	3 oz	271	24	17	0	0	0	60	96
Boston (steaks), lean and fat, broiled	3 oz	220	22	13	0	0	0	59	81
Boston (steaks), lean only, braised	3 oz	232	26	12	0	0	0	64	99
Boston (steaks), lean only, broiled	3 oz	193	23	9	0	0	0	63	80

WHOLE

Description	Serving Size	Cal	Prot (g)	Fat (g)	Carbs (g)	Net Carb(g)	Fiber (g)	Sod (mg)	Chol (mg)
Lean and fat, raw	1 oz	67	5	5	0	0	0	18	20
Lean and fat, roasted	1 cup, diced	394	31	26	0	0	0	92	122
Lean and fat, roasted	3 oz	248	20	16	0	0	0	58	77
Lean only, raw	1 oz	42	6	2	0	0	0	22	19
Lean only, roasted	1 cup, diced	311	34	16	0	0	0	101	122
Lean only, roasted	3 oz	196	22	10	0	0	0	64	77
Separable fat, cooked	1 oz	178	3	17	0	0	0	10	26
Separable fat, cooked	4 oz	711	14	66	0	0	0	38	105

Description	Serving Size	Cal	Prot (g)	Fat (g)	Carbs (g)	Net Carb(g)	Fiber (g)	Sod (mg)	Chol (mg)
SHOULDER (continued)									
Separable fat, raw	1 oz	181	2	17	0	0	0	5	26
Separable fat, raw	4 oz	721	7	69	0	0	0	20	105

Sirloin

Description	Serving Size	Cal	Prot (g)	Fat (g)	Carbs (g)	Net Carb(g)	Fiber (g)	Sod (mg)	Chol (mg)
Chops or roasts, bone-in, lean and fat, raw	1 chop, exclud. refuse	219	21	13	0	0	0	58	72
Chops or roasts, bone-in, lean only, raw	1 chop, exclud. refuse	133	20	5	0	0	0	48	59
Chops or roasts, boneless, lean and fat, raw	1 chop, exclud. refuse	151	21	6	0	0	0	52	67
Chops or roasts, boneless, lean only, raw	1 chop, exclud. refuse	129	21	4	0	0	0	52	64
Chops, bone-in, lean and fat, braised	3 oz	208	22	11	0	0	0	43	70
Chops, bone-in, lean and fat, braised	1 chop, exclud. refuse	196	20	11	0	0	0	41	66
Chops, bone-in, lean and fat, broiled	3 oz	220	23	12	0	0	0	58	73
Chops, bone-in, lean and fat, broiled	1 chop, exclud. refuse	194	20	11	0	0	0	51	65
Chops, bone-in, lean only, braised	3 oz	167	23	7	0	0	0	45	69
Chops, bone-in, lean only, braised	1 chop, exclud. refuse	142	19	6	0	0	0	38	58
Chops, bone-in, lean only, broiled	3 oz	181	24	8	0	0	0	61	72
Chops, bone-in, lean only, broiled	1 chop, exclud. refuse	143	19	6	0	0	0	48	57
Chops, boneless, lean and fat, braised	3 oz	161	23	6	0	0	0	39	69
Chops, boneless, lean and fat, braised	1 chop, exclud. refuse	155	22	6	0	0	0	38	66
Chops, boneless, lean and fat, broiled	3 oz	177	26	6	0	0	0	48	77
Chops, boneless, lean and fat, broiled	1 chop, exclud. refuse	154	23	5	0	0	0	41	67
Chops, boneless, lean only, braised	3 oz	149	23	5	0	0	0	39	69
Chops, boneless, lean only, braised	1 chop, exclud. refuse	140	22	5	0	0	0	37	65
Chops, boneless, lean only, broiled	3 oz	164	26	5	0	0	0	48	78
Chops, boneless, lean only, broiled	1 chop, exclud. refuse	137	22	4	0	0	0	40	65
Roasts, bone-in, lean and fat, roasted	3 oz	222	23	12	0	0	0	51	74
Roasts, bone-in, lean only, roasted	3 oz	184	24	8	0	0	0	54	73

Description	Serving Size	Cal	Prot (g)	Fat (g)	Carbs (g)	Net Carb(g)	Fiber (g)	Sod (mg)	Chol (mg)
Roasts, boneless, lean and fat, roasted	3 oz	176	24	7	0	0	0	48	73
Roasts, boneless, lean only, roasted	3 oz	168	25	6	0	0	0	48	73

Spareribs

Description	Serving Size	Cal	Prot (g)	Fat (g)	Carbs (g)	Net Carb(g)	Fiber (g)	Sod (mg)	Chol (mg)
Lean and fat, braised	3 oz	337	25	23	0	0	0	79	103
Lean and fat, raw	1 oz	81	5	6	0	0	0	22	22

Tenderloin

Description	Serving Size	Cal	Prot (g)	Fat (g)	Carbs (g)	Net Carb(g)	Fiber (g)	Sod (mg)	Chol (mg)
Lean and fat, broiled	3 oz	171	25	6	0	0	0	54	80
Lean and fat, broiled	1 chop, exclud. refuse	153	23	5	0	0	0	49	71
Lean and fat, raw	1 oz	39	6	1	0	0	0	14	19
Lean and fat, roasted	3 oz	147	24	4	0	0	0	47	67
Lean only, broiled	3 oz	159	26	5	0	0	0	55	80
Lean only, broiled	1 chop, exclud. refuse	137	22	4	0	0	0	47	69
Lean only, raw	1 oz	34	6	1	0	0	0	14	18
Lean only, roasted	3 oz	139	24	3	0	0	0	48	67

Top Loin

Description	Serving Size	Cal	Prot (g)	Fat (g)	Carbs (g)	Net Carb(g)	Fiber (g)	Sod (mg)	Chol (mg)
Chops, boneless, lean and fat, braised	3 oz	198	24	10	0	0	0	36	64
Chops, boneless, lean and fat, broiled	3 oz	195	25	8	0	0	0	54	69
Chops, boneless, lean and fat, broiled	1 chop, exclud. refuse	163	21	7	0	0	0	45	58
Chops, boneless, lean and fat, pan-fried	3 oz	218	25	11	0	0	0	47	66
Chops, boneless, lean and fat, pan-fried	1 chop, exclud. refuse	177	20	9	0	0	0	38	54
Chops, boneless, lean and fat, raw	1 chop, exclud. refuse	189	21	10	0	0	0	44	59
Chops, boneless, lean only, braised	3 oz	172	25	7	0	0	0	36	62
Chops, boneless, lean only, braised	1 chop, exclud. refuse	149	22	6	0	0	0	31	54
Chops, boneless, lean only, broiled	3 oz	173	26	6	0	0	0	55	68
Chops, boneless, lean only, broiled	1 chop, exclud. refuse	134	21	4	0	0	0	43	53
Chops, boneless, lean only, pan-fried	3 oz	191	26	8	0	0	0	48	65
Chops, boneless, lean only, pan-fried	1 chop, exclud. refuse	142	19	6	0	0	0	36	49
Chops, boneless, lean only, raw	1 chop, exclud. refuse	131	20	4	0	0	0	42	51
Roasts, boneless, lean and fat, raw	1 oz	54	6	3	0	0	0	12	17
Roasts, boneless, lean and fat, roasted	3 oz	192	24	9	0	0	0	37	66

Description	Serving Size	Cal	Prot (g)	Fat (g)	Carbs (g)	Net Carb(g)	Fiber (g)	Sod (mg)	Chol (mg)
TOP LOIN (continued)									
Roasts, boneless, lean only, raw	1 oz	40	6	1	0	0	0	13	16
Roasts, boneless, lean only, roasted	3 oz	165	26	5	0	0	0	38	66

Variety Meats & By-products

Description	Serving Size	Cal	Prot (g)	Fat (g)	Carbs (g)	Net Carb(g)	Fiber (g)	Sod (mg)	Chol (mg)
Brain, braised	3 oz	117	10	5	0	0	0	77	2169
Brain, raw	1 oz	36	3	1	0	0	0	34	622
Brain, raw	4 oz	144	12	6	0	0	0	136	2480
Chitterlings, raw	1 oz	71	3	6	0	0	0	10	45
Chitterlings, raw	1 pc., cooked, exclud. refuse	912	36	78	1	1	0	127	576
Chitterlings, simmered	3 oz	258	9	23	0	0	0	33	122
Ears, frozen, raw	1 oz	66	6	4	0	0	0	54	23
Ears, frozen, raw	1 ear	264	25	16	1	1	0	216	93
Ears, frozen, simmered	1 ear	184	18	11	0	0	0	185	100
Feet, raw	1 oz	75	6	5	0	0	0	18	30
Feet, raw	1/2 foot	251	21	17	0	0	0	59	101
Feet, simmered	3 oz	165	16	10	0	0	0	26	85
Heart, braised	1 cup	215	34	6	1	1	0	51	320
Heart, braised	1 heart	191	30	5	1	1	0	45	285
Heart, raw	1 oz	33	5	1	0	0	0	16	37
Heart, raw	1 heart	267	39	7	3	3	0	127	296
Jowl, raw	1 oz	186	2	19	0	0	0	7	26
Jowl, raw	4 oz	740	7	75	0	0	0	28	102
Kidneys, braised	1 cup	211	36	5	0	0	0	112	672
Kidneys, braised	3 oz	128	22	3	0	0	0	68	408
Kidneys, raw	1 oz	28	5	1	0	0	0	34	90
Kidneys, raw	1 kidney	233	38	6	0	0	0	282	743
Leaf fat, raw	1 oz	243	0	25	0	0	0	1	31
Leaf fat, raw	4 oz	968	2	101	0	0	0	6	124
Liver, braised	3 oz	140	22	3	3	3	0	42	302
Liver, raw	1 oz	38	6	1	1	1	0	25	85
Liver, raw	4 oz	151	24	3	3	3	0	98	340
Lungs, braised	3 oz	84	14	2	0	0	0	69	329
Lungs, raw	1 oz	24	4	1	0	0	0	43	91
Mechanically separated, raw	1 oz	86	4	7	0	0	0	14	22
Pancreas, braised	3 oz	186	24	8	0	0	0	36	268
Pancreas, raw	1 oz	56	5	3	0	0	0	12	55

Description	Serving Size	Cal	Prot (g)	Fat (g)	Carbs (g)	Net Carb(g)	Fiber (g)	Sod (mg)	Chol (mg)
Pancreas, raw	4 oz	225	21	13	0	0	0	50	218
Spleen, braised	3 oz	127	24	2	0	0	0	91	428
Spleen, raw	1 oz	28	5	0	0	0	0	28	103
Spleen, raw	4 oz	113	20	2	0	0	0	111	410
Stomach, raw	1 oz	45	5	2	0	0	0	15	55
Stomach, raw	4 oz	177	19	10	0	0	0	59	218
Tail, raw	1 oz	107	5	9	0	0	0	18	27
Tail, raw	4 oz	427	20	35	0	0	0	71	110
Tail, simmered	3 oz	337	14	28	0	0	0	21	110
Tongue, braised	3 oz	230	20	15	0	0	0	93	124
Tongue, raw	1 oz	64	5	4	0	0	0	31	29
Tongue, raw	4 oz	254	18	18	0	0	0	124	114

Whole Loin

Description	Serving Size	Cal	Prot (g)	Fat (g)	Carbs (g)	Net Carb(g)	Fiber (g)	Sod (mg)	Chol (mg)
Lean and fat, braised	3 oz	203	23	10	0	0	0	41	68
Lean and fat, braised	1 chop, exclud. refuse	213	24	11	0	0	0	43	71
Lean and fat, broiled	3 oz	206	23	11	0	0	0	53	68
Lean and fat, broiled	1 chop, exclud. refuse	211	24	11	0	0	0	54	70
Lean and fat, raw	1 chop, exclud. refuse	232	23	13	0	0	0	59	74
Lean and fat, roasted	3 oz	211	23	11	0	0	0	50	70
Lean and fat, roasted	1 chop, exclud. refuse	221	24	12	0	0	0	53	73
Lean only, braised	3 oz	173	24	7	0	0	0	43	67
Lean only, braised	1 chop, exclud. refuse	163	23	7	0	0	0	40	63
Lean only, broiled	3 oz	179	24	8	0	0	0	54	67
Lean only, broiled	1 chop, exclud. refuse	166	23	7	0	0	0	51	62
Lean only, raw	1 chop, exclud. refuse	152	23	5	0	0	0	55	63
Lean only, roasted	3 oz	178	24	7	0	0	0	49	69
Lean only, roasted	1 chop, exclud. refuse	169	23	7	0	0	0	47	66
Back fat, raw	1 oz	230	1	24	0	0	0	3	16
Back ribs, lean and fat, raw	1 oz	80	5	6	0	0	0	21	23
Back ribs, lean and fat, roasted	3 oz	315	21	23	0	0	0	86	100
Belly, raw	1 oz	147	3	14	0	0	0	9	20

Description	Serving Size	Cal	Prot (g)	Fat (g)	Carbs (g)	Net Carb(g)	Fiber (g)	Sod (mg)	Chol (mg)
WHOLE LOIN (continued)									
Carcass, lean and fat, raw	1 oz	107	4	9	0	0	0	12	21
Composite of trimmed leg, loin, shoulder, and spareribs, (includes cuts to be cured), lean and fat, raw	1 oz	64	5	4	0	0	0	15	20
Composite of trimmed retail cuts (leg, loin, and shoulder), lean only, cooked	3 oz	180	25	7	0	0	0	50	73
Composite of trimmed retail cuts (leg, loin, shoulder), lean only, raw	1 oz	41	6	2	0	0	0	16	17
Composite of trimmed retail cuts (leg, loin, shoulder, and spareribs), lean and fat, cooked	3 oz	232	23	13	0	0	0	53	77
Composite of trimmed retail cuts (leg, loin, shoulder, and spareribs), lean and fat, raw	1 oz	61	5	4	0	0	0	16	19
Composite of trimmed retail cuts (loin and shoulder blade), lean and fat, cooked	3 oz	214	24	11	0	0	0	48	73
Composite of trimmed retail cuts (loin and shoulder blade), lean and fat, raw	1 oz	57	6	3	0	0	0	14	18
Composite of trimmed retail cuts (loin and shoulder blade), lean only, cooked	3 oz	179	25	7	0	0	0	48	72
Composite of trimmed retail cuts (loin and shoulder blade), lean only, raw	1 oz	41	6	2	0	0	0	15	17

Description	Serving Size	Cal	Prot (g)	Fat (g)	Carbs (g)	Net Carb(g)	Fiber (g)	Sod (mg)	Chol (mg)
Chicken									
BROILERS OR FRYERS									
Back, meat and skin, fried, batter	1/2 back, bone removed	397	26	24	12	12	0	380	106
Back, meat and skin, fried, flour	1/2 back, bone removed	238	20	13	5	5	0	65	64
Back, meat and skin, raw	1/2 back, bone removed	316	14	26	0	0	0	63	78
Back, meat and skin, roasted	1/2 back, bone removed	159	14	10	0	0	0	46	47
Back, meat and skin, stewed	1 cup, chop. or diced	413	35	26	0	0	0	102	125
Back, meat only, fried	1/2 back, bone & skin rem.	167	17	8	3	3	0	57	54
Back, meat only, raw	1/2 back, bone & skin rem.	70	10	2	0	0	0	42	41
Back, meat only, roasted	1/2 back, bone & skin rem.	96	11	5	0	0	0	38	36
Back, meat only, stewed	1/2 back, bone & skin rem.	88	11	4	0	0	0	28	36
Breast, meat and skin, fried, batter	1/2 breast, bone rem.	364	35	17	13	12	0	385	119
Breast, meat and skin, fried, flour	1/2 breast, bone rem.	218	31	8	2	2	0	74	87
Breast, meat and skin, raw	1/2 breast, bone rem.	249	30	12	0	0	0	91	93
Breast, meat and skin, roasted	1 cup, chop. or diced	276	42	10	0	0	0	99	118
Breast, meat and skin, stewed	1 cup, chop. or diced	258	38	9	0	0	0	87	105
Breast, meat only, fried	1/2 breast, bone rem.	161	29	4	0	0	0	68	78
Breast, meat only, raw	1/2 breast, bone rem.	130	27	1	0	0	0	77	68
Breast, meat only, roasted	1 cup, chop. or diced	231	43	4	0	0	0	104	119
Breast, meat only, stewed	1 cup, chop. or diced	211	41	4	0	0	0	88	108
Dark meat, meat and skin, fried, batter	1/2 chicken, bone rem.	828	61	47	26	26	0	820	247
Dark meat, meat and skin, fried, flour	1/2 chicken, bone rem.	524	50	28	8	8	0	164	169

Description	Serving Size	Cal	Prot (g)	Fat (g)	Carbs (g)	Net Carb(g)	Fiber (g)	Sod (mg)	Chol (mg)
CHICKEN (continued)									
Dark meat, meat and skin, raw	1/2 chicken, bone rem.	630	44	45	0	0	0	194	215
Dark meat, meat and skin, roasted	1/2 chicken, bone rem.	423	43	23	0	0	0	145	152
Dark meat, meat and skin, stewed	1/2 chicken, bone rem.	429	43	24	0	0	0	129	151
Dark meat, meat only, fried	1 cup	335	41	14	4	4	0	136	134
Dark meat, meat only, raw	1/2 chicken, bone & skin removed	228	37	6	0	0	0	155	146
Dark meat, meat only, roasted	1 cup, chop. or diced	287	38	12	0	0	0	130	130
Dark meat, meat only, stewed	1 cup, chop. or diced	269	36	11	0	0	0	104	123
Drumstick, meat and skin, fried, batter	1 drumstick, bone rem.	193	16	10	6	6	0	194	62
Drumstick, meat and skin, fried, flour	1 drumstick, bone rem.	120	13	6	1	1	0	44	44
Drumstick, meat and skin, raw	1 drumstick, bone rem.	118	14	6	0	0	0	61	59
Drumstick, meat and skin, roasted	1 cup, chop. or diced	302	38	14	0	0	0	126	127
Drumstick, meat and skin, stewed	1 cup, chop. or diced	286	35	13	0	0	0	106	116
Drumstick, meat only, fried	1 drumstick, bone & skin removed	82	12	3	0	0	0	40	39
Drumstick, meat only, raw	1 drumstick, bone & skin removed	74	13	2	0	0	0	55	48
Drumstick, meat only, roasted	1 cup, chop. or diced	241	40	7	0	0	0	133	130
Drumstick, meat only, stewed	1 cup, chop. or diced	270	44	8	0	0	0	128	141
Giblets, fried	1 cup, chop. or diced	402	47	17	6	6	0	164	647
Giblets, raw	1 giblets	93	13	3	1	1	0	58	197
Giblets, simmered	1 cup, chop. or diced	228	37	5	1	1	0	84	570
Leg, meat and skin, fried, batter	1 leg, bone removed	431	34	23	14	13	0	441	142
Leg, meat and skin, fried, flour	1 leg, bone removed	284	30	14	3	3	0	99	105

Description	Serving Size	Cal	Prot (g)	Fat (g)	Carbs (g)	Net Carb(g)	Fiber (g)	Sod (mg)	Chol (mg)
Leg, meat and skin, raw	1 leg, bone removed	312	30	18	0	0	0	132	139
Leg, meat and skin, roasted	1 cup, chop. or diced	325	36	17	0	0	0	122	129
Leg, meat and skin, stewed	1 cup, chop. or diced	308	34	16	0	0	0	102	118
Leg, meat only, fried	1 leg, bone & skin rem.	196	27	8	1	1	0	90	93
Leg, meat only, raw	1 leg, bone & skin rem.	156	26	4	0	0	0	112	104
Leg, meat only, roasted	1 cup, chop. or diced	267	38	10	0	0	0	127	132
Leg, meat only, stewed	1 cup, chop. or diced	296	42	11	0	0	0	125	142
Light meat, meat and skin, fried, batter	1/2 chicken, bone rem.	521	44	26	18	18	0	540	158
Light meat, meat and skin, fried, flour	1/2 chicken, bone rem.	320	40	14	2	2	0	100	113
Light meat, meat and skin, raw	1/2 chicken, bone rem.	361	39	19	0	0	0	126	130
Light meat, meat and skin, roasted	1/2 chicken, bone rem.	293	38	13	0	0	0	99	111
Light meat, meat and skin, stewed	1/2 chicken, bone rem.	302	39	13	0	0	0	95	111
Light meat, meat only, fried	1 cup	269	46	7	1	1	0	113	126
Light meat, meat only, raw	1/2 chicken, bone & skin removed	168	34	2	0	0	0	100	85
Light meat, meat only, roasted	1 cup, chop. or diced	242	43	5	0	0	0	108	119
Light meat, meat only, stewed	1 cup, chop. or diced	223	40	5	0	0	0	91	108
Meat and skin, fried, batter	1/2 chicken, bone rem.	1347	105	74	44	42	1	1361	405
Meat and skin, fried, flour	1/2 chicken, bone rem.	845	90	42	10	10	0	264	283
Meat and skin, raw	1/2 chicken, bone rem.	989	86	63	0	0	0	322	345
Meat and skin, roasted	1 cup, chop. or diced	335	38	17	0	0	0	115	123
Meat and skin, stewed	1 cup, chop. or diced	307	35	16	0	0	0	94	109
Meat only, fried	1 cup, chop. or diced	307	43	11	2	2	0	127	132

Description	Serving Size	Cal	Prot (g)	Fat (g)	Carbs (g)	Net Carb(g)	Fiber (g)	Sod (mg)	Chol (mg)
CHICKEN (continued)									
Meat only, raw	1/2 chicken, bone & skin removed	392	70	8	0	0	0	253	230
Meat only, roasted	1 cup, chop. or diced	266	41	9	0	0	0	120	125
Meat only, roasted	1 tbsp	17	3	1	0	0	0	7	8
Meat only, stewed	1 cup, chop. or diced	248	38	8	0	0	0	98	116
Meat only, stewed	1 tbsp	15	2	1	0	0	0	6	7
Neck, meat and skin, cooked simmered	1 neck, bone removed	94	7	6	0	0	0	20	27
Neck, meat and skin, fried, batter	1 neck, bone removed	172	10	11	5	5	0	144	47
Neck, meat and skin, fried, flour	1 neck, bone removed	120	9	8	2	2	0	30	34
Neck, meat and skin, raw	1 neck, bone removed	149	7	12	0	0	0	32	50
Neck, meat only, fried	1 neck, bone & skin rem.	50	6	2	0	0	0	22	23
Neck, meat only, raw	1 neck, bone & skin rem.	31	4	1	0	0	0	16	17
Neck, meat only, simmered	1 neck, bone & skin rem.	32	4	1	0	0	0	12	14
Separable fat, raw	1 tbsp	81	0	8	0	0	0	4	7
Skin only, fried, batter	1/2 chicken, skin only	749	20	51	44	44	0	1104	141
Skin only, fried, flour	1/2 chicken, skin only	281	11	22	5	5	0	30	41
Skin only, raw	1/2 chicken, skin only	276	11	23	0	0	0	50	86
Skin only, roasted	1/2 chicken, skin only	254	11	21	0	0	0	36	46
Skin only, stewed	1/2 chicken, skin only	261	11	22	0	0	0	40	45
Thigh, meat and skin, fried, batter	1 thigh, bone rem.	238	19	13	8	8	0	248	80
Thigh, meat and skin, fried, flour	1 thigh, bone rem.	162	17	8	2	2	0	55	60
Thigh, meat and skin, raw	1 thigh, bone rem.	198	16	13	0	0	0	71	79
Thigh, meat and skin, roasted	1 cup, chop. or diced	346	35	19	0	0	0	118	130

Description	Serving Size	Cal	Prot (g)	Fat (g)	Carbs (g)	Net Carb(g)	Fiber (g)	Sod (mg)	Chol (mg)
Thigh, meat and skin, stewed	1 thigh, bone rem.	158	16	9	0	0	0	48	57
Thigh, meat only, fried	1 thigh, bone & skin rem.	113	15	5	1	1	0	49	53
Thigh, meat only, raw	1 thigh, bone & skin rem.	82	14	2	0	0	0	59	57
Thigh, meat only, roasted	1 cup, chop. or diced	293	36	14	0	0	0	123	133
Thigh, meat only, stewed	1 cup, chop. or diced	273	35	12	0	0	0	105	126
Wing, meat and skin, fried, batter	1 wing, bone rem.	159	10	10	5	5	0	157	39
Wing, meat and skin, fried, flour	1 wing, bone rem.	103	8	6	1	1	0	25	26
Wing, meat and skin, raw	1 wing, bone removed	109	9	7	0	0	0	36	38
Wing, meat and skin, roasted	1 cup, chop. or diced	406	38	24	0	0	0	115	118
Wing, meat and skin, stewed	1 cup, chop. or diced	349	32	21	0	0	0	94	98
Wing, meat only, fried	1 wing, bone & skin rem.	42	6	2	0	0	0	18	17
Wing, meat only, raw	1 wing, bone & skin rem.	37	6	1	0	0	0	23	17
Wing, meat only, roasted	1 wing, bone & skin rem.	43	6	1	0	0	0	19	18
Wing, meat only, stewed	1 cup, chop. or diced	253	38	8	0	0	0	102	104
CAPONS									
Giblets, raw	1 giblets	150	21	5	2	2	0	89	336
Giblets, simmered	1 cup, chop. or diced	238	38	6	1	1	0	80	629
Meat and skin and giblets and neck, raw	1 capon	4993	398	337	2	2	0	1011	1872
Meat and skin and giblets and neck, roasted	1 capon	3205	402	149	1	1	0	709	1461
Meat and skin, raw	1/2 capon, bone rem.	2256	181	153	0	0	0	434	723
Meat and skin, roasted	1/2 capon, bone rem.	1459	184	67	0	0	0	312	548
CORNISH GAME HENS									
Meat and skin, raw	1/2 bird	336	29	22	0	0	0	102	170
Meat and skin, roasted	1/2 bird	335	29	21	0	0	0	83	169

Description	Serving Size	Cal	Prot (g)	Fat (g)	Carbs (g)	Net Carb(g)	Fiber (g)	Sod (mg)	Chol (mg)
CHICKEN (continued)									
Meat only, raw	1/2 bird	139	24	3	0	0	0	82	109
Meat only, roasted	1/2 bird	147	26	3	0	0	0	69	117
Canned, meat only, with broth	1 can	234	31	10	0	0	0	714	88
Gizzard, all classes, raw	1 gizzard	44	7	1	0	0	0	28	48
Gizzard, all classes, simmered	1 cup, chop. or diced	222	39	4	2	2	0	97	281
Heart, all classes, raw	1 heart	9	1	0	0	0	0	5	8
Heart, all classes, simmered	1 cup, chop. or diced	268	38	10	0	0	0	70	351
Liver, all classes, raw	1 liver	40	6	1	1	1	0	25	140
Liver, all classes, simmered	1 cup, chop. or diced	220	34	6	1	1	0	71	883
Roasting, dark meat, meat only, raw	1/2 chicken, bone & skin removed	292	48	8	0	0	0	245	186
Roasting, dark meat, meat only, roasted	1 cup, chop. or diced	249	33	11	0	0	0	133	105
Roasting, giblets, raw	1 giblets	144	20	5	1	1	0	87	267
Roasting, giblets, simmered	1 cup, chop. or diced	239	39	6	1	1	0	87	518
Roasting, light meat, meat only, raw	1/2 chicken, bone & skin removed	240	49	3	0	0	0	112	125
Roasting, light meat, meat only, roasted	1 cup, chop. or diced	214	38	5	0	0	0	71	105
Roasting, meat and skin, raw	1/2 chicken, bone rem.	1443	114	97	0	0	0	454	488
Roasting, meat and skin, roasted	1/2 chicken, bone rem.	1070	115	58	0	0	0	350	365
Roasting, meat only, raw	1/2 chicken, bone & skin removed	529	97	10	0	0	0	358	310
Roasting, meat only, roasted	1 cup, chop. or diced	234	35	8	0	0	0	105	105
Stewing, dark meat, meat only, raw	1/2 chicken, bone & skin removed	242	30	10	0	0	0	156	119
Stewing, dark meat, meat only, stewed	1 cup, chop. or diced	361	39	18	0	0	0	133	133
Stewing, giblets, raw	1 giblets	136	14	6	2	2	0	62	194

Description	Serving Size	Cal	Prot (g)	Fat (g)	Carbs (g)	Net Carb(g)	Fiber (g)	Sod (mg)	Chol (mg)
Stewing, giblets, simmered	1 cup, chop. or diced	281	37	11	0	0	0	81	515
Stewing, light meat, meat only, raw	1/2 chicken, bone & skin removed	178	30	4	0	0	0	69	61
Stewing, light meat, meat only, stewed	1 cup, chop. or diced	298	46	9	0	0	0	81	98
Stewing, meat and skin, and giblets and neck, stewed	1 cup, chop. or diced	442	42	25	0	0	0	114	163
Stewing, meat and skin, raw	1/2 chicken, bone rem.	1027	70	73	0	0	0	283	283
Stewing, meat and skin, stewed	1/2 chicken, bone rem.	744	70	43	0	0	0	191	206
Stewing, meat only, raw	1/2 chicken, bone & skin removed	420	60	14	0	0	0	224	179
Stewing, meat only, stewed	1 cup, chop. or diced	332	43	14	0	0	0	109	116

Duck

DOMESTICATED

Description	Serving Size	Cal	Prot (g)	Fat (g)	Carbs (g)	Net Carb(g)	Fiber (g)	Sod (mg)	Chol (mg)
Liver, raw	1 liver	60	8	1	2	2	0	62	227
Meat and skin, raw	1/2 duck	2561	73	235	0	0	0	399	482
Meat and skin, roasted	1 cup, chop. or diced	472	27	37	0	0	0	83	118
Meat only, raw	1/2 duck	400	55	14	0	0	0	224	233
Meat only, roasted	1 cup, chop. or diced	281	33	13	0	0	0	91	125

WHITE PEKIN

Description	Serving Size	Cal	Prot (g)	Fat (g)	Carbs (g)	Net Carb(g)	Fiber (g)	Sod (mg)	Chol (mg)
Breast, meat and skin, boneless, roasted	3 oz	172	21	8	0	0	0	71	116
Breast, meat only, boneless, cooked without skin, broiled	1 cup, chop. or diced	244	48	3	0	0	0	183	249
Leg, meat and skin, bone in, roasted	1 leg, bone removed	200	25	10	0	0	0	101	105
Leg, meat only, bone in, cooked without skin, braised	1 cup, chop. or diced, cooked	310	51	8	0	0	0	188	183

WILD

Description	Serving Size	Cal	Prot (g)	Fat (g)	Carbs (g)	Net Carb(g)	Fiber (g)	Sod (mg)	Chol (mg)
Breast, meat only, raw	1/2 breast, bone & skin removed	102	16	3	0	0	0	47	64

Description	Serving Size	Cal	Prot (g)	Fat (g)	Carbs (g)	Net Carb(g)	Fiber (g)	Sod (mg)	Chol (mg)
DUCK (continued)									
Meat and skin, raw	1/2 duck	570	47	37	0	0	0	151	216

Goose

DOMESTICATED

Meat and skin, raw	1/2 goose	4893	209	413	0	0	0	963	1055
Meat and skin, roasted	1 cup, chop. or diced	427	35	27	0	0	0	98	127
Meat only, raw	1/2 goose	1233	174	42	0	0	0	666	643
Meat only, roasted	1/2 goose	1407	171	62	0	0	0	449	567
Liver, raw	1 liver	125	15	3	6	6	0	132	484
Pate de foie gras, canned (goose liver pate), smoked	1 tbsp	60	1	5	1	1	0	91	20
Pate de foie gras, canned (goose liver pate), smoked	1 oz	131	3	12	1	1	0	198	43

Guinea Hen

Meat and skin, raw	1/2 guinea	545	81	19	0	0	0	231	255
Meat only, raw	1/2 guinea	290	54	5	0	0	0	182	166

Pheasant

Breast, meat only, raw	1/2 breast, bone & skin removed	242	44	5	0	0	0	60	106
Leg, meat only, raw	1 leg, bone & skin rem.	143	24	4	0	0	0	48	86
Meat and skin, raw	1/2 pheasant	724	91	33	0	0	0	160	284
Meat only, raw	1/2 pheasant	468	83	11	0	0	0	130	232

Quail

Breast, meat only, raw	1 breast	69	13	1	0	0	0	31	32
Meat and skin, raw	1 quail	209	21	11	0	0	0	58	83
Meat only, raw	1 quail	123	20	3	0	0	0	47	64

Squab (pigeon)

Light meat without skin, raw	1 breast, bone rem.	135	22	4	0	0	0	56	91
Meat and skin, raw	1 unit	873	55	63	0	0	0	160	282
Meat only, raw	1 unit	356	44	16	0	0	0	128	226

Turkey

ALL CLASSES

Description	Serving Size	Cal	Prot (g)	Fat (g)	Carbs (g)	Net Carb(g)	Fiber (g)	Sod (mg)	Chol (mg)
Back, meat and skin, raw	1/2 back, bone rem.	708	65	43	0	0	0	238	267
Back, meat and skin, roasted	1 cup, chop. or diced	340	37	18	0	0	0	102	127
Back, meat and skin, roasted	1/2 back, bone rem.	637	70	34	0	0	0	191	238
Breast, meat and skin, raw	1/2 breast, bone rem.	1777	248	71	0	0	0	668	736
Breast, meat and skin, roasted	1/2 breast, bone rem.	1633	248	55	0	0	0	544	639
Dark meat, meat and skin, raw	1/2 turkey, bone rem.	1882	222	92	0	0	0	835	847
Dark meat, meat and skin, roasted	1 cup, chop. or diced	309	38	14	0	0	0	106	125
Dark meat, raw	1/2 turkey, bone & skin removed	1271	204	38	0	0	0	783	702
Dark meat, roasted	1 cup, chop. or diced	262	40	9	0	0	0	111	119
Giblets, raw	1 giblets	315	47	8	5	5	0	212	688
Giblets, simmered, some giblet fat	1 cup, chop. or diced	242	39	6	3	3	0	86	606
Leg, meat and skin, raw	1 leg, bone removed	1175	159	49	0	0	0	604	579
Leg, meat and skin, roasted	1 leg, bone removed	1136	152	47	0	0	0	420	464
Light meat, meat and skin, raw	1/2 turkey, bone rem.	2207	300	91	0	0	0	819	902
Light meat, meat and skin, roasted	1 cup, chop. or diced	276	40	10	0	0	0	88	106
Light meat, raw	1/2 turkey, bone & skin removed	1329	272	14	0	0	0	728	694
Light meat, roasted	1 cup, chop. or diced	220	42	3	0	0	0	90	97
Meat and skin and giblets and neck, raw	1 turkey	8720	1131	383	4	4	0	3721	4332
Meat and skin and giblets and neck, roasted	1 turkey	8247	1126	331	3	3	0	2695	3822
Meat and skin, raw	1/2 turkey, bone rem.	4104	524	183	0	0	0	1667	1744

Description	Serving Size	Cal	Prot (g)	Fat (g)	Carbs (g)	Net Carb(g)	Fiber (g)	Sod (mg)	Chol (mg)
TURKEY (continued)									
Meat and skin, roasted	1 cup, chop. or diced	291	39	12	0	0	0	95	115
Meat only, raw	1/2 turkey, bone & skin removed	2587	473	52	0	0	0	1522	1413
Meat only, roasted	1 cup, chop. or diced	238	41	6	0	0	0	98	106
Neck, meat only, raw	1 neck, bone & skin rem.	243	36	8	0	0	0	167	142
Neck, meat only, simmered	1 neck, bone & skin rem.	274	41	10	0	0	0	85	185
Skin only, raw	1/2 turkey, skin only	1517	50	133	0	0	0	141	357
Skin only, roasted	1/2 turkey, skin only	1096	49	90	0	0	0	131	280
Wing, meat and skin, raw	1 wing, bone removed	504	52	28	0	0	0	141	179
Wing, meat and skin, roasted	1 wing, bone removed	426	51	20	0	0	0	113	151
FRYER-ROASTERS									
Back, meat and skin, raw	1/2 back, bone rem.	276	36	12	0	0	0	110	157
Back, meat and skin, roasted	1/2 back, bone rem.	265	34	12	0	0	0	91	140
Back, meat only, raw	1/2 back, bone & skin removed	180	31	5	0	0	0	98	111
Back, meat only, roasted	1/2 back, bone & skin removed	168	28	5	0	0	0	72	94
Breast, meat and skin, raw	1/2 breast, bone rem.	541	103	10	0	0	0	208	303
Breast, meat and skin, roasted	1/2 breast, bone rem.	526	100	10	0	0	0	182	310
Breast, meat only, raw	1/2 breast, bone & skin removed	433	96	2	0	0	0	191	242
Breast, meat only, roasted	1/2 breast, bone & skin removed	413	92	2	0	0	0	159	254
Dark meat, meat and skin, raw	1/2 turkey, bone rem.	686	107	23	0	0	0	351	463

Description	Serving Size	Cal	Prot (g)	Fat (g)	Carbs (g)	Net Carb(g)	Fiber (g)	Sod (mg)	Chol (mg)
Dark meat, meat and skin, roasted	1/2 turkey, bone rem.	681	104	23	0	0	0	284	438
Dark meat, meat only, raw	1/2 turkey, bone & skin removed	532	98	11	0	0	0	331	388
Dark meat, meat only, roasted	1 cup, chop. or diced	227	40	5	0	0	0	111	157
Leg, meat and skin, raw	1 leg, bone removed	412	70	11	0	0	0	241	304
Leg, meat and skin, roasted	1 leg, bone removed	417	70	12	0	0	0	196	172
Leg, meat only, raw	1 leg, bone & skin rem.	355	67	7	0	0	0	234	276
Leg, meat only, roasted	1 leg, bone & skin rem.	356	65	7	0	0	0	181	267
Light meat, meat and skin, raw	1/2 turkey, bone rem.	746	130	19	0	0	0	281	426
Light meat, meat and skin, roasted	1/2 turkey, bone rem.	710	125	17	0	0	0	247	411
Light meat, meat only, raw	1/2 turkey, bone & skin removed	519	116	2	0	0	0	250	317
Light meat, meat only, roasted	1 cup, chop. or diced	196	42	1	0	0	0	78	120
Meat and skin and giblets and neck, raw	1 turkey	3205	534	91	1	1	0	1470	2217
Meat and skin and giblets and neck, roasted	1 turkey	3030	498	88	1	1	0	1152	2091
Meat and skin, raw	1/2 turkey, bone rem.	1465	245	41	0	0	0	634	885
Meat and skin, roasted	1/2 turkey, bone rem.	1390	228	41	0	0	0	533	848
Meat only, raw	1/2 turkey, bone & skin removed	1089	221	13	0	0	0	604	723
Meat only, roasted	1 cup, chop. or diced	210	41	3	0	0	0	94	137
Skin only, raw	1/2 turkey, skin only	376	22	29	0	0	0	47	185
Skin only, roasted	1/2 turkey, skin only	362	25	26	0	0	0	74	174
Wing, meat and skin, raw	1 wing, bone rem.	204	27	9	0	0	0	72	125
Wing, meat and skin, roasted	1 wing, bone rem.	186	25	8	0	0	0	66	104

Description	Serving Size	Cal	Prot (g)	Fat (g)	Carbs (g)	Net Carb(g)	Fiber (g)	Sod (mg)	Chol (mg)
TURKEY (continued)									
Wing, meat only, raw	1 wing, bone & skin rem.	95	20	1	0	0	0	59	73
Wing, meat only, roasted	1 wing, bone & skin rem.	98	19	2	0	0	0	47	61
YOUNG HEN									
Back, meat and skin, raw	1/2 back, bone rem.	650	52	43	0	0	0	182	203
Back, meat and skin, roasted	1/2 back, bone rem.	551	57	30	0	0	0	150	184
Breast, meat and skin, raw	1/2 breast, bone rem.	1460	189	65	0	0	0	481	542
Breast, meat and skin, roasted	1/2 breast, bone rem.	1331	198	46	0	0	0	398	494
Dark meat, meat and skin, raw	1/2 turkey, bone & skin removed	1639	178	87	0	0	0	639	619
Dark meat, meat and skin, roasted	1/2 turkey, bone & skin removed	1543	182	75	0	0	0	479	559
Dark meat, meat only, raw	1/2 turkey, bone & skin removed	1056	163	34	0	0	0	601	503
Dark meat, meat only, roasted	1 cup, chop. or diced	269	40	9	0	0	0	105	112
Leg, meat and skin, raw	1 leg, bone removed	991	128	43	0	0	0	459	413
Leg, meat and skin, roasted	1 leg, bone removed	954	124	41	0	0	0	327	367
Light meat, meat and skin, raw	1/2 turkey, bone rem.	1813	236	79	0	0	0	604	681
Light meat, meat and skin, roasted	1/2 turkey, bone rem.	1778	246	69	0	0	0	498	636
Light meat, meat only, raw	1/2 turkey, bone & skin removed	1066	217	12	0	0	0	551	533
Light meat, meat only, roasted	1 cup, chop. or diced	225	42	4	0	0	0	84	95
Meat and skin and giblets and neck, raw	1 turkey	7399	898	348	5	5	0	2808	3254
Meat and skin and giblets and neck, roasted	1 turkey	7095	924	303	2	2	0	2079	3102
Meat and skin, raw	1/2 turkey, bone rem.	3447	414	166	0	0	0	1252	1293

Description	Serving Size	Cal	Prot (g)	Fat (g)	Carbs (g)	Net Carb(g)	Fiber (g)	Sod (mg)	Chol (mg)
Meat and skin, roasted	1/2 turkey, bone rem.	3322	428	145	0	0	0	975	1189
Meat only, raw	1/2 turkey, bone & skin removed	2112	377	46	0	0	0	1142	1039
Meat only, roasted	1 cup, chop. or diced	245	41	6	0	0	0	94	102
Skin only, raw	1/2 turkey, skin only	1339	38	119	0	0	0	103	260
Skin only, roasted	1/2 turkey, skin only	945	37	80	0	0	0	86	208
Wing, meat and skin, raw	1 wing, bone rem.	470	45	28	0	0	0	114	146
Wing, meat and skin, roasted	1 wing, bone rem.	414	48	21	0	0	0	97	134
YOUNG TOM									
Back, meat and skin, raw	1/2 back, bone rem.	938	97	53	0	0	0	372	414
Back, meat and skin, roasted	1/2 back, bone rem.	904	102	46	0	0	0	293	357
Breast, meat and skin, raw	1/2 breast, bone rem.	2701	393	100	0	0	0	1127	1199
Breast, meat and skin, roasted	1/2 breast, bone rem.	2512	380	85	0	0	0	890	997
Dark meat, meat and skin, raw	1/2 turkey, bone rem.	2672	335	124	0	0	0	1319	1354
Dark meat, meat and skin, roasted	1/2 turkey, bone rem.	2557	327	114	0	0	0	947	1077
Dark meat, meat only, raw	1/2 turkey, bone & skin removed	1884	307	54	0	0	0	1226	1149
Dark meat, meat only, roasted	1 cup, chop. or diced	259	40	8	0	0	0	115	123
Leg, meat and skin, raw	1 leg, bone removed	1740	241	69	0	0	0	950	938
Leg, meat and skin, roasted	1 leg, bone removed	1658	225	68	0	0	0	644	725
Light meat, meat and skin, raw	1/2 turkey, bone rem.	3334	462	134	0	0	0	1346	1432
Light meat, meat and skin, roasted	1/2 turkey, bone rem.	2991	446	104	0	0	0	1049	1175
Light meat, meat only, raw	1/2 turkey, bone & skin removed	2019	415	21	0	0	0	1187	1098

Description	Serving Size	Cal	Prot (g)	Fat (g)	Carbs (g)	Net Carb(g)	Fiber (g)	Sod (mg)	Chol (mg)
TURKEY (continued)									
Light meat, meat only, roasted	1 cup, chop. or diced	216	42	3	0	0	0	95	97
Meat and skin and giblets and neck, raw	1 turkey	12766	1713	537	7	7	0	5879	6803
Meat and skin and giblets and neck, roasted	1 turkey	11854	1666	459	6	6	0	4289	5719
Meat and skin, raw	1/2 turkey, bone rem.	5998	797	258	0	0	0	2649	2804
Meat and skin, roasted	1/2 turkey, bone rem.	5555	772	218	0	0	0	1980	2255
Meat only, raw	1/2 turkey, bone & skin removed	3863	717	74	0	0	0	2410	2245
Meat only, roasted	1 cup, chop. or diced	235	41	5	0	0	0	104	108
Skin only, raw	1/2 turkey, skin only	2179	78	187	0	0	0	237	562
Skin only, roasted	1/2 turkey, skin only	1578	75	128	0	0	0	224	438
Wing, meat and skin, raw	1 wing, bone rem.	654	71	35	0	0	0	209	251
Wing, meat and skin, roasted	1 wing, bone rem.	524	65	24	0	0	0	156	192
Breast, pre-basted, meat and skin, roasted	1/2 breast, bone rem.	1089	191	26	0	0	0	3430	363
Canned, meat only, with broth	1 cup	220	32	8	0	0	0	630	89
Canned, meat only, with broth	1 can	231	34	9	0	0	0	663	94
Diced, light and dark meat, seasoned	1 oz	39	5	1	0	0	0	241	16
Diced, light and dark meat, seasoned	1/2 lb	313	42	12	2	2	0	1930	125
Gizzard, all classes, raw	1 gizzard	132	22	3	1	1	0	90	179
Gizzard, all classes, simmered	1 cup, chop. or diced	236	43	4	1	1	0	78	336
Ground turkey, cooked	1 patty	193	22	9	0	0	0	88	84
Ground turkey, raw	1 patty	170	20	8	0	0	0	107	90
Heart, all classes, raw	1 heart	41	5	2	0	0	0	25	33
Heart, all classes, simmered	1 cup, chop. or diced	257	39	7	3	3	0	80	328
Liver, all classes, raw	1 liver	140	20	3	4	4	0	98	475
Liver, all classes, simmered	1 cup, chop. or diced	237	34	6	5	5	0	90	876

Description	Serving Size	Cal	Prot (g)	Fat (g)	Carbs (g)	Net Carb(g)	Fiber (g)	Sod (mg)	Chol (mg)
Patties, breaded, battered, fried	1 med. slice	79	4	5	4	4	0	224	17
Patties, breaded, battered, fried	1 thick slice	119	6	7	7	6	0	336	26
Roast, boneless, frozen, seasoned, light and dark meat, raw	1/4 box	341	50	5	18	18	0	1926	151
Roast, boneless, frozen, seasoned, light and dark meat, roasted	1 cup, chop. or diced	209	29	6	4	4	0	918	72
Roast, boneless, frozen, seasoned, light and dark meat, roasted	1 box	1212	167	37	24	24	0	5318	414
Thigh, pre-basted, meat and skin, roasted	1 thigh, bone rem.	493	59	24	0	0	0	1372	195
Turkey sticks, breaded, battered, fried	1 stick	179	9	10	11	11	0	536	41
USDA commodity, turkey ham, dark meat, smoked, frozen	1 oz	33	5	1	1	1	0	258	18
USDA commodity, turkey ham, dark meat, smoked, frozen	1 serving	33	5	1	1	1	0	258	18

Description	Serving Size	Cal	Prot (g)	Fat (g)	Carbs (g)	Net Carb(g)	Fiber (g)	Sod (mg)	Chol (mg)
Custard									
Egg custards, dry mix	1 portion	86	1	1	17	82	0	102	53
Egg custards, dry mix, prepared with 2% milk	1/2 cup	149	6	3	24	18	0	200	74
Egg custards, dry mix, prepared with whole milk	1/2 cup	162	5	5	23	18	0	198	81
Flan									
Flan, caramel custard, dry mix	1 portion	73	0	0	19	92	0	91	0
Flan, caramel custard, dry mix, prepared with 2% milk	1/2 cup	136	4	2	26	19	0	67	9
Flan, caramel custard, dry mix, prepared with whole milk	1/2 cup	150	4	4	25	19	0	65	16
Mousse									
ALSA Mousse Mix, powder, dark chocolate	1/2 tbsp	105	2	4	13	NA	NA	83	0
Pudding									
JELL-O BRAND									
Fat Free Cook & Serve Reduced Calorie Pudding & Pie Filling Chocolate, regular, powder	1 serving	90	0	0	23	90	0	107	0
Fat Free Cook & Serve Reduced Calorie Pudding & Pie Filling Vanilla, regular, powder	1 serving	86	0	0	22	94	0	138	0
Fat Free Pudding Snacks Chocolate, ready-to-eat	1 serving	102	3	0	23	19	1	192	2
Fat Free Pudding Snacks Vanilla, ready-to-eat	1 serving	104	2	0	23	20	1	241	2
Fat Free Sugar Free Instant Reduced Calorie Pudding & Pie Filling Chocolate, with aspartame and acesulfame potassium sweetener, powder	1 serving	34	1	0	8	67	1	318	0
Fat Free Sugar Free Instant Reduced Calorie Pudding & Pie Filling Vanilla, with aspartame and acesulfame potassium sweetener, powder	1 serving	26	0	0	6	77	0	332	0
Instant Pudding & Pie Filling Chocolate, powder	1 serving	99	0	0	25	88	1	414	0
Instant Pudding & Pie Filling Vanilla, powder	1 serving	94	0	0	23	93	0	353	0

Description	Serving Size	Cal	Prot (g)	Fat (g)	Carbs (g)	Net Carb(g)	Fiber (g)	Sod (mg)	Chol (mg)
PUDDING (continued)									
Sugar Free Cook & Serve Reduced Calorie Pudding & Pie Filling Chocolate, regular, with aspartame and acesulfame potassium sweetener, powder	1 serving	31	1	0	7	65	1	109	0
Sugar Free Cook & Serve Reduced Calorie Pudding & Pie Filling Vanilla, regular, with aspartame and acesulfame potassium sweetener, powder	1 serving	21	0	0	5	81	0	113	0
GENERIC PUDDINGS									
Banana, dry mix, instant	1 portion	92	0	0	23	93	0	375	0
Banana, dry mix, instant, prepared with 2% milk	1/2 cup	153	4	2	29	20	0	435	9
Banana, dry mix, instant, prepared with whole milk	1/2 cup	166	4	4	29	20	0	434	16
Banana, dry mix, instant, with added oil	1 portion	97	0	1	22	89	0	375	0
Banana, dry mix, regular	1 portion	83	0	0	20	93	0	173	0
Banana, dry mix, regular, prepared with 2% milk	1/2 cup	143	4	2	25	18	0	232	10
Banana, dry mix, regular, prepared with whole milk	1/2 cup	157	4	4	25	18	0	231	17
Banana, dry mix, regular, with added oil	1 package	341	0	4	78	88	0	693	0
Banana, ready-to-eat	1 oz	36	1	1	6	21	0	56	0
Chocolate, dry mix, instant	1 portion	89	1	0	22	85	1	357	0
Chocolate, dry mix, instant, prepared with 2% milk	1/2 cup	150	5	3	28	19	1	417	9
Chocolate, dry mix, regular	1 portion	90	1	0	22	87	0	88	0
Chocolate, dry mix, regular, prepared with 2% milk	1/2 cup	151	5	3	28	19	0	149	10
Chocolate, dry mix, regular, prepared with whole milk	1/2 cup	158	5	5	26	17	1	146	17
Chocolate, ready-to-eat	1 can	189	4	5	32	22	1	183	4
Coconut cream, dry mix, instant	1 portion	97	0	1	22	89	0	302	0
Coconut cream, dry mix, instant, prepared with 2% milk	1/2 cup	157	4	3	28	19	0	362	9
Coconut cream, dry mix, instant, prepared with whole milk	1/2 cup	172	4	5	28	19	0	362	16
Coconut cream, dry mix, regular	1 portion	98	0	1	22	86	0	260	0
Coconut cream, dry mix, regular, prepared with 2% milk	1/2 cup	146	4	3	25	18	0	228	10

Description	Serving Size	Cal	Prot (g)	Fat (g)	Carbs (g)	Net Carb(g)	Fiber (g)	Sod (mg)	Chol (mg)
Coconut cream, dry mix, regular, prepared with whole milk	1/2 cup	160	4	5	25	18	0	227	17
Lemon, dry mix, instant	1 portion	95	0	0	24	95	0	333	0
Lemon, dry mix, instant, prepared with 2% milk	1/2 cup	154	4	2	30	20	0	394	9
Lemon, dry mix, instant, prepared with whole milk	1/2 cup	169	4	4	30	20	0	392	16
Lemon, dry mix, regular	1 portion	77	0	0	19	92	0	107	0
Lemon, dry mix, regular, prepared with sugar, egg yolk and water	1/2 cup	164	1	2	36	25	0	93	77
Lemon, ready-to-eat	1 can	178	0	4	36	25	0	199	0
Rice, dry mix	1 portion	102	1	0	25	91	0	99	0
Rice, dry mix, prepared with 2% milk	1/2 cup	161	5	2	30	21	0	158	9
Rice, dry mix, prepared with whole milk	1/2 cup	176	5	4	30	21	0	157	16
Rice, ready-to-eat	1 can	231	3	10	31	22	0	121	1
Tapioca, dry mix	1 portion	85	0	0	22	94	0	110	0
Tapioca, dry mix, prepared with 2% milk	1/2 cup	147	4	2	28	20	0	172	8
Tapioca, dry mix, prepared with whole milk	1/2 cup	161	4	4	28	20	0	171	17
Tapioca, dry mix, with no added salt	1 portion	85	0	0	22	94	0	2	0
Tapioca, ready-to-eat	1 can	169	3	5	28	20	0	226	1
Vanilla, dry mix, instant	1 portion	92	0	0	23	93	0	360	0
Vanilla, dry mix, regular	1 portion	81	0	0	21	93	0	166	0
Vanilla, dry mix, regular, prepared with 2% milk	1/2 cup	141	4	2	26	19	0	224	10
Vanilla, dry mix, regular, prepared with whole milk	1/2 cup	155	4	4	26	19	0	224	17
Vanilla, dry mix, regular, with added oil	1 portion	81	0	0	20	92	0	166	0
Vanilla, ready-to-eat	1 snack size	147	3	4	25	22	0	153	8

Rennin

Description	Serving Size	Cal	Prot (g)	Fat (g)	Carbs (g)	Net Carb(g)	Fiber (g)	Sod (mg)	Chol (mg)
Chocolate, dry mix	1 tbsp	33	0	0	8	86	0	6	0
Tablets, unsweetened	1 package	8	0	0	2	20	0	2579	0
Vanilla, dry mix	1 tbsp	41	0	0	11	99	0	1	0

Description	Serving Size	Cal	Prot (g)	Fat (g)	Carbs (g)	Net Carb(g)	Fiber (g)	Sod (mg)	Chol (mg)
Beerwurst									
Beer salami, pork	1 slice	55	3	4	0	0	0	285	14
Beer salami, pork and beef	1 slice	76	3	6	0	0	0	236	14
Bockwurst									
Pork, Raw	1 oz	87	4	7	0	0	0	313	17
Pork, Raw	1 link	200	9	17	0	0	0	718	38
Bologna									
Beef	1 slice	88	3	8	0	0	0	278	16
Beef and pork	1 slice	90	3	8	1	1	0	289	16
Pork	1 slice	70	4	5	0	0	0	336	17
Turkey	1 oz	56	4	4	0	0	0	249	28
Turkey	2 slices	113	8	8	1	1	0	498	56
Bratwurst									
Pork, beef, link	1 oz	92	4	7	1	1	0	315	18
Pork, beef, link	1 link	226	10	18	2	2	0	778	44
Pork, cooked	1 oz	85	4	7	1	1	0	158	17
Pork, cooked	1 link	256	12	21	2	2	0	473	51
CARL BUDDIG									
Cooked Corned Beef, Chopped, Pressed	2 oz	81	11	2	1	1	0	761	37
Cooked Smoked Beef Pastrami, Chopped, Pressed	2 oz	80	11	2	1	1	0	599	37
Smoked Sliced Beef	2 oz	79	11	2	0	0	0	811	38
Smoked Sliced Chicken, light and dark meat	2 oz	94	10	3	0	0	0	541	30
Smoked Sliced Ham	2 oz	92	10	2	1	1	0	783	31
Smoked Sliced Turkey, light and dark meat	2 oz	91	10	3	1	1	0	621	32
HORMEL									
Pillow Pak Sliced Turkey Pepperoni	1 serving	74	9	3	1	1	0	557	37
SPAM, Lite Luncheon Meat, Pork and chicken	1 oz	54	4	4	0	0	0	289	21
SPAM, Lite Luncheon Meat, Pork and chicken	1 serving	108	9	7	1	1	0	578	42
SPAM, Luncheon Meat, pork with ham	1 oz	86	4	8	0	0	0	395	19
SPAM, Luncheon Meat, pork with ham	1 serving	172	7	15	1	1	0	789	39
WRANGLER Beef Franks	1 frankfurter	162	7	14	1	NA	NA	557	38

Description	Serving Size	Cal	Prot (g)	Fat (g)	Carbs (g)	Net Carb(g)	Fiber (g)	Sod (mg)	Chol (mg)
HORMEL (continued)									
WRANGLER Beef Franks	4 oz	325	14	27	2	NA	NA	1113	75

LOUIS RICH

Description	Serving Size	Cal	Prot (g)	Fat (g)	Carbs (g)	Net Carb(g)	Fiber (g)	Sod (mg)	Chol (mg)
Chicken (white, oven roasted)	1 serving	36	5	1	1	1	0	335	17
Chicken Breast (oven roasted deluxe)	1 serving	28	5	0	1	1	0	333	14
Chicken Breast Classic Baked /Grill (carving board)	1 serving	44	9	0	2	2	0	514	23
Chicken Breast Classic Baked /Grill (carving board)	1 slice	22	4	0	1	1	0	251	11
Franks (turkey and chicken cheese)	1 serving	90	6	6	2	2	0	482	42
Franks (turkey and chicken)	1 serving	85	5	6	2	2	0	511	41
Turkey (honey roasted, fat free)	1 serving	57	11	0	3	3	0	661	22
Turkey Bacon	1 serving	34	2	2	0	0	0	184	12
Turkey Bologna	1 serving	52	3	4	1	1	0	270	19
Turkey Breast (oven roasted fat free)	1 serving	24	4	0	1	1	0	334	9
Turkey Breast (oven roasted, portion fat free)	1 serving	50	11	0	1	1	0	659	22
Turkey Breast (Smoked, Carving Board)	1 serving	42	9	0	1	1	0	540	19
Turkey Breast (Smoked, Carving Board)	1 slice	21	4	0	0	1	0	264	9
Turkey Breast (smoked, portion fat free)	1 serving	52	11	0	1	1	0	721	23
Turkey Breast and White Turkey (oven roasted)	1 serving	27	5	0	1	1	0	309	11
Turkey Breast and White Turkey (smoked sliced)	1 serving	28	5	1	1	1	0	257	12
Turkey Ham (10% water added)	1 serving	32	5	1	0	0	0	316	19
Turkey Nuggets/Sticks (breaded)	1 serving	235	12	15	13	13	0	577	34
Turkey Salami	1 serving	41	4	2	0	0	0	281	21
Turkey Salami Cotto	1 serving	42	4	3	0	0	0	285	22
Turkey Smoked Sausage	1 serving	90	8	5	2	2	0	515	36

OSCAR MAYER

Description	Serving Size	Cal	Prot (g)	Fat (g)	Carbs (g)	Net Carb(g)	Fiber (g)	Sod (mg)	Chol (mg)
Bologna (beef light)	1 serving	55	3	4	2	2	0	314	13
Bologna (beef)	1 serving	89	3	8	1	1	0	310	20
Bologna (chicken, pork, beef)	1 serving	89	3	8	1	1	0	289	29
Bologna (fat free)	1 serving	22	4	0	2	2	0	274	7
Bologna (Wisconsin made ring)	1 serving	175	7	15	1	1	0	463	35
Bologna Light (pork, chicken, beef)	1 serving	56	3	4	2	2	0	312	15
Braunschweiger Liver Sausage (saren tube)	1 serving	191	8	17	1	1	0	626	90

Description	Serving Size	Cal	Prot (g)	Fat (g)	Carbs (g)	Net Carb(g)	Fiber (g)	Sod (mg)	Chol (mg)
Braunschweiger Liver Sausage (sliced)	1 serving	94	4	8	1	1	0	324	49
Chicken Breast (honey glazed)	1 slice	14	3	0	1	1	0	180	7
Chicken Breast (oven roasted, fat free)	1 slice	11	2	0	0	0	0	161	6
Ham (40% ham/water product, smoked, fat free)	1 slice	12	2	0	0	0	0	173	6
Ham (chopped with natural juice)	1 serving	52	5	3	1	1	0	327	0
Ham (water added, baked cooked 96% fat free)	1 slice	22	3	1	0	0	0	255	10
Ham (water added, boiled)	1 slice	22	3	1	0	0	0	283	10
Ham (water added, honey)	1 slice	23	4	1	1	1	0	262	9
Ham (water added, smoked, cooked)	1 slice	21	3	1	0	0	0	255	10
Ham and Cheese Loaf	1 serving	64	4	5	1	1	0	351	18
Head Cheese	1 serving	52	4	4	0	0	0	300	25
Honey Loaf	1 serving	33	5	1	1	1	0	378	15
Liver Cheese, pork fat wrapped	1 serving	114	6	10	1	1	0	419	80
Luncheon Loaf (spiced)	1 serving	66	4	4	2	2	0	343	19
Old Fashioned Loaf	1 serving	65	4	5	2	2	0	332	17
Olive Loaf (chicken, pork, turkey)	1 serving	74	3	6	2	2	0	369	20
Pickle Pimiento Loaf (with chicken)	1 serving	75	3	6	3	3	0	357	22
Pork Sausage Links (cooked)	1 link	82	4	7	0	0	0	201	18
Salami (for beer)	1 slice	52	3	4	0	0	0	283	16
Salami (Genoa)	1 slice	35	2	3	0	0	0	164	9
Salami (hard)	1 slice	36	2	3	0	0	0	169	9
Salami Beef Cotto	1 slice	47	3	3	0	0	0	301	19
Salami Cotto (beef, pork, chicken)	1 slice	56	3	5	1	1	0	252	18
Sandwich Spread (pork, chicken, beef)	1 serving	71	2	5	5	5	0	246	14
Smokie Links Sausage	1 serving	130	5	11	1	1	0	433	27
Smokies (beef)	1 serving	128	5	11	1	1	0	425	28
Smokies (cheese)	1 serving	130	6	11	1	1	0	450	30
Smokies Sausage Little (pork, turkey)	1 link	27	1	2	0	0	0	92	6
Smokies Sausage Little Cheese (pork, turkey)	1 link	28	1	2	0	0	0	93	6
Summer Sausage Beef Thuringer Cervelat	1 slice	71	3	6	0	0	0	328	18
Summer Sausage Thuringer Cervalat	1 slice	70	3	6	0	0	0	329	19
Turkey Breast (smoked, fat free)	1 slice	10	2	0	0	0	0	142	4
Wieners (beef franks)	1 serving	143	5	13	1	1	0	458	29
Wieners (beef franks, bun length)	1 serving	184	6	16	2	2	0	576	32

Description	Serving Size	Cal	Prot (g)	Fat (g)	Carbs (g)	Net Carb(g)	Fiber (g)	Sod (mg)	Chol (mg)
OSCAR MAYER (continued)									
Wieners (beef franks, fat free)	1 serving	39	7	0	3	3	0	464	15
Wieners (beef franks, light)	1 serving	110	6	8	2	2	0	615	28
Wieners (cheese hot dogs with turkey)	1 serving	143	5	12	1	1	0	514	33
Wieners (fat free hot dogs)	1 serving	37	6	0	2	2	0	487	15
Wieners (light pork, turkey, beef)	1 serving	111	7	8	2	2	0	591	35
Wieners (pork, turkey)	1 serving	145	5	12	1	1	0	435	32
Wieners Little (pork, turkey)	1 serving	177	6	16	1	1	0	592	31
Barbecue loaf, pork, beef	1 oz	49	4	2	2	2	0	378	10
Barbecue loaf, pork, beef	1 slice	40	4	2	1	1	0	307	9
Blood sausage	1 oz	107	4	9	0	0	0	193	34
Blood sausage	1 slice	95	4	8	0	0	0	170	30
Braunschweiger (a liver sausage), pork	1 oz	102	4	8	1	1	0	324	44
Braunschweiger (a liver sausage), pork	1 slice	65	2	5	1	1	0	206	28
Cheesefurter, cheese smokie, pork, beef	1 oz	93	4	8	0	0	0	307	19
Cheesefurter, cheese smokie, pork, beef	1 cheesefurter	141	6	12	1	1	0	465	29
Chicken roll, light meat	2 slices	90	11	4	1	1	0	331	28
Chicken spread	1 tbsp	25	2	1	1	1	0	50	7
Chicken spread	1 oz	54	4	3	2	2	0	109	15
Chorizo, pork and beef	1 oz	129	7	10	1	1	0	350	25
Chorizo, pork and beef	1 link	273	14	22	1	1	0	741	53
Corned beef loaf, jellied	1 slice	43	6	2	0	0	0	270	13
Dutch brand loaf, chicken, pork and beef	1 slice	68	4	5	2	2	0	354	13
Frankfurter, beef	1 frankfurter	142	5	12	1	1	0	462	27
Frankfurter, beef and pork	1 frankfurter	144	5	12	1	1	0	504	23
Frankfurter, chicken	1 oz	73	4	5	2	2	0	388	29
Frankfurter, chicken	1 frankfurter	116	6	8	3	3	0	617	45
Frankfurter, turkey	1 oz	64	4	5	0	0	0	404	30
Frankfurter, turkey	1 frankfurter	102	6	7	1	1	0	642	48
Ham and cheese loaf or roll	1 slice	73	5	5	0	0	0	381	16
Ham and cheese spread	1 tbsp	37	2	3	0	0	0	180	9
Ham and cheese spread	1 oz	69	5	5	1	1	0	339	17
Ham salad spread	1 tbsp	32	1	2	2	2	0	137	6
Ham salad spread	1 oz	61	2	4	3	3	0	259	10
Ham, chopped, canned	1 oz	68	5	5	0	0	0	387	14

Description	Serving Size	Cal	Prot (g)	Fat (g)	Carbs (g)	Net Carb(g)	Fiber (g)	Sod (mg)	Chol (mg)
Ham, chopped, canned	1 slice	50	3	4	0	0	0	287	10
Ham, chopped, not canned	1 slice	65	5	5	0	0	0	389	14
Ham, minced	1 oz	75	5	5	1	1	0	353	20
Ham, minced	1 slice	55	3	4	0	0	0	261	15
Ham, sliced, extra lean	1 cup, diced	177	26	6	1	1	0	1929	63
Ham, sliced, extra lean	1 slice	37	5	1	0	0	0	405	13
Ham, sliced, regular (approximately 11% fat)	1 cup, diced	246	24	13	4	4	0	1778	77
Ham, sliced, regular (approximately 11% fat)	1 slice	52	5	3	1	1	0	373	16
Headcheese, pork	1 slice	60	5	4	0	0	0	356	23
Honey loaf, pork, beef	1 slice	36	4	1	2	2	0	374	10
Honey roll sausage, beef	1 oz	52	5	3	1	1	0	375	14
Honey roll sausage, beef	1 slice	42	4	2	1	1	0	304	12
Kielbasa, Kolbassy, pork, beef, nonfat dry milk added	1 oz	88	4	7	1	1	0	305	19
Kielbasa, Kolbassy, pork, beef, nonfat dry milk added	1 slice	81	3	7	1	1	0	280	17
Knackwurst, knockwurst, pork, beef	1 oz	87	3	7	0	0	0	286	16
Knackwurst, knockwurst, pork, beef	1 link	209	8	18	1	1	0	687	39
Lebanon bologna, beef	1 oz	60	5	4	1	1	0	379	20
Lebanon bologna, beef	1 slice	49	4	3	1	1	0	308	16
Liver cheese, pork	1 oz	86	4	7	1	1	0	347	49
Liver cheese, pork	1 slice	116	6	9	1	1	0	466	66
Liver sausage, liverwurst, pork	1 oz	92	4	8	1	1	0	244	45
Liver sausage, liverwurst, pork	1 slice	59	3	5	0	0	0	155	28
Luncheon meat, beef, loaved	1 slice	87	4	7	1	1	0	377	18
Luncheon meat, beef, thin sliced	1 oz	50	8	1	2	2	0	408	12
Luncheon meat, beef, thin sliced	5 slices	37	6	1	1	1	0	302	9
Luncheon meat, pork, beef	1 slice	100	4	9	1	1	0	367	16
Luncheon meat, pork, canned	1 oz	95	4	8	1	1	0	365	18
Luncheon meat, pork, canned	1 slice	70	3	6	0	0	0	271	13
Luncheon sausage, pork and beef	1 oz	74	4	6	0	0	0	335	18
Luncheon sausage, pork and beef	1 slice	60	4	5	0	0	0	272	15
Luxury loaf, pork	1 slice	40	5	1	1	1	0	347	10
Mortadella, beef, pork	1 oz	88	5	7	1	1	0	353	16
Mortadella, beef, pork	1 slice	47	2	4	1	1	0	187	8
Mother's loaf, pork	1 oz	80	3	6	2	2	0	320	13
Mother's loaf, pork	1 slice	59	3	4	2	2	0	237	9

Description	Serving Size	Cal	Prot (g)	Fat (g)	Carbs (g)	Net Carb(g)	Fiber (g)	Sod (mg)	Chol (mg)
New England brand sausage, pork, beef	1 oz	46	5	2	1	1	0	346	14
New England brand sausage, pork, beef	1 slice	37	4	2	1	1	0	281	11
Olive loaf, pork	1 slice	67	3	4	3	3	0	421	11
Pastrami, turkey	2 slices	80	10	3	1	1	0	593	31
Pate, chicken liver, canned	1 tbsp	26	2	2	1	1	0	50	51
Pate, chicken liver, canned	1 oz	57	4	3	2	2	0	109	111
Pate, goose liver, smoked, canned	1 tbsp	60	1	5	1	1	0	91	20
Pate, goose liver, smoked, canned	1 oz	131	3	12	1	1	0	198	43
Pate, liver, not specified, canned	1 tbsp	41	2	3	0	0	0	91	33
Pate, liver, not specified, canned	1 oz	90	4	7	0	0	0	198	72
Peppered loaf, pork, beef	1 slice	42	5	2	1	1	0	432	13
Pepperoni, pork, beef	1 sausage	1247	53	104	7	7	0	5120	198
Pepperoni, pork, beef	1 slice	27	1	2	0	0	0	112	4
Pickle and pimiento loaf, pork	1 slice	74	3	6	2	2	0	394	10
Picnic loaf, pork, beef	1 slice	66	4	4	1	1	0	330	11
Polish sausage, pork	1 oz	92	4	8	0	0	0	248	20
Polish sausage, pork	1 sausage	740	32	61	4	4	0	1989	159
Pork and beef sausage, fresh, cooked	1 link	51	2	4	0	0	0	105	9
Pork and beef sausage, fresh, cooked	1 patty	107	4	9	1	1	0	217	19
Pork sausage, fresh, cooked	1 link	48	3	4	0	0	0	168	11
Pork sausage, fresh, cooked	1 patty	100	5	8	0	0	0	349	22
Pork sausage, fresh, raw	1 link	117	3	11	0	0	0	187	19
Pork sausage, fresh, raw	1 patty	238	7	22	1	1	0	380	39
Poultry salad sandwich spread	1 tbsp	26	2	2	1	1	0	49	4
Poultry salad sandwich spread	1 oz	57	3	4	2	2	0	107	9
Salami, beef	1 oz	74	4	6	1	1	0	333	18
Salami, beef	1 slice	60	3	4	1	1	0	270	15
Salami, beef and pork	1 oz	71	4	5	1	1	0	302	18
Salami, beef and pork	1 slice	58	3	4	1	1	0	245	15
Salami, dry or hard, pork	1 slice	41	2	3	0	0	0	226	8
Salami, dry or hard, pork, beef	1 slice	42	2	3	0	0	0	186	8
Salami, turkey	2 slices	111	9	7	0	0	0	569	46
Sandwich spread, pork, beef	1 tbsp	35	1	2	2	2	0	152	6
Sandwich spread, pork, beef	1 oz	67	2	5	3	3	0	287	11
Sausage, Berliner, pork, beef	1 oz	65	4	4	1	1	0	368	13
Sausage, Berliner, pork, beef	1 slice	53	4	4	1	1	0	298	11
Sausage, Italian, pork, cooked	1 link	268	17	20	1	1	0	765	65
Sausage, Italian, pork, cooked	1 link	216	13	16	1	1	0	618	52

Description	Serving Size	Cal	Prot (g)	Fat (g)	Carbs (g)	Net Carb(g)	Fiber (g)	Sod (mg)	Chol (mg)
Sausage, Italian, pork, raw	1 link	391	16	33	1	1	0	826	86
Sausage, Italian, pork, raw	1 link	315	13	27	1	1	0	665	69
Sausage, smoked link sausage, pork and beef	1 reg. link	228	9	19	1	1	0	643	48
Sausage, smoked link sausage, pork and beef	1 little link	54	2	4	0	0	0	151	11
Sausage, Vienna, canned, chicken, beef, pork	1 sausage	45	2	4	0	0	0	152	8
Sausage, Vienna, canned, chicken, beef, pork	7 sausages	315	12	27	2	2	0	1077	59
Smoked link sausage, pork	1 reg. link	265	15	20	1	1	0	1020	46
Smoked link sausage, pork	1 little link	62	4	5	0	0	0	240	11
Smoked link sausage, pork and beef, flour and nonfat dry milk added	1 reg. link	182	9	14	3	3	0	741	59
Smoked link sausage, pork and beef, flour and nonfat dry milk added	1 little link	43	2	3	1	1	0	174	14
Smoked link sausage, pork and beef, nonfat dry milk added	1 reg. link	213	9	17	1	1	0	798	44
Smoked link sausage, pork and beef, nonfat dry milk added	1 little link	50	2	4	0	0	0	188	10
Thuringer, cervelat, summer sausage, beef, pork	1 oz	95	4	7	0	0	0	352	21
Thuringer, cervelat, summer sausage, beef, pork	1 slice	77	4	6	0	0	0	286	17
Turkey breast meat	2 slices	47	10	1	0	0	0	608	17
Turkey breast meat	1 slice	23	5	0	0	0	0	301	9
Turkey ham, cured turkey thigh meat	2 slices	73	11	2	0	0	0	565	32
Turkey roll, light and dark meat	1 oz	42	5	2	1	1	0	166	16
Turkey roll, light and dark meat	2 slices	84	10	3	1	1	0	332	31
Turkey roll, light meat	1 oz	42	5	2	0	0	0	139	12
Turkey roll, light meat	2 slices	83	11	4	0	0	0	277	24

Description	Serving Size	Cal	Prot (g)	Fat (g)	Carbs (g)	Net Carb(g)	Fiber (g)	Sod (mg)	Chol (mg)
Chips									
POTATO CHIPS									
Barbecue-flavor	1 oz	139	2	9	15	48	1	213	0
Canned, cheese-flavor	1 oz	156	2	10	14	47	1	214	1
Canned, light	1 oz	142	2	7	18	61	1	121	0
Canned, plain	1 oz	158	2	10	14	47	1	186	0
Canned, sour-cream and onion-flavor	1 oz	155	2	10	15	50	0	204	1
Cheese-flavor	1 oz	141	2	7	16	53	1	225	1
Plain, made with partially hydrogenated soybean oil, salted	1 oz	152	2	9	15	48	1	168	0
Plain, made with partially hydrogenated soybean oil, unsalted	1 oz	152	2	9	15	48	1	2	0
Plain, salted	1 oz	152	2	9	15	48	1	168	0
Plain, unsalted	1 oz	152	2	9	15	48	1	2	0
Reduced fat	1 oz	134	2	6	19	61	2	139	0
Sour-cream-and-onion-flavor	1 oz	151	2	9	15	46	1	177	2
TORTILLA CHIPS									
Corn-based, extruded, chips, barbecue-flavor	1 oz	148	2	9	16	51	1	216	0
Corn-based, extruded, chips, plain	1 oz	153	2	9	16	52	1	179	0
Corn-based, extruded, cones, nacho-flavor	1 oz	152	2	8	16	56	0	270	1
Corn-based, extruded, cones, plain	1 oz	145	2	7	18	62	0	290	0
Corn-based, extruded, onion-flavor	1 oz	142	2	6	18	61	0	278	0
Corn-based, extruded, puffs or twists, cheese-flavor	1 oz	157	2	9	15	53	0	298	1
Nacho-flavor	1 oz	141	2	7	18	57	2	201	1
Nacho-flavor, made with enriched masa flour	1 oz	141	2	7	18	57	2	201	1
Nacho-flavor, reduced fat	1 oz	126	2	4	20	67	1	284	1
Plain	1 oz	142	2	7	18	56	2	150	0
Ranch-flavor	1 oz	139	2	6	18	61	1	174	0
Taco-flavor	1 oz	136	2	6	18	58	2	223	1
Taro chips	1 oz	141	1	7	19	61	2	97	0
Cookies									
ARCHWAY HOME STYLE									
Apple Filled Oatmeal	1 serving	99	1	2	16	64	1	103	2

Description	Serving Size	Cal	Prot (g)	Fat (g)	Carbs (g)	Net Carb(g)	Fiber (g)	Sod (mg)	Chol (mg)
COOKIES (continued)									
Apricot Filled	1 serving	100	1	3	16	63	0	80	7
Aunt Bea's Pound Cake Cookie	1 serving	105	1	3	16	60	0	83	15
Black Walnut Ice Box	1 serving	119	1	4	15	61	0	77	10
Cherry Filled	1 serving	100	1	3	16	63	0	83	7
Chocolate Chip Drop	1 serving	101	1	3	15	61	0	78	14
Chocolate Chip Ice Box	1 serving	117	1	4	15	63	0	59	8
Cinnamon Apple	1 serving	106	1	2	17	65	0	132	0
Coconut Macaroon	1 serving	106	1	6	12	54	1	38	0
Cookies Jar Hermits	1 serving	95	1	2	17	64	1	147	5
Dark Molasses	1 serving	115	1	2	20	71	0	154	0
Date Filled Oatmeal	1 serving	99	1	2	17	64	1	98	3
Dutch Cocoa	1 serving	98	1	2	17	67	1	87	3
Fat Free Cinnamon Honey Hearts	1 serving	106	1	0	25	81	0	123	0
Fat Free Devil's Food Cookie	1 serving	68	1	0	16	76	1	79	0
Fat Free Lemon Nuggets	1 serving	115	1	0	27	83	0	117	0
Fat Free Oatmeal Raisin	1 serving	106	1	0	24	76	1	165	0
Fat Free Oatmeal Raspberry	1 serving	109	1	0	25	77	1	166	0
Fat Free Sugar Cookies	1 serving	71	1	0	17	82	0	80	0
Frosty Lemon	1 serving	112	1	3	17	64	0	95	0
Frosty Orange	1 serving	113	1	3	17	64	0	94	0
Fruit & Honey Bar	1 serving	103	1	2	18	65	0	107	6
Gourmet Apple'n Raisin	1 serving	111	1	3	17	63	1	121	5
Gourmet Carrot Cake	1 serving	120	1	4	18	62	1	176	4
Gourmet Chocolate Chip n' Toffee	1 serving	131	1	5	18	62	1	124	6
Gourmet Oatmeal Pecan	1 serving	134	2	6	16	55	1	103	5
Gourmet Ol'Fashion Peanut Butter	1 serving	117	2	5	14	54	1	118	9
Gourmet Rocky Road	1 serving	127	2	5	18	60	1	71	11
Gourmet Ruth's Golden Oatmeal	1 serving	122	2	4	18	60	1	107	4
Iced Ginger Snaps	1 serving	172	1	5	26	70	0	132	0
Iced Molasses	1 serving	114	1	3	20	69	0	130	0
Iced Oatmeal	1 serving	123	1	4	18	64	1	92	3
Lemon Drop	1 serving	93	1	2	15	60	0	95	9
Lemon Snaps	1 serving	152	2	5	20	64	0	117	7
Molasses	1 serving	103	1	2	18	69	0	144	8
Mud Pie	1 serving	107	1	4	15	57	1	103	5
Oatmeal	1 serving	106	2	3	17	64	1	87	3
Oatmeal Raisin	1 serving	107	1	2	17	64	1	98	3

Description	Serving Size	Cal	Prot (g)	Fat (g)	Carbs (g)	Net Carb(g)	Fiber (g)	Sod (mg)	Chol (mg)
Old Fashioned Molasses	1 serving	105	1	2	18	70	0	138	8
Old Fashioned Windmill Cookies	1 serving	91	1	3	14	68	1	93	0
Peanut Butter	1 serving	101	2	4	12	56	1	85	8
Peanut Jumble	1 serving	116	2	5	13	53	1	77	4
Pecan Ice Box	1 serving	120	1	4	15	61	0	75	6
Raspberry Filled	1 serving	101	1	3	16	64	0	84	7
Reduced Fat Ginger Snaps	1 serving	136	1	3	25	76	0	141	0
Ruth's Oatmeal	1 serving	111	2	3	17	64	1	114	4
Strawberry Filled	1 serving	100	1	3	16	63	0	84	7
Sugar	1 serving	98	1	2	17	68	0	162	5
Sugar Free Chocolate Chip	1 serving	108	1	4	16	66	0	64	0
Sugar Free Oatmeal	1 serving	106	1	3	16	65	0	74	0
Sugar Free Rocky Road	1 serving	101	1	4	15	62	1	66	0
Sugar Free Shortbread	1 serving	107	1	4	16	65	0	47	0
KEEBLER									
Chocolate Graham SELECTS	1 serving	144	2	1	22	NA	NA	111	0
GOLDEN Vanilla Wafers, Artificially Flavored	1 serving	147	2	1	22	NA	NA	120	0
LITTLE DEBBIE									
NUTTY BARS, Wafers with Peanut Butter, Chocolate Covered	1 serving	312	5	4	31	NA	NA	127	0
NABISCO									
SNACKWELL'S Caramel Delights Cookies	1 serving	69	1	1	13	68	0	33	0
SNACKWELL'S Fat Free Devil's Food Cookie Cakes	1 serving	49	1	0	12	73	0	28	0
SNACKWELL'S Mint Creme Cookies	1 serving	108	1	2	19	73	1	72	0
PILLSBURY									
Chocolate Chip Cookies, refrigerated dough	1 serving	127	1	5	18	62	1	88	0
GENERIC COOKIES									
Animal crackers (includes arrowroot, tea biscuits)	1 cracker	22	0	1	4	73	0	19	0
Butter cookies, commercially prepared	1 cookie	23	0	1	3	68	0	18	6
Chocolate chip, commercially prepared, regular, higher fat	1 cookie	58	1	3	8	64	0	38	0
Chocolate chip, commercially prepared, regular, lower fat	1 cookie	45	1	1	7	70	0	38	0

Description	Serving Size	Cal	Prot (g)	Fat (g)	Carbs (g)	Net Carb(g)	Fiber (g)	Sod (mg)	Chol (mg)
COOKIES (continued)									
Chocolate chip, commercially prepared, soft-type	1 cookie	69	1	4	9	56	0	49	0
Chocolate chip, commercially prepared, special dietary	1 cookie	32	0	1	5	72	0	1	0
Chocolate chip, dry mix	1 oz	141	1	7	19	NA	NA	82	0
Chocolate chip, prepared from recipe, made with butter	1 cookie	78	1	4	9	NA	NA	55	11
Chocolate chip, prepared from recipe, made with margarine	1 bar	156	2	9	19	56	1	116	10
Chocolate chip, refrigerated dough	1 portion	128	1	6	18	60	0	61	7
Chocolate chip, refrigerated dough, baked	1 cookie	59	1	3	8	67	0	28	3
Chocolate sandwich, with creme filling, regular	1 cookie	47	0	2	7	67	0	60	0
Chocolate sandwich, with creme filling, regular, chocolate-coated	1 cookie	82	0	4	11	61	1	55	0
Chocolate sandwich, with creme filling, special dietary	1 cookie	46	0	2	7	64	0	24	0
Chocolate sandwich, with extra creme filling	1 cookie	65	0	3	9	66	0	64	0
Chocolate wafers	1 oz	123	2	4	21	69	1	164	1
Coconut macaroons, prepared from recipe	1 cookie	97	1	3	17	70	0	59	0
Fig bars	1 Figaroo	150	2	3	30	66	2	151	0
Fortune cookies	1 cookie	30	0	0	7	82	0	22	0
Gingersnaps	1 cookie	29	0	1	5	75	0	46	0
Graham crackers, chocolate-coated	1 cracker	68	1	3	9	63	0	41	0
Graham crackers, plain or honey (includes cinnamon)	1 cup, crush.	355	6	8	65	74	2	508	0
Graham crackers, plain or honey (includes cinnamon)	1 oz	120	2	3	22	74	1	172	0
Ladyfingers, with lemon juice and rind	1 anisette sponge	47	1	1	8	59	0	19	47
Ladyfingers, without lemon juice and rind	1 anisette sponge	47	1	1	8	59	0	19	47
Marshmallow, chocolate-coated (includes marshmallow pies)	1 Fudge Mashmallow	118	1	4	19	66	1	47	0
Molasses	1 large	138	2	4	24	73	0	147	0
Oatmeal, commercially prepared, fat-free	1 oz	92	2	0	22	71	2	84	0

Description	Serving Size	Cal	Prot (g)	Fat (g)	Carbs (g)	Net Carb(g)	Fiber (g)	Sod (mg)	Chol (mg)
Oatmeal, commercially prepared, regular	1 cookie	113	2	4	17	66	1	96	0
Oatmeal, commercially prepared, soft-type	1 cookie	61	1	2	10	63	0	52	1
Oatmeal, commercially prepared, special dietary	1 cookie	31	0	1	5	67	0	1	0
Oatmeal, prepared from recipe, with raisins	1 cookie	65	1	2	10	NA	NA	81	5
Oatmeal, prepared from recipe, without raisins	1 cookie	67	1	3	10	NA	NA	90	5
Oatmeal, refrigerated dough	1 portion	68	1	3	9	57	0	47	4
Oatmeal, refrigerated dough, baked	1 cookie	57	1	2	8	63	0	39	3
Peanut butter sandwich, regular	1 cookie	67	1	3	9	64	0	52	0
Peanut butter sandwich, special dietary	1 cookie	54	1	3	5	NA	NA	41	0
Peanut butter, commercially prepared, regular	1 cookie	72	1	3	9	57	0	62	0
Peanut butter, commercially prepared, soft-type	1 cookie	69	1	3	9	56	0	50	0
Peanut butter, prepared from recipe	1 cookie	95	2	4	12	NA	NA	104	6
Peanut butter, refrigerated dough	1 portion	73	1	4	8	51	0	64	4
Peanut butter, refrigerated dough, baked	1 cookie	60	1	3	7	56	0	52	4
Raisin, soft-type	1 cookie	60	1	2	10	67	0	51	0
Shortbread cookies, commercially prepared, pecan	1 cookie	76	1	4	8	57	0	39	5
Shortbread cookies, commercially prepared, plain	1 cookie	40	0	2	5	63	0	36	2
Sugar cookies, commercially prepared, regular (includes vanilla)	1 cookie	72	1	3	10	67	0	54	8
Sugar cookies, commercially prepared, special dietary	1 cookie	30	0	1	5	76	0	0	0
Sugar cookies, prepared from recipe, made with margarine	1 cookie	66	1	3	8	59	0	69	4
Sugar cookies, refrigerated dough	1 cookie	113	1	5	15	58	0	110	8
Sugar cookies, refrigerated dough, baked	1 cookie	111	1	5	15	65	0	108	7
Sugar wafers with creme filling, regular	1 wafer	46	0	2	6	70	0	13	0
Sugar wafers with creme filling, special dietary	1 wafer	20	0	1	3	NA	NA	0	0
Vanilla sandwich with creme filling	1 cookie, oval	72	1	3	11	71	0	52	0
Vanilla wafers, higher fat	1 wafer	28	0	1	4	69	0	18	0

Description	Serving Size	Cal	Prot (g)	Fat (g)	Carbs (g)	Net Carb(g)	Fiber (g)	Sod (mg)	Chol (mg)
Corn Cakes									
Corn cakes	1 cake	35	1	0	8	82	0	44	0
Corn cakes, very low sodium	1 cake	35	1	0	8	NA	NA	3	0
Cornnuts									
Cornnuts, barbecue-flavor	1 oz	124	3	4	20	63	2	277	0
Cornnuts, nacho-flavor	1 oz	124	3	4	20	64	2	180	1
Plain	1 oz	124	2	4	21	66	2	156	0
Crackers									
NABISCO									
GRAHAMS Crackers	1 serving	119	2	2	21	73	1	185	0
ORIGINAL PREMIUM Saltine Crackers	1 serving	59	2	1	10	69	0	178	0
RITZ Crackers	1 serving	79	1	4	10	62	0	124	0
SNACKWELL'S Cracked Pepper Cracker	1 serving	61	1	1	10	72	0	117	0
SNACKWELL'S French Onion Snack Crackers	1 serving	128	2	2	23	75	1	275	1
SNACKWELL'S Italian Ranch Snack Crackers	1 serving	128	2	2	23	76	1	311	1
SNACKWELL'S Salsa Snack Crackers	1 serving	128	2	2	23	76	1	321	1
SNACKWELL'S Wheat Cracker	1 serving	62	1	0	12	73	1	150	0
SNACKWELL'S Zesty Cheese Crackers	1 serving	129	2	2	23	75	1	315	1
WHEAT THINS Crackers, baked	1 serving	136	2	3	20	66	1	168	0
GENERIC CRACKERS									
Cheese crackers, low sodium	1 cup	312	6	15	36	56	1	284	8
Cheese crackers, regular	1 cup, bite size	312	6	15	36	56	1	617	8
Cheese crackers, sandwich-type with peanut butter filling	1 sandwich	34	1	2	4	54	0	69	0
Crispbread crackers, rye	1 crispbread	37	1	0	8	66	2	26	0
Matzo crackers, egg	1 matzo	111	3	0	22	76	1	6	24
Matzo crackers, egg and onion	1 matzo	111	3	1	22	72	1	81	13
Matzo crackers, plain	1 matzo	112	3	0	24	81	1	1	0
Matzo crackers, whole-wheat	1 matzo	100	4	0	22	67	3	1	0
Melba toast, rye (includes pumpernickel)	1 toast	19	1	0	4	69	0	45	0
Melba toast, wheat	1 toast	19	1	0	4	69	0	42	0
Milk crackers	1 cracker	50	1	2	8	68	0	65	1
Rusk toast	1 rusk	41	1	1	7	NA	NA	25	8

Description	Serving Size	Cal	Prot (g)	Fat (g)	Carbs (g)	Net Carb(g)	Fiber (g)	Sod (mg)	Chol (mg)
Rye crackers, sandwich-type with cheese filling	1 cracker	34	1	1	4	57	0	73	1
Rye wafers, plain	1 cracker	37	1	0	9	58	3	87	0
Rye wafers, seasoned	1 cracker	84	2	2	16	53	5	195	0
Saltines (includes oyster, soda, soup)	1 cup	195	4	5	32	69	1	586	0
Saltines, fat-free, low-sodium	3 saltines	59	2	0	12	80	0	95	0
Saltines, low salt (includes oyster, soda, soup)	1 cup	195	4	5	32	69	1	286	0
Saltines, low salt (includes oyster, soda, soup)	1 cracker	13	0	0	2	69	0	19	0
Saltines, unsalted tops (includes oyster, soda, soup)	1 cracker	13	0	0	2	69	0	23	0
Standard snack crackers, regular	1 cup, bite size	311	5	15	38	59	1	525	0
Standard snack crackers, regular, low salt	1 cup, bite size	311	5	15	38	59	1	231	0
Standard snack crackers, sandwich, with cheese filling	1 cracker	33	1	1	4	60	0	98	0
Standard snack crackers, sandwich, with peanut butter filling	1 cracker	34	1	2	4	56	0	66	0
Wheat, low salt	1 cup, crushed	14	0	1	2	60	0	8	0
Wheat, regular	1 cup, crushed	393	7	16	54	60	4	660	0
Wheat, sandwich, with cheese filling	1 cracker	35	1	2	4	55	0	64	0
Wheat, sandwich, with peanut butter filling	1 cracker	35	1	2	4	49	0	56	0
Whole-wheat	1 cracker	18	0	1	3	58	0	26	0
Whole-wheat, low salt	1 cracker	18	0	1	3	58	0	10	0

Frozen Desserts

FROZEN YOGURT

Description	Serving Size	Cal	Prot (g)	Fat (g)	Carbs (g)	Net Carb(g)	Fiber (g)	Sod (mg)	Chol (mg)
Frozen yogurts, chocolate, soft-serve	1/2 cup	115	3	4	18	23	2	71	4
Frozen yogurts, vanilla, soft-serve	1/2 cup	114	3	4	17	24	0	63	1

ICE CREAM

Description	Serving Size	Cal	Prot (g)	Fat (g)	Carbs (g)	Net Carb(g)	Fiber (g)	Sod (mg)	Chol (mg)
Chocolate	1 individual	125	2	6	16	27	1	44	20
ESKIMO PIE BAR, Vanilla Ice Cream, with dark chocolate coating	1 bar	166	2	7	12	25	0	34	14
French vanilla, soft-serve	1/2 cup	185	4	10	19	22	0	52	78
HEALTHY CHOICE Praline and Caramel	1/2 cup	129	3	2	25	35	0	70	4
KLONDIKE BAR vanilla ice cream with chocolate coating	1 bar	488	6	19	36	24	0	108	40
Sherbet, orange	1/2 cup	102	1	1	22	30	0	34	4
Sherbet, orange	1 bar	91	1	1	20	30	0	30	4

Description	Serving Size	Cal	Prot (g)	Fat (g)	Carbs (g)	Net Carb(g)	Fiber (g)	Sod (mg)	Chol (mg)
FROZEN DESSERTS (continued)									
Strawberry	1/2 cup	127	2	3	18	27	0	40	19
Vanilla	1 serving	117	2	6	14	24	0	46	26
Vanilla, light	1 serving	90	2	3	15	23	0	55	9
Vanilla, light, no sugar added	1/2 cup	99	3	4	12	19	0	58	11
Vanilla, light, soft-serve	1/2 cup	111	4	2	19	22	0	62	11
Vanilla, rich	1/2 cup	178	3	11	17	22	0	41	45
ICE NOVELTIES									
Frozen ice novelties, fruit, no sugar added	1 bar	12	0	0	3	6	0	3	0
Italian, restaurant-prepared	1/2 cup	61	0	0	16	14	0	5	0
Lime	1/2 cup	127	0	0	32	33	0	22	0
Pineapple-coconut	1/2 cup	112	0	2	24	23	1	35	0
Pop	1 bar	37	0	0	10	19	0	6	0
Frozen juice novelties, fruit and juice bars	1 bar	63	1	0	16	20	0	3	0
FRUIT SNACKS									
Apricot	1 tbsp	48	0	0	13	63	0	8	0
Banana chips	1 oz	147	1	9	17	51	2	2	0
BETTY CROCKER Fruit Roll Ups, berry flavored, with vitamin C	2 rolls	104	0	1	24	NA	NA	89	0
FARLEY Fruit Snacks, with vitamins A, C, and E	1 pouch	89	1	0	21	NA	NA	9	0
Fruit leather, bars	1 bar	81	0	1	18	75	1	18	0
Fruit leather, pieces	1 package	92	0	2	21	75	1	109	0
Fruit leather, rolls	1 large	74	0	1	18	81	1	13	0
Fruit leather, rolls	1 small	49	0	0	12	81	1	9	0
SUNKIST Fruit Roll, strawberry, with vitamins A, C, and E	1 roll	72	0	0	17	75	2	23	0

Granola Bars

Description	Serving Size	Cal	Prot (g)	Fat (g)	Carbs (g)	Net Carb(g)	Fiber (g)	Sod (mg)	Chol (mg)
HARD									
Almond	1 bar	117	2	6	15	57	1	60	0
Chocolate chip	1 bar	103	2	4	17	68	1	81	0
Peanut	1 bar	113	3	5	15	59	1	66	0
Peanut butter	1 bar	114	2	5	15	59	1	67	0
Plain	1 bar	134	3	5	18	59	2	83	0

Description	Serving Size	Cal	Prot (g)	Fat (g)	Carbs (g)	Net Carb(g)	Fiber (g)	Sod (mg)	Chol (mg)
SOFT									
Coated, milk chocolate coating, chocolate chip	1 bar	132	2	7	18	60	1	57	1
Coated, milk chocolate coating, peanut butter	1 bar	187	4	9	20	51	1	71	4
Uncoated, chocolate chip	1 bar	119	2	4	20	64	1	77	0
Uncoated, chocolate chip, graham and marshmallow	1 bar	121	2	4	20	67	1	90	0
Uncoated, nut and raisin	1 bar	129	2	5	18	58	2	72	0
Uncoated, peanut butter	1 bar	121	3	4	18	60	1	116	0
Uncoated, peanut butter and chocolate chip	1 bar	122	3	5	18	58	1	93	0
Uncoated, plain	1 bar	126	2	5	19	63	1	79	0
Uncoated, raisin	1 bar	127	2	4	19	62	1	80	0

Gum

Description	Serving Size	Cal	Prot (g)	Fat (g)	Carbs (g)	Net Carb(g)	Fiber (g)	Sod (mg)	Chol (mg)
Chewing gum	1 stick	10	0	0	3	97	0	0	0
Chewing gum	10 Chiclets	55	0	0	15	97	0	1	0

Ice Cream Cones

Description	Serving Size	Cal	Prot (g)	Fat (g)	Carbs (g)	Net Carb(g)	Fiber (g)	Sod (mg)	Chol (mg)
Cake or wafer-type	1 cone	17	0	0	3	76	0	6	0
Sugar, rolled-type	1 cone	40	1	0	8	82	0	32	0

Popcorn

Description	Serving Size	Cal	Prot (g)	Fat (g)	Carbs (g)	Net Carb(g)	Fiber (g)	Sod (mg)	Chol (mg)
Air-popped	1 cup	31	1	0	6	63	1	0	0
Air-popped, white popcorn	1 cup	31	1	0	6	63	1	0	0
Caramel-coated, with peanuts	1 oz	113	2	2	23	77	1	84	0
Caramel-coated, without peanuts	1 oz	122	1	3	22	74	1	58	1
Cheese-flavor	1 cup	58	1	3	6	42	1	98	1
Oil-popped	1 cup	55	1	3	6	47	1	97	0
Oil-popped, white popcorn	1 cup	55	1	3	6	47	1	97	0
Popcorn, cakes	1 cake	38	1	0	8	77	0	29	0

Pork Skins

Description	Serving Size	Cal	Prot (g)	Fat (g)	Carbs (g)	Net Carb(g)	Fiber (g)	Sod (mg)	Chol (mg)
Barbecue-flavor	1 oz	153	16	9	0	NA	NA	756	33
Plain	1 oz	155	17	8	0	0	0	521	27

Pretzels

Description	Serving Size	Cal	Prot (g)	Fat (g)	Carbs (g)	Net Carb(g)	Fiber (g)	Sod (mg)	Chol (mg)
Hard, confectioner's coating, chocolate-flavor	1 oz	130	2	4	20	NA	NA	161	0
Hard, plain, salted	1 oz	108	3	1	22	76	1	486	0

Description	Serving Size	Cal	Prot (g)	Fat (g)	Carbs (g)	Net Carb(g)	Fiber (g)	Sod (mg)	Chol (mg)
PRETZELS (continued)									
Hard, plain, unsalted	1 oz	108	3	1	22	76	1	82	0
Hard, whole-wheat	1 oz	103	3	1	23	74	2	58	0

Rice Cakes

Description	Serving Size	Cal	Prot (g)	Fat (g)	Carbs (g)	Net Carb(g)	Fiber (g)	Sod (mg)	Chol (mg)
Brown rice, buckwheat	1 cake	34	1	0	7	76	0	10	0
Brown rice, buckwheat, unsalted	1 cake	34	1	0	7	NA	NA	0	0
Brown rice, corn	1 cake	35	1	0	7	78	0	26	0
Brown rice, multigrain	1 cake	35	1	0	7	77	0	23	0
Brown rice, multigrain, unsalted	1 cake	35	1	0	7	NA	NA	0	0
Brown rice, plain	1 cake	35	1	0	7	77	0	29	0
Brown rice, plain, unsalted	1 cake	35	1	0	7	77	0	2	0
Brown rice, rye	1 cake	35	1	0	7	76	0	10	0
Brown rice, sesame seed	1 cake	35	1	0	7	76	0	20	0
Brown rice, sesame seed, unsalted	1 cake	35	1	0	7	NA	NA	0	0

Trail Mix

Description	Serving Size	Cal	Prot (g)	Fat (g)	Carbs (g)	Net Carb(g)	Fiber (g)	Sod (mg)	Chol (mg)
Regular	1 cup	693	21	42	67	NA	NA	344	0
Regular	1 oz	131	4	8	13	NA	NA	65	0
Regular, unsalted	1 cup	693	21	42	67	NA	NA	15	0
Regular, unsalted	1 oz	131	4	8	13	NA	NA	3	0
Regular, with chocolate chips, salted nuts and seeds	1 cup	707	21	45	66	NA	NA	177	6
Regular, with chocolate chips, salted nuts and seeds	1 oz	137	4	9	13	NA	NA	34	1
Regular, with chocolate chips, unsalted nuts and seeds	1 cup	707	21	45	66	NA	NA	39	6
Regular, with chocolate chips, unsalted nuts and seeds	1 oz	137	4	9	13	NA	NA	8	1
Tropical	1 cup	570	9	23	92	NA	NA	14	0
Tropical	1 oz	115	2	5	19	NA	NA	3	0
Beef jerky, chopped and formed	1 piece	81	7	5	2	9	0	438	10
Beef sticks, smoked	1 stick	109	4	9	1	NA	NA	293	26
CHEX mix	1 oz	120	3	2	18	60	2	288	0
COMBOS Snacks Cheddar Cheese Pretzel	1 oz	131	3	0	19	NA	NA	317	1
Crisped rice bar, chocolate chip	1 bar	115	1	4	21	71	1	79	0
DOO DADS snack mix, original flavor	1 cup	259	6	2	36	58	4	721	1
Oriental mix, rice-based	1 oz	156	5	7	15	38	4	117	0

Description	Serving Size	Cal	Prot (g)	Fat (g)	Carbs (g)	Net Carb(g)	Fiber (g)	Sod (mg)	Chol (mg)
Potato sticks	1/2 cup	94	1	6	10	50	1	45	0
Sesame sticks, wheat-based, salted	1 oz	153	3	10	13	44	1	422	0
Sesame sticks, wheat-based, unsalted	1 oz	153	3	10	13	NA	NA	8	0

Gravies

Description	Serving Size	Cal	Prot (g)	Fat (g)	Carbs (g)	Net Carb(g)	Fiber (g)	Sod (mg)	Chol (mg)
CUSTOM FOODS									
RED LABEL Au Jus Base, dry	1 serving	19	2	0	2	2	0	1862	1
SUPERB Country Gravy Mix, dry	1 serving	47	1	3	5	5	0	217	0
SUPERB Instant Au Jus Mix, dry	1 serving	20	1	0	3	2	0	741	0
SUPERB Instant Beef Gravy Mix, dry	1 serving	25	1	1	4	4	0	349	1
SUPERB Instant Brown Gravy Mix, dry	1 serving	25	1	1	4	4	0	339	1
SUPERB Instant Chicken Gravy Mix, dry	1 serving	26	1	1	4	4	0	309	2
SUPERB Instant Pork Gravy Mix, dry	1 serving	24	1	1	4	4	0	299	1
SUPERB Instant Turkey Gravy Mix, dry	1 serving	27	1	1	4	4	0	274	2
SUPERB Old-Fashioned BISCUIT Gravy Mix, dry	1 serving	48	1	3	5	5	0	191	0
SUPERB Peppered Old-Fashioned Biscuit Gravy Mix, dry	1 serving	49	1	3	5	5	0	241	0
NESTLE									
CHEF-MATE Country Sausage Gravy, ready-to-serve	1 serving	96	3	7	4	3	0	236	13
TRIO Au Jus Gravy Mix, dry	1 tsp	8	0	0	2	2	0	399	0
TRIO Brown Gravy Mix, dry	1 tbsp	24	1	1	3	3	0	262	0
TRIO Chicken Gravy Mix, dry	1 tbsp	32	1	1	5	5	0	260	2
TRIO Country Gravy Mix, dry	1 tbsp	35	1	1	5	4	1	205	0
TRIO Southern Gravy Mix, dry	1 serving	48	0	2	6	6	0	290	0
TRIO Turkey Gravy Mix, dry	1 serving	29	1	0	6	6	0	271	1
Au jus, canned	1 cup	38	3	0	6	6	0	119	0
Au jus, dry	1 tsp	9	0	0	1	NA	NA	348	0
Beef, canned	1 cup	123	9	5	11	10	1	1305	7
Brown, dry	1 tbsp	22	1	0	4	3	0	291	0
Chicken, canned	1 cup	188	5	13	13	12	1	1373	5
Chicken, dry	1 tbsp	30	1	1	5	NA	NA	332	2
HEINZ Home Style Savory Brown Gravy, canned	1/4 cup	25	1	1	3	NA	NA	352	2
Mushroom, canned	1 cup	119	3	6	13	12	1	1359	0
Mushroom, dehydrated, dry	1 cup	70	2	1	14	13	1	1402	1
Onion, dehydrated, dry	1 cup	77	2	1	16	15	1	1005	0
Pork, dry	1 serving	25	1	1	4	4	0	359	1
Turkey, canned	1 cup	122	6	5	12	11	1	1376	5
Turkey, dry	1 serving	26	1	0	5	NA	NA	307	1

Description	Serving Size	Cal	Prot (g)	Fat (g)	Carbs (g)	Net Carb(g)	Fiber (g)	Sod (mg)	Chol (mg)
Sauces									
BARBECUE SAUCE									
Barbecue sauce	1 cup	188	5	4	32	29	3	2038	0
KRAFT Barbecue Sauce Hickory Smoke	2 tbsp	39	0	0	9	9	0	418	0
KRAFT Barbecue Sauce Original	2 tbsp	39	0	0	9	9	0	424	0
MARZETTI, TEXAS BEST Barbecue Sauce Original Recipe	2 tbsp	42	1	1	4	NA	NA	315	0
RIDG'S, BULLS-EYE Original Barbecue Sauce	2 tbsp	63	0	0	15	NA	NA	302	0
CHEESE SAUCE									
Cheese, dehydrated, dry	1 packet	157	8	8	12	11	0	1439	18
Cheese, ready-to-serve	1/4 cup	110	4	8	4	4	0	522	18
CHEF-MATE Basic Cheddar Cheese Sauce, ready-to-serve	1 cup	327	7	6	32	32	0	1885	25
CHEF-MATE Golden Cheese Sauce, ready-to-serve	1 cup	554	27	43	9	6	3	2006	116
CHEF-MATE Sharp Cheddar Cheese Sauce, ready-to-serve	1 cup	532	22	39	7	5	3	1893	91
LA VICTORIA, Cheddar Cheese Sauce	1/4 cup	105	1	8	6	6	0	633	2
LA VICTORIA, Nacho Cheese Sauce with Jalapeno Peppers, Medium	1/4 cup	122	1	9	7	7	0	547	4
ORTEGA Mild Nacho Cheese Sauce, ready-to-serve	1 cup	476	18	38	10	8	2	1968	81
ORTEGA Nacho Cheese Sauce, ready-to-serve	1 cup	512	21	41	16	14	2	2318	116
QUE BUENO Jalapeno Cheese Sauce, ready-to-serve	1 serving	81	2	4	8	8	0	571	6
SUPERB Instant Cheddar Cheese Sauce Mix, dry	1 serving	60	1	3	8	7	1	685	4
SUPERB Instant Nacho Cheese Sauce Mix, dry	1 serving	60	1	3	8	8	0	733	3
TRIO Cheese Sauce Mix, dry	1 serving	54	1	2	7	7	0	310	2
TRIO Nacho Cheese Sauce Mix, dry	1 serving	51	1	2	8	7	0	338	2
SALSA & TACO SAUCE									
LA VICTORIA Enchilada Sauce	1/4 cup	20	0	0	3	2	0	397	0
LA VICTORIA Green Chile Salsa, Mild	2 tbsp	8	0	0	1	1	0	175	0
LA VICTORIA Green Taco Sauce, Medium	1 tbsp	5	0	0	1	1	0	96	0
LA VICTORIA Green Taco Sauce, Mild	1 tbsp	5	0	0	1	1	0	96	0
LA VICTORIA Red Taco Sauce, Medium	1 tbsp	7	0	0	1	1	0	103	0

Description	Serving Size	Cal	Prot (g)	Fat (g)	Carbs (g)	Net Carb(g)	Fiber (g)	Sod (mg)	Chol (mg)
LA VICTORIA Red Taco Sauce, mild	1 tbsp	7	0	0	1	1	0	103	0
LA VICTORIA Salsa Picante, Medium	2 tbsp	8	0	0	1	1	0	150	0
LA VICTORIA Salsa Picante, Mild	2 tbsp	8	0	0	1	1	0	182	0
LA VICTORIA Salsa Ranchera, Hot	2 tbsp	9	0	0	2	2	0	171	0
LA VICTORIA Salsa Suprema, Medium	2 tbsp	8	0	0	1	1	0	166	0
LA VICTORIA Salsa Suprema, Mild	2 tbsp	8	0	0	2	1	0	179	0
LA VICTORIA Salsa Victoria, Hot	2 tbsp	7	0	0	1	1	0	163	0
LA VICTORIA Thick 'N Chunky Salsa, Hot	2 tbsp	9	0	0	1	1	0	133	0
LA VICTORIA Thick 'N Chunky Salsa, Medium	2 tbsp	8	0	0	1	1	0	160	0
LA VICTORIA Thick 'N Chunky Salsa, Mild	2 tbsp	8	0	0	1	1	0	157	0
LA VICTORIA, Green Salsa Jalapena	2 tbsp	10	0	0	1	1	0	181	0
LA VICTORIA, LA VICTORIA Chunky Chili Dip, salsa, canned	2 tbsp	9	0	0	2	2	0	148	0
LA VICTORIA, Red Salsa Jalapena	2 tbsp	12	0	0	2	2	0	148	0
LA VICTORIA, Salsa Brava, Hot	1 tbsp	2	0	0	0	0	0	33	0
ORTEGA Enchilada Sauce, ready-to-serve	1 serving	15	0	1	2	2	0	77	0
ORTEGA Picante Sauce, ready-to-serve	1 serving	10	0	0	2	2	0	252	0
Salsa	1 cup	73	3	0	16	12	4	1124	0
TOMATO SAUCE									
LJ MINOR Italian Sauce, ready-to-serve	1 cup	125	2	2	24	22	2	627	0
Pasta, spaghetti/marinara, ready-to-serve	1 cup	143	4	5	21	17	4	1030	0
PREGO 100% Natural Spaghetti Sauce, Traditional, jar	2 tbsp	136	2	1	21	17	4	557	0
RAGU Old World Style Smooth Pasta Sauce, Traditional, jar	1/2 cup	80	2	2	12	9	3	756	0
RED LABEL All Purpose Italian Sauce Mix, dry	1 serving	19	0	0	4	4	0	359	0
Spaghetti with mushrooms, dehydrated, dry	1 serving	30	1	1	5	NA	NA	942	3
Spaghetti, dehydrated, dry	1 serving	28	1	0	6	6	0	848	0
Alfredo Sauce, dry mix, KNORR	2 tbsp	62	2	3	7	NA	NA	730	5
Béarnaise, dehydrated, dry	1 cup	60	2	1	10	NA	NA	559	0
CHEF-MATE Hot Dog Chili Sauce, ready-to-serve	1 serving	69	3	2	9	8	2	399	4
Curry, dehydrated, dry	1 cup	121	3	6	14	NA	NA	1155	0

Description	Serving Size	Cal	Prot (g)	Fat (g)	Carbs (g)	Net Carb(g)	Fiber (g)	Sod (mg)	Chol (mg)
SAUCES (continued)									
Fish, ready-to-serve	1 tbsp	6	1	0	1	1	0	1390	0
Hoisin, ready-to-serve	1 tbsp	35	1	1	7	7	0	258	0
Hollandaise, with butter fat, dehydrated, dry	1 cup	249	5	19	14	14	0	1639	53
Hollandaise, with vegetable oil, dehydrated, dry	1 cup	62	2	1	10	10	0	429	0
LA VICTORIA, Mole Poblano	2 oz	240	8	0	28	19	9	1847	0
LJ MINOR All Purpose Stir Fry Sauce, ready-to-serve	1 tbsp	16	0	1	2	2	0	233	0
LJ MINOR Creole Sauce, ready-to-serve	1 cup	99	4	2	15	12	3	1357	0
LJ MINOR Lemon Sauce, ready-to-serve	1 serving	43	0	0	10	10	0	3	0
LJ MINOR Sweet N' Sour Glaze, ready-to-serve	1 serving	51	0	0	12	12	0	229	0
LJ MINOR Sweet N' Sour Sauce, ready-to-serve	1 serving	40	0	0	8	8	0	116	0
LJ MINOR Teriyaki Sauce, ready-to-serve	1 tbsp	21	0	1	4	4	0	159	0
Mole poblano, dry mix, single brand	1 cup, sauce	1512	20	0	110	84	27	3082	0
Mole poblano, prepared from recipe	1 cup, sauce	398	9	0	31	21	10	325	0
Mushroom, dehydrated, dry	1 cup	79	3	2	12	NA	NA	1414	0
Oyster, ready-to-serve	1 tbsp	2	0	0	0	0	0	109	0
Pepper or hot sauce	1 tsp	1	0	0	0	0	0	124	0
Pepper, TABASCO	1 tsp	1	0	0	0	0	0	30	0
Plum, ready-to-serve	1 cup	561	3	3	131	128	2	1641	0
Sofrito, prepared from recipe	1 tbsp	35	2	0	1	1	0	171	0
Sour cream, dehydrated, dry	1 cup	360	11	21	34	NA	NA	887	56
Stroganoff, dehydrated, dry	1 cup	195	7	5	32	31	1	2252	14
Sweet and sour, dehydrated, dry	1 cup	294	1	0	73	71	1	779	0
Teriyaki, dehydrated, dry	1 packet	130	4	1	28	27	1	4784	0
Teriyaki, ready-to-serve	1 cup	242	17	0	46	46	0	11039	0
White, dehydrated, dry	1 cup	92	2	5	10	9	1	675	0
White, homemade, medium	1 cup	368	10	25	23	22	1	885	18
White, homemade, thick	1 cup	465	10	33	29	28	1	933	15
White, homemade, thin	1 cup	263	9	16	19	18	0	820	20

Soups

LIPTON

Description	Serving Size	Cal	Prot (g)	Fat (g)	Carbs (g)	Net Carb(g)	Fiber (g)	Sod (mg)	Chol (mg)
CUP-A-SOUP BROCCOLI & CHEESE, Mix, Dry	1 serving	67	2	1	9	8	1	545	3

Description	Serving Size	Cal	Prot (g)	Fat (g)	Carbs (g)	Net Carb(g)	Fiber (g)	Sod (mg)	Chol (mg)
CUP-A-SOUP CHICKEN BROTH FAT FREE, Mix, Dry	1 serving	18	1	0	3	3	0	442	0
CUP-A-SOUP CHICKEN FLAVOR VEGETABLE	1 serving	52	1	0	10	9	0	518	10
CUP-A-SOUP CHICKEN NOODLE WITH MEAT	1 serving	381	16	3	62	60	2	4177	88
CUP-A-SOUP CHICKEN/PASTA FAT FREE, Mix, Dry	1 serving	44	2	0	8	8	0	449	0
CUP-A-SOUP CREAM OF CHICKEN, Mix, Dry	1 envelope	68	1	0	12	11	1	636	1
CUP-A-SOUP CREAM OF MUSHROOM, Mix, Dry	1 serving	60	1	0	10	9	0	608	1
CUP-A-SOUP GREEN PEA, Mix, Dry	1 serving	75	4	0	12	9	3	520	0
CUP-A-SOUP HEARTY CHICKEN NOODLE, Mix, Dry	1 envelope	61	3	0	10	10	0	591	14
CUP-A-SOUP HEARTY CHICKEN SUPREME, Mix, Dry	1 serving	90	1	1	14	13	1	635	1
CUP-A-SOUP RING NOODLE, Mix, Dry	1 serving	53	2	0	9	9	0	557	12
CUP-A-SOUP SPRING VEGETABLE, Mix, Dry	1 envelope	47	2	0	8	8	1	497	8
CUP-A-SOUP TOMATO, Mix, Dry	1 envelope	95	2	0	20	19	1	506	2
KETTLE CREATIONS CHICKEN WITH PASTA & BEAN, Mix, Dry	1 serving	106	5	0	19	17	3	699	6
KETTLE CREATIONS HOMESTYLE LENTIL, Mix, Dry	1 serving	127	7	0	22	17	5	753	0
KETTLE CREATIONS PASTA & BEAN, Mix, Dry	1 serving	125	6	0	23	18	4	693	0
RECIPE SECRETS BEEFY MUSHROOM, Mix, Dry	1 serving	33	1	0	7	7	0	645	0
RECIPE SECRETS BEEFY ONION, Mix, Dry	1 serving	25	1	0	5	4	0	607	0
RECIPE SECRETS FIESTA HERB WITH RED, Mix, Dry	1 serving	29	1	0	6	5	0	559	1
RECIPE SECRETS ONION MUSHROOM, Mix, Dry	1 serving	32	1	0	6	5	0	626	0
RECIPE SECRETS ONION, Mix, Dry	1 serving	18	0	0	4	4	0	610	0
RECIPE SECRETS SAVORY HERB WITH GARLIC, Mix, Dry	1 serving	31	1	0	6	6	0	477	1
RECIPE SECRETS VEGETABLE, Mix, Dry	1 serving	28	1	0	6	5	1	603	0
SOUP SECRETS CHICKEN NOODLE, Mix, Dry	1 serving	77	3	1	11	11	0	690	15

Description	Serving Size	Cal	Prot (g)	Fat (g)	Carbs (g)	Net Carb(g)	Fiber (g)	Sod (mg)	Chol (mg)
SOUPS (continued)									
SOUP SECRETS EXTRA NOODLE, Mix, Dry	1 serving	86	3	1	15	14	1	681	23
SOUP SECRETS GIGGLE NOODLE, Mix, Dry	1 serving	74	3	1	11	11	0	736	18
SOUP SECRETS NOODLE WITH REAL CHICKEN BROTH, Mix, Dry	1 serving	62	2	1	9	9	0	724	14
SOUP SECRETS RING-O-NOODLE	1 serving	66	2	1	10	10	0	724	16
SOUP SECRETS SPIRAL PASTA SOUP, Mix, Dry	1 serving	64	2	0	11	11	0	657	2
PROGRESSO HEALTHY CLASSICS									
BEEF BARLEY, canned, ready-to-serve	1 cup	142	11	2	20	17	3	470	19
BEEF VEGETABLE, canned, ready-to-serve	1 cup	154	10	1	25	19	6	403	14
CHICKEN NOODLE, canned, ready-to-serve	1 cup	76	6	1	9	8	1	460	19
CHICKEN RICE WITH VEGETABLES, canned, ready-to-serve	1 cup	88	6	1	12	12	1	459	17
CREAM OF BROCCOLI, canned, ready-to-serve	1 cup	88	2	2	13	11	2	578	5
GARLIC AND PASTA, canned, ready-to-serve	1 cup	100	4	1	18	15	3	450	5
LENTIL, canned, ready-to-serve	1 cup	126	8	1	20	15	6	443	0
MINESTRONE, canned, ready-to-serve	1 cup	123	5	2	20	19	1	470	0
NEW ENGLAND CLAM CHOWDER, canned, ready-to-serve	1 cup	117	5	2	20	19	1	529	5
SPLIT PEA, canned, ready-to-serve	1 cup	180	10	2	30	25	5	420	5
TOMATO GARDEN, canned, ready-to-serve	1 cup	98	3	1	19	15	4	480	0
VEGETABLE, canned, ready-to-serve	1 cup	81	4	1	13	12	1	466	5
GENERIC SOUPS									
Bean with bacon, condensed, single brand	1 serving	158	9	2	24	18	6	994	4
Bean with bacon, dehydrated, dry mix	1 cup	105	5	2	16	8	9	928	3
Bean with bacon, dehydrated, prepared with water	1 cup	106	5	2	16	7	9	927	3
Bean with frankfurters, canned, condensed, commercial	1 cup	373	20	13	44	32	12	2186	24
Bean with frankfurters, canned, prepared with equal volume water, commercial	1 cup	188	10	7	22	NA	NA	1093	13

Description	Serving Size	Cal	Prot (g)	Fat (g)	Carbs (g)	Net Carb(g)	Fiber (g)	Sod (mg)	Chol (mg)
Bean with ham, canned, chunky, ready-to-serve, commercial	1 cup	231	13	8	27	16	11	972	22
Bean with pork, canned, condensed, commercial	1 cup	347	16	11	46	30	16	1907	5
Bean with pork, canned, prepared with equal volume water, commercial	1 cup	172	8	6	23	14	9	951	3
Beef broth bouillon and consommé, canned, condensed, commercial	1 cup	59	11	0	4	4	0	1279	0
Beef broth or bouillon canned, ready-to-serve	1 cup	17	3	1	0	0	0	782	0
Beef broth or bouillon, powder, dry	1 cube	9	1	0	1	1	0	611	0
Beef broth or bouillon, powder, prepared with water	1 cup	20	1	1	2	2	0	1362	0
Beef broth, bouillon, consommé, prepared with equal volume water, commercial	1 cup	29	5	0	2	2	0	636	0
Beef broth, canned, condensed, single brand	1 serving	23	3	0	0	NA	NA	969	1
Beef broth, cubed, dry	1 cube	6	1	0	1	1	0	864	0
Beef broth, cubed, prepared with water	1 cup	7	1	0	1	1	0	1158	0
Beef mushroom, canned, condensed, commercial	1 cup	153	12	6	13	13	1	1940	13
Beef mushroom, canned, prepared with equal volume water, commercial	1 cup	73	6	3	6	6	0	942	7
Beef noodle mix, dehydrated, dry form	1 cup	47	3	1	7	7	0	1194	2
Beef noodle, canned, condensed, commercial	1 cup	168	10	6	18	16	2	1905	10
Beef noodle, canned, prepared with equal volume water, commercial	1 cup	83	5	3	9	8	1	952	5
Beef noodle, dehydrated, prepared with water	1 cup	40	2	1	6	5	1	1042	3
Beef with country vegetables, chunky, ready-to-serve, single brand	1 serving	153	12	4	16	NA	NA	868	24
Beef with vegetables and barley, canned, condensed, single brand	1 serving	77	5	1	10	NA	NA	898	8
Beef, canned, chunky, ready-to-serve	1 cup	170	12	5	20	18	1	866	14
Black bean, canned, condensed, commercial	1 cup	234	12	3	40	22	17	2493	0
Black bean, canned, prepared with equal volume water, commercial	1 cup	116	6	1	20	15	4	1198	0
Cauliflower, dehydrated, dry mix	1 cup	68	3	2	11	NA	NA	841	0
Cauliflower, dehydrated, prepared with water	1 cup	69	3	2	11	NA	NA	843	0

Description	Serving Size	Cal	Prot (g)	Fat (g)	Carbs (g)	Net Carb(g)	Fiber (g)	Sod (mg)	Chol (mg)
SOUPS (continued)									
Cheese, canned, condensed, commercial	1 cup	311	11	20	21	19	2	1920	59
Cheese, canned, prepared with equal volume milk, commercial	1 cup	231	9	14	16	15	1	1019	48
Cheese, canned, prepared with equal volume water, commercial	1 cup	156	5	10	11	10	1	958	30
Chicken broth cubes, dehydrated, dry	1 cube	10	1	0	1	1	0	1152	1
Chicken broth cubes, dehydrated, prepared with water	1 cube	9	1	0	1	NA	NA	593	0
Chicken broth or bouillon, dehydrated, dry	1 tsp	5	0	0	0	0	0	372	0
Chicken broth or bouillon, dehydrated, prepared with water	1 cup	22	1	1	1	1	0	1484	0
Chicken broth, canned, condensed, commercial	1 cup	78	11	3	2	2	0	1571	3
Chicken broth, canned, prepared with equal volume water, commercial	1 cup	38	5	1	1	1	0	763	0
Chicken corn chowder, chunky, ready-to-serve, single brand	1 serving	238	7	12	18	16	2	718	26
Chicken gumbo, canned, condensed, commercial	1 cup	113	5	3	17	13	4	1910	8
Chicken gumbo, canned, prepared with equal volume water, commercial	1 cup	56	3	1	8	6	2	954	5
Chicken mushroom chowder, chunky, ready-to-serve, single brand	1 serving	192	7	9	17	14	3	814	14
Chicken mushroom, canned, condensed, commercial	1 cup	274	9	18	19	19	1	1940	20
Chicken mushroom, canned, prepared with equal volume water, commercial	1 cup	132	4	9	9	9	0	942	10
Chicken noodle mix, dehydrated, dry form	1 packet	286	10	6	45	43	2	2804	55
Chicken noodle with celery and carrots, home-style, ready-to-serve, single brand	1 serving	95	6	3	9	NA	NA	985	21
Chicken noodle, canned, chunky, ready-to-serve	1 cup	175	13	6	17	13	4	850	19
Chicken noodle, canned, condensed, commercial	1 cup	150	8	4	19	17	1	1862	12
Chicken noodle, canned, prepared with equal volume water, commercial	1 cup	75	4	2	9	9	1	1106	7
Chicken noodle, chunky, ready-to-serve, single brand	1 serving	114	8	3	14	NA	NA	875	24

Description	Serving Size	Cal	Prot (g)	Fat (g)	Carbs (g)	Net Carb(g)	Fiber (g)	Sod (mg)	Chol (mg)
Chicken noodle, dehydrated, prepared with water	1 cup	55	2	1	9	9	0	550	10
Chicken noodle, with meatballs, canned, chunky, ready-to-serve	1 cup	99	8	3	8	NA	NA	1039	10
Chicken rice mix, dehydrated, dry form	1 cup	60	2	1	9	9	0	980	3
Chicken rice, canned, chunky, ready-to-serve	1 cup	127	12	3	13	12	1	888	12
Chicken rice, dehydrated, prepared with water	1 cup	58	2	1	9	8	1	931	2
Chicken vegetable, canned, chunky, ready-to-serve	1 cup	166	12	5	19	NA	NA	1068	17
Chicken vegetable, canned, condensed, commercial	1 cup	150	7	5	17	16	2	1897	17
Chicken vegetable, canned, prepared with equal volume water, commercial	1 cup	75	4	3	9	8	1	945	10
Chicken vegetable, chunky, reduced fat, reduced sodium, ready-to-serve, single brand	1 serving	96	6	1	15	NA	NA	461	10
Chicken vegetable, dehydrated, dry	1 cup	49	3	1	8	7	0	803	3
Chicken vegetable, dehydrated, prepared with water	1 cup	50	3	1	8	NA	NA	807	3
Chicken with dumplings, canned, condensed, commercial	1 cup	194	11	10	12	11	1	1729	66
Chicken with dumplings, canned, prepared with equal volume water, commercial	1 cup	96	6	5	6	6	0	860	34
Chicken with rice, canned, condensed, commercial	1 cup	121	7	4	14	13	1	1636	12
Chicken with rice, canned, prepared with equal volume water, commercial	1 cup	60	4	2	7	6	1	815	7
Chicken with star-shaped pasta, canned, condensed, single brand	1 serving	63	3	1	9	NA	NA	915	5
Chicken, canned, chunky, ready-to-serve, commercial	1 cup	170	12	6	17	15	1	850	29
Chili beef, canned, condensed, commercial	1 cup	339	13	13	43	24	19	2072	26
Chili beef, canned, prepared with equal volume water, commercial	1 cup	170	7	6	21	12	10	1035	13
Clam chowder, Manhattan style, canned, chunky, ready-to-serve	1 cup	134	7	3	19	16	3	1001	14
Clam chowder, Manhattan style, dehydrated, dry	1 cup	65	2	1	11	NA	NA	1336	0
Clam chowder, Manhattan, canned, condensed, commercial	1 cup	153	4	4	24	21	3	1147	5

Description	Serving Size	Cal	Prot (g)	Fat (g)	Carbs (g)	Net Carb(g)	Fiber (g)	Sod (mg)	Chol (mg)
Clam chowder, Manhattan, canned, prepared with equal volume water	1 cup	78	2	2	12	11	1	578	2
Clam chowder, New England, canned, condensed, commercial	1 cup	176	11	5	22	20	2	1865	10
Clam chowder, New England, canned, prepared with equal volume milk, commercial	1 cup	164	9	6	17	15	1	992	22
Clam chowder, New England, canned, prepared with equal volume water, commercial	1 cup	95	5	3	12	11	1	915	5
Clam chowder, New England, dehydrated, dry	1 cup	95	3	3	13	12	1	745	1
Consommé with gelatin, dehydrated, dry	1 cup	17	2	0	2	2	0	3301	0
Consommé with gelatin, dehydrated, prepared with water	1 cup	17	2	0	2	2	0	3299	0
Crab, canned, ready-to-serve	1 cup	76	5	1	10	10	1	1235	10
Cream of asparagus, canned, condensed, commercial	1 cup	173	5	8	21	20	1	1963	10
Cream of asparagus, canned, prepared with equal volume milk, commercial	1 cup	161	6	8	16	16	1	1042	22
Cream of asparagus, canned, prepared with equal volume water, commercial	1 cup	85	2	4	11	10	0	981	5
Cream of asparagus, dehydrated, dry mix	1 cup	52	2	1	8	8	0	707	0
Cream of asparagus, dehydrated, prepared with water	1 cup	58	2	1	9	NA	NA	800	0
Cream of celery, canned, condensed, commercial	1 cup	181	3	10	18	16	2	1900	28
Cream of celery, canned, prepared with equal volume milk, commercial	1 cup	164	6	9	15	14	1	1009	32
Cream of celery, canned, prepared with equal volume water, commercial	1 cup	90	2	5	9	8	1	949	15
Cream of celery, dehydrated, dry	1 cup	62	3	2	10	9	0	837	1
Cream of celery, dehydrated, prepared with water	1 cup	64	3	2	10	NA	NA	838	0
Cream of chicken, canned, condensed, commercial	1 cup	233	7	14	19	18	1	1973	20
Cream of chicken, canned, condensed, single brand	1 serving	125	3	7	10	NA	NA	993	9
Cream of chicken, canned, prepared with equal volume water, commercial	1 cup	117	3	7	9	9	0	986	10

Description	Serving Size	Cal	Prot (g)	Fat (g)	Carbs (g)	Net Carb(g)	Fiber (g)	Sod (mg)	Chol (mg)
Cream of chicken, dehydrated, dry	1 cup	106	2	5	13	13	0	1176	3
Cream of chicken, dehydrated, prepared with water	1 cup	107	2	5	13	13	0	1185	3
Cream of chicken, prepared with equal volume milk, commercial	1 cup	191	7	11	15	15	0	1047	27
Cream of mushroom, canned, condensed, commercial	1 cup	259	4	18	19	18	1	1737	3
Cream of mushroom, canned, prepared with equal volume milk, commercial	1 cup	203	6	13	15	15	0	918	20
Cream of mushroom, canned, prepared with equal volume water, commercial	1 cup	129	2	8	9	9	0	881	2
Cream of onion, canned, condensed, commercial	1 cup	221	6	10	26	25	1	1908	30
Cream of onion, canned, prepared with equal volume milk, commercial	1 cup	186	7	9	18	18	1	1004	32
Cream of onion, canned, prepared with equal volume water, commercial	1 cup	107	3	5	13	12	1	927	15
Cream of potato, canned, condensed	1 cup	148	3	4	23	22	1	2000	13
Cream of potato, canned, prepared with equal volume milk, commercial	1 cup	149	6	6	17	17	0	1061	22
Cream of potato, canned, prepared with equal volume water, commercial	1 cup	73	2	2	11	11	0	1000	5
Cream of shrimp, canned, condensed	1 cup	181	6	10	16	16	1	1953	33
Cream of shrimp, canned, prepared with equal volume milk, commercial	1 cup	164	7	9	14	14	0	1037	35
Cream of shrimp, canned, prepared with equal volume water, commercial	1 cup	90	3	5	8	8	0	976	17
Cream of vegetable, dehydrated, dry	1 cup	105	2	5	12	12	1	1170	0
Cream of vegetable, dehydrated, prepared with water	1 cup	107	2	5	12	12	1	1170	0
Escarole, canned, ready-to-serve	1 cup	27	2	2	2	NA	NA	3864	2
Gazpacho, canned, ready-to-serve	1 cup	46	7	0	4	4	0	739	0
Leek, dehydrated, dry	1 cup	65	2	2	11	10	1	889	2
Leek, dehydrated, prepared with water	1 cup	71	2	2	11	8	3	965	3
Lentil with ham, canned, ready-to-serve	1 cup	139	9	3	20	NA	NA	1319	7
Minestrone, canned, chunky, ready-to-serve	1 cup	127	5	3	21	15	6	864	5
Minestrone, canned, condensed, commercial	1 cup	167	9	5	23	21	2	1830	2
Minestrone, canned, prepared with equal volume water, commercial	1 cup	82	4	2	11	10	1	911	2

Description	Serving Size	Cal	Prot (g)	Fat (g)	Carbs (g)	Net Carb(g)	Fiber (g)	Sod (mg)	Chol (mg)
SOUPS (continued)									
Minestrone, dehydrated, dry	1 cup	62	3	1	9	9	1	799	1
Minestrone, dehydrated, prepared with water	1 cup	79	4	2	12	NA	NA	1026	3
Mushroom barley, canned, condensed, commercial	1 cup	153	4	4	24	NA	NA	1832	0
Mushroom barley, canned, prepared with equal volume water, commercial	1 cup	73	2	2	12	11	1	891	0
Mushroom with beef stock, canned, condensed, commercial	1 cup	171	6	7	19	18	0	1940	15
Mushroom with beef stock, canned, prepared with equal volume water, commercial	1 cup	85	3	4	9	9	1	969	7
Mushroom, dehydrated, dry	1 packet	328	8	16	38	35	3	3483	1
Mushroom, dehydrated, prepared with water	1 cup	96	2	5	11	10	1	1020	0
NISSIN, CUP NOODLES, Ramen Noodle, chicken flavor, dry mix	1 container	296	6	6	37	NA	NA	1434	0
NISSIN, OODLES OF NOODLES TOP RAMEN Ramen Noodle, Oriental flavor, dry form	1 serving	190	4	6	28	NA	NA	487	0
Onion mix, dehydrated, dry form	1 packet	115	5	2	21	17	4	3493	2
Onion, canned, condensed, commercial	1 cup	113	8	3	16	15	2	2116	0
Onion, canned, prepared with equal volume water, commercial	1 cup	58	4	2	8	7	1	1053	0
Onion, dehydrated, prepared with water	1 cup	27	1	1	5	4	1	849	0
Oxtail, dehydrated, dry	1 cup	62	2	2	8	8	0	1066	2
Oxtail, dehydrated, prepared with water	1 cup	68	3	2	9	8	0	1166	2
Oyster stew, canned, condensed, commercial	1 cup	118	4	7	8	8	0	1968	27
Oyster stew, canned, prepared with equal volume milk, commercial	1 cup	135	6	7	10	10	0	1041	32
Oyster stew, canned, prepared with equal volume water, commercial	1 cup	58	2	4	4	NA	NA	981	14
Pea, green, canned, condensed, commercial	1 cup	329	17	6	53	47	6	1836	0
Pea, green, canned, prepared with equal volume milk, commercial	1 cup	239	13	7	32	29	3	970	18
Pea, green, canned, prepared with equal volume water, commercial	1 cup	165	9	3	27	24	3	918	0
Pea, green, mix, dehydrated, dry form	1 packet	402	23	6	69	57	11	3687	1
Pea, green, mix, dehydrated, prepared with water	1 cup	133	8	1	23	20	3	1220	3

Description	Serving Size	Cal	Prot (g)	Fat (g)	Carbs (g)	Net Carb(g)	Fiber (g)	Sod (mg)	Chol (mg)
Pea, split with ham, canned, chunky, ready-to-serve	1 cup	185	11	4	27	23	4	965	7
Pea, split with ham, canned, condensed, commercial	1 cup	379	21	8	56	51	5	2018	16
Pea, split with ham, canned, prepared with equal volume water, commercial	1 cup	190	10	4	28	26	2	1007	8
Pepper pot, canned, condensed, commercial	1 cup	207	13	9	19	18	1	1948	20
Pepper pot, canned, prepared with equal volume water, commercial	1 cup	104	6	4	9	9	0	971	10
Potato ham chowder, chunky, ready-to-serve, single brand	1 serving	192	6	11	13	12	1	874	22
Scotch broth, canned, condensed, commercial	1 cup	162	10	5	19	17	2	2032	10
Scotch broth, canned, prepared with equal volume water, commercial	1 cup	80	5	2	9	8	1	1012	5
Shark fin, restaurant-prepared	1 cup	99	7	3	8	8	0	1082	4
Sirloin burger with vegetables, ready-to-serve, single brand	1 serving	185	10	8	16	11	6	866	26
Split pea with ham and bacon, canned, condensed, single brand	1 serving	189	12	3	29	25	4	984	4
Split pea with ham, chunky, reduced fat, reduced sodium, ready-to-serve, single brand	1 serving	185	13	2	27	NA	NA	833	15
Stock, fish, home-prepared	1 cup	40	5	1	0	0	0	363	2
Stockpot, canned, condensed, commercial	1 cup	200	10	7	23	NA	NA	2097	8
Stockpot, canned, prepared with equal volume water, commercial	1 cup	99	5	4	11	NA	NA	1047	5
Tomato beef with noodle, canned, condensed, commercial	1 cup	281	9	8	42	39	3	1835	8
Tomato beef with noodle, canned, prepared with equal volume water, commercial	1 cup	139	4	4	21	20	1	917	5
Tomato bisque, canned, condensed, commercial	1 cup	247	5	5	47	45	2	2097	10
Tomato bisque, canned, prepared with equal volume milk, commercial	1 cup	198	6	6	29	29	1	1109	23
Tomato bisque, canned, prepared with equal volume water, commercial	1 cup	124	2	2	24	23	0	1047	5
Tomato rice, canned, condensed, commercial	1 cup	239	4	5	44	41	3	1632	3
Tomato rice, canned, prepared with equal volume water, commercial	1 cup	119	2	2	22	20	1	815	2

Description	Serving Size	Cal	Prot (g)	Fat (g)	Carbs (g)	Net Carb(g)	Fiber (g)	Sod (mg)	Chol (mg)
SOUPS (continued)									
Tomato vegetable mix, dry form	1 tbsp	4	0	0	1	1	0	81	0
Tomato vegetable, prepared with water	1 cup	53	2	1	10	9	0	1092	0
Tomato, canned, condensed, commercial	1 cup	171	4	3	33	32	1	1391	0
Tomato, canned, prepared with equal volume milk, commercial	1 cup	161	6	6	22	20	3	744	17
Tomato, canned, prepared with equal volume water, commercial	1 cup	85	2	2	17	16	0	695	0
Tomato, dehydrated, prepared with water	1 cup	103	2	2	19	19	1	943	0
Turkey noodle, canned, condensed, commercial	1 cup	138	8	4	17	16	2	1632	10
Turkey noodle, canned, prepared with equal volume water, commercial	1 cup	68	4	2	9	8	1	815	5
Turkey vegetable, canned, condensed, commercial	1 cup	148	6	6	17	16	1	1818	2
Turkey vegetable, canned, prepared with equal volume water, commercial	1 cup	72	3	3	9	8	0	906	2
Turkey, chunky, ready-to-serve	1 cup	135	10	4	14	NA	NA	923	9
Vegetable beef, canned, condensed, commercial	1 cup	158	11	4	20	16	4	1584	10
Vegetable beef, dehydrated, dry	1 cup	57	3	1	9	8	0	1066	1
Vegetable beef, dehydrated, prepared with water	1 cup	53	3	1	8	8	1	1002	0
Vegetable beef, microwavable, ready-to-serve, single brand	1 serving	128	18	2	10	5	4	1098	9
Vegetable beef, prepared with equal volume water, commercial	1 cup	78	6	2	10	10	0	791	5
Vegetable with beef broth, canned, condensed, commercial	1 cup	162	6	4	26	23	3	1626	2
Vegetable with beef broth, canned, prepared with equal volume water, commercial	1 cup	82	3	2	13	13	0	810	2
Vegetable, canned, chunky, ready-to-serve, commercial	1 cup	122	4	4	19	18	1	1010	0
Vegetarian vegetable, canned, condensed, commercial	1 cup	145	4	4	24	23	1	1653	0
Vegetarian vegetable, canned, prepared with equal volume water, commercial	1 cup	72	2	2	12	11	0	822	0

Description	Serving Size	Cal	Prot (g)	Fat (g)	Carbs (g)	Net Carb(g)	Fiber (g)	Sod (mg)	Chol (mg)
Allspice, ground	1 tsp	5	0	0	1	1	0	1	0
Allspice, ground	1 tbsp	16	0	1	4	3	1	5	0
Anise seed	1 tsp	7	0	0	1	1	0	0	0
Anise seed	1 tbsp	23	1	1	3	2	1	1	0
Basil, dried	1 tsp	4	0	0	1	0	1	0	0
Basil, dried	1 tbsp	11	1	0	3	1	2	2	0
Basil, fresh	5 leaves	1	0	0	0	0	0	0	0
Basil, fresh	2 tbsp	1	0	0	0	0	0	0	0
Bay leaf	1 tsp, crumbled	2	0	0	0	0	0	0	0
Bay leaf	1 tbsp, crumbled	6	0	0	1	1	0	0	0
Capers, canned	1 tbsp	2	0	0	0	0	0	255	0
Caraway seed	1 tsp	7	0	0	1	0	1	0	0
Caraway seed	1 tbsp	22	1	1	3	1	3	1	0
Cardamom	1 tsp	6	0	0	1	1	1	0	0
Cardamom	1 tbsp	18	1	0	4	2	2	1	0
Celery seed	1 tsp	8	0	1	1	1	0	3	0
Celery seed	1 tbsp	25	1	2	3	2	1	10	0
Chervil, dried	1 tsp	1	0	0	0	0	0	0	0
Chervil, dried	1 tbsp	5	0	0	1	1	0	2	0
Chili powder	1 tsp	8	0	0	1	1	1	26	0
Chili powder	1 tbsp	24	1	1	4	2	3	76	0
Cinnamon, ground	1 tsp	6	0	0	2	1	1	1	0
Cinnamon, ground	1 tbsp	18	0	0	5	2	4	2	0
Cloves, ground	1 tsp	7	0	0	1	1	1	5	0
Cloves, ground	1 tbsp	21	0	1	4	2	2	16	0
Coriander leaf, dried	1 tsp	2	0	0	0	0	0	1	0
Coriander leaf, dried	1 tbsp	5	0	0	1	1	0	4	0
Coriander seed	1 tsp	5	0	0	1	0	1	1	0
Coriander seed	1 tbsp	15	1	1	3	1	2	2	0
Cumin seed	1 tsp	8	0	0	1	1	0	4	0
Cumin seed	1 tbsp	23	1	1	3	2	1	10	0
Curry powder	1 tsp	7	0	0	1	0	1	1	0
Curry powder	1 tbsp	20	1	1	4	2	2	3	0
Dill seed	1 tsp	6	0	0	1	1	0	0	0
Dill seed	1 tbsp	20	1	1	4	2	1	1	0
Dill weed, dried	1 tsp	3	0	0	1	0	0	2	0

Description	Serving Size	Cal	Prot (g)	Fat (g)	Carbs (g)	Net Carb(g)	Fiber (g)	Sod (mg)	Chol (mg)
Dill weed, dried	1 tbsp	8	1	0	2	1	0	6	0
Dill weed, fresh	5 sprigs	0	0	0	0	0	0	1	0
Dill weed, fresh	1 cup, sprigs	4	0	0	1	0	0	5	0
Fennel seed	1 tsp	7	0	0	1	0	1	2	0
Fennel seed	1 tbsp	20	1	1	3	1	2	5	0
Fenugreek seed	1 tsp	12	1	0	2	1	1	2	0
Fenugreek seed	1 tbsp	36	3	1	6	4	3	7	0
Garlic powder	1 tsp	9	0	0	2	2	0	1	0
Garlic powder	1 tbsp	28	1	0	6	5	1	2	0
Ginger, ground	1 tsp	6	0	0	1	1	0	1	0
Ginger, ground	1 tbsp	19	0	0	4	3	1	2	0
Horseradish, prepared	1 tsp	2	0	0	1	0	0	16	0
Horseradish, prepared	1 tbsp	7	0	0	2	1	0	47	0
Mace, ground	1 tsp	8	0	1	1	1	0	1	0
Mace, ground	1 tbsp	25	0	2	3	2	1	4	0
Marjoram, dried	1 tsp	2	0	0	0	0	0	0	0
Marjoram, dried	1 tbsp	5	0	0	1	0	1	1	0
Mustard seed, yellow	1 tsp	15	1	1	1	1	0	0	0
Mustard seed, yellow	1 tbsp	53	3	3	4	2	2	1	0
Mustard, prepared, yellow	1 tsp	3	0	0	0	0	0	56	0
Mustard, prepared, yellow	1 cup	165	10	8	19	11	8	2800	0
Nutmeg, ground	1 tsp	12	0	1	1	1	0	0	0
Nutmeg, ground	1 tbsp	37	0	3	3	2	1	1	0
Onion powder	1 tsp	7	0	0	2	2	0	1	0
Onion powder	1 tbsp	23	1	0	5	5	0	4	0
Oregano, dried	1 tsp	5	0	0	1	0	1	1	0
Oregano, dried	1 tbsp	14	0	0	3	1	2	1	0
Paprika	1 tsp	6	0	0	1	1	0	1	0
Paprika	1 tbsp	20	1	1	4	2	1	2	0
Parsley, dried	1 tsp	1	0	0	0	0	0	1	0
Parsley, dried	1 tbsp	4	0	0	1	0	0	6	0
Pepper, black	1 tsp	5	0	0	1	1	1	1	0
Pepper, black	1 tbsp	16	1	0	4	2	2	3	0
Pepper, red or cayenne	1 tsp	6	0	0	1	1	0	1	0
Pepper, red or cayenne	1 tbsp	17	1	1	3	2	1	2	0
Pepper, white	1 tsp	7	0	0	2	1	1	0	0
Pepper, white	1 tbsp	21	1	0	5	3	2	0	0
Peppermint, fresh	2 leaves	0	0	0	0	0	0	0	0

Description	Serving Size	Cal	Prot (g)	Fat (g)	Carbs (g)	Net Carb(g)	Fiber (g)	Sod (mg)	Chol (mg)
Peppermint, fresh	2 tbsp	2	0	0	0	0	0	1	0
Poppy seed	1 tsp	15	1	1	1	0	0	1	0
Poppy seed	1 tbsp	47	2	4	2	1	1	2	0
Poultry seasoning	1 tsp	5	0	0	1	1	0	0	0
Poultry seasoning	1 tbsp	11	0	0	2	2	0	1	0
Pumpkin pie spice	1 tsp	6	0	0	1	1	0	1	0
Pumpkin pie spice	1 tbsp	19	0	1	4	3	1	3	0
Rosemary, dried	1 tsp	4	0	0	1	0	1	1	0
Rosemary, dried	1 tbsp	11	0	1	2	1	1	2	0
Rosemary, fresh	1 tsp	1	0	0	0	0	0	0	0
Rosemary, fresh	1 tbsp	2	0	0	0	0	0	0	0
Saffron	1 tsp	2	0	0	0	0	0	1	0
Saffron	1 tbsp	7	0	0	1	1	0	3	0
Sage, ground	1 tsp	2	0	0	0	0	0	0	0
Sage, ground	1 tbsp	6	0	0	1	0	1	0	0
Salt, table	1 tbsp	0	0	0	0	0	0	0	0
Salt, table	1 cup	0	0	0	0	0	0	0	0
Savory, ground	1 tsp	4	0	0	1	0	1	0	0
Savory, ground	1 tbsp	12	0	0	3	1	2	1	0
Spearmint, dried	1 tsp	1	0	0	0	0	0	2	0
Spearmint, dried	1 tbsp	5	0	0	1	0	0	6	0
Spearmint, fresh	2 tbsp	5	0	0	1	0	1	3	0
Tarragon, dried	1 tsp	5	0	0	1	1	0	1	0
Tarragon, dried	1 tbsp	14	1	0	2	2	0	3	0
Thyme, dried	1 tsp	4	0	0	1	0	1	1	0
Thyme, dried	1 tbsp	12	0	0	3	1	2	2	0
Thyme, fresh	1/2 tsp	0	0	0	0	0	0	0	0
Thyme, fresh	1 tsp	1	0	0	0	0	0	0	0
Turmeric, ground	1 tsp	8	0	0	1	1	0	1	0
Turmeric, ground	1 tbsp	24	1	1	4	3	1	3	0
Vanilla extract	1 tbsp	37	0	0	2	2	0	1	0
Vanilla extract	1 cup	599	0	0	26	26	0	19	0
Vanilla extract, imitation, alcohol	1 tsp	10	0	0	0	0	0	0	0
Vanilla extract, imitation, alcohol	1 tbsp	31	0	0	0	0	0	1	0
Vanilla extract, imitation, no alcohol	1 tsp	2	0	0	1	1	0	0	0
Vanilla extract, imitation, no alcohol	1 tbsp	7	0	0	2	2	0	0	0
Vinegar, cider	1 tbsp	2	0	0	1	1	0	0	0
Vinegar, cider	1 cup	34	0	0	14	14	0	2	0

Description	Serving Size	Cal	Prot (g)	Fat (g)	Carbs (g)	Net Carb(g)	Fiber (g)	Sod (mg)	Chol (mg)
Alfalfa Seeds									
Sprouted, raw	1 cup	10	1	0	1	0	1	2	0
Sprouted, raw	1 tbsp	1	0	0	0	0	0	0	0
Amaranth Leaves									
Boiled, drained	1 cup	28	3	0	5	NA	NA	28	0
Raw	1 cup	6	1	0	1	NA	NA	6	0
Raw	1 leaf	3	0	0	1	NA	NA	3	0
Arrowhead									
Boiled, drained	1 medium	9	1	0	2	NA	NA	2	0
Raw	1 large	25	1	0	5	NA	NA	6	0
Raw	1 medium	12	1	0	2	NA	NA	3	0
Artichokes									
Globe or French, boiled, drained	1/2 cup, hearts	42	3	0	9	5	5	80	0
Globe or French, boiled, drained	1 artichoke	60	4	0	13	7	6	114	0
Globe or French, raw	1 artichoke	60	4	0	13	7	7	120	0
Jerusalem-artichokes, raw	1 cup, sliced	114	3	0	26	24	2	6	0
Arugula									
Raw	1/2 cup	3	0	0	0	0	0	3	0
Raw	1 leaf	1	0	0	0	0	0	1	0
Asparagus									
Boiled, drained	1/2 cup	22	2	0	4	2	1	10	0
Boiled, drained	4 spears	14	2	0	3	2	1	7	0
Canned, drained solids	1 cup	46	5	1	6	2	4	695	0
Canned, drained solids	1 spear	3	0	0	0	0	0	52	0
Canned, no salt added, solids and liquids	1/2 cup	18	2	0	3	2	1	32	0
Canned, regular pack, solids and liquids	1/2 cup	18	2	0	3	2	1	346	0
Raw	1 cup	31	3	0	6	3	3	3	0
Raw	1 spear	3	0	0	1	0	0	0	0
Balsam-pear									
Boiled, drained	1 cup	20	2	0	4	3	1	8	0
Leafy tips, raw	1/2 cup	7	1	0	1	NA	NA	3	0
Leafy tips, raw	1 leaf	1	0	0	0	NA	NA	0	0
Pods, boiled, drained	1 cup	24	1	0	5	3	2	7	0

Description	Serving Size	Cal	Prot (g)	Fat (g)	Carbs (g)	Net Carb(g)	Fiber (g)	Sod (mg)	Chol (mg)
BALSAM-PEAR (continued)									
Pods, raw	1 cup	16	1	0	3	1	3	5	0

Bamboo Shoots

Description	Serving Size	Cal	Prot (g)	Fat (g)	Carbs (g)	Net Carb(g)	Fiber (g)	Sod (mg)	Chol (mg)
Boiled, drained	1 cup	14	2	0	2	1	1	5	0
Boiled, drained	1 shoot	17	2	0	3	1	1	6	0
Canned, drained solids	1 cup	25	2	0	4	2	2	9	0
Raw	1 cup	41	4	0	8	5	3	6	0

Beans

Description	Serving Size	Cal	Prot (g)	Fat (g)	Carbs (g)	Net Carb(g)	Fiber (g)	Sod (mg)	Chol (mg)
Fava, in pod, raw	1 cup	111	10	1	22	NA	NA	32	0
Lima	1/2 cup	88	5	0	17	12	4	312	0
Mung	1 cup	15	2	0	3	2	1	175	0
Navy	1 cup	70	6	1	14	NA	NA	14	0
Pinto	1 package	460	26	1	88	63	24	236	0
Shellie, canned	1 cup	74	4	0	15	7	8	818	0
Snap, canned, all styles	1/2 cup	18	1	0	4	2	2	425	0
Snap, green variety, canned	1/2 cup	18	1	0	4	2	2	311	0
Snap, green, raw	1 cup	34	2	0	8	4	4	7	0

Beets

Description	Serving Size	Cal	Prot (g)	Fat (g)	Carbs (g)	Net Carb(g)	Fiber (g)	Sod (mg)	Chol (mg)
Boiled, drained	1/2 cup, sliced	37	1	0	8	7	2	65	0
Boiled, drained	2 beets	44	2	0	10	8	2	77	0
Canned, drained solids	1 cup, diced	49	1	0	11	9	3	305	0
Greens, raw	1 cup	7	1	0	2	0	1	76	0
Greens, raw	1 leaf	6	1	0	1	0	1	64	0
Harvard, canned, solids and liquids	1 cup, sliced	180	2	0	45	39	6	399	0
Pickled, canned, solids and liquids	1 cup, sliced	148	2	0	37	31	6	599	0
Raw	1 beet	35	1	0	8	6	2	64	0
Raw	1 cup	58	2	0	13	9	4	106	0

Borage

Description	Serving Size	Cal	Prot (g)	Fat (g)	Carbs (g)	Net Carb(g)	Fiber (g)	Sod (mg)	Chol (mg)
Raw	1 cup	19	2	0	3	NA	NA	71	0

Broccoli

Description	Serving Size	Cal	Prot (g)	Fat (g)	Carbs (g)	Net Carb(g)	Fiber (g)	Sod (mg)	Chol (mg)
Boiled	1 stalk	78	8	1	14	6	8	73	0
Broccoli, raw	1 cup, chop.	25	3	0	5	2	3	24	0
Broccoli, raw	1 stalk	32	3	0	6	3	3	31	0
Chinese, cooked	1 cup	19	1	0	3	1	2	6	0
Frozen, chopped, boiled	1 cup	52	6	0	10	4	6	44	0

Description	Serving Size	Cal	Prot (g)	Fat (g)	Carbs (g)	Net Carb(g)	Fiber (g)	Sod (mg)	Chol (mg)
Brudock Root									
Boiled, drained	1 cup	110	3	0	26	24	2	5	0
Raw	1 cup	85	2	0	20	17	4	6	0
Brussel Sprouts									
Boiled, drained	1/2 cup	30	2	0	7	5	2	16	0
Boiled, drained	1 sprout	8	1	0	2	1	1	4	0
Frozen, boiled, drained	1 cup	65	6	0	13	7	6	36	0
Frozen, unprepared	1 package	116	11	1	22	12	11	28	0
Raw	1 cup	38	3	0	8	5	3	22	0
Raw	1 sprout	8	1	0	2	1	1	5	0
Butterbur									
Canned	1 cup, chop.	4	0	0	0	NA	NA	5	0
Raw	1 cup	13	0	0	3	NA	NA	7	0
Cabbage									
Chinese (pak-choi), boiled, drained	1 cup, shred.	20	3	0	3	0	3	58	0
Chinese (pak-choi), raw	1 cup, shred.	9	1	0	2	1	1	46	0
Chinese (pe-tsai), boiled, drained	1 cup, shred.	17	2	0	3	0	3	11	0
Chinese (pe-tsai), raw	1 cup, shred.	12	1	0	2	0	2	7	0
Coleslaw, home-prepared	1/2 cup	41	1	1	7	7	1	14	5
Napa, cooked	1 cup	13	1	0	2	NA	NA	12	0
Raw	1/2 cup, shred.	8	0	0	2	1	1	6	0
Raw	1 head	218	11	1	49	28	21	163	0
Red, boiled, drained	1/2 cup, shred.	16	1	0	3	2	2	6	0
Red, boiled, drained	1 leaf	5	0	0	1	1	0	2	0
Red, raw	1 cup, chop.	24	1	0	5	4	2	10	0
Sauerkraut, canned, solids and liquids	1 cup	27	1	0	6	3	4	939	0
Savoy, boiled, drained	1 cup, shred.	35	3	0	8	4	4	35	0
Savoy, raw	1 cup, shred.	19	1	0	4	2	2	20	0
Swamp (skunk cabbage), raw	1 cup, chop.	11	1	0	2	1	1	63	0
Swamp cabbage, boiled, drained	1 cup, chop.	20	2	0	4	2	2	120	0
Cardoon									
Raw	1 cup, shred.	36	1	0	9	6	3	303	0
Carrots									
Baby, raw	1 large	6	0	0	1	1	0	5	0
Baby, raw	1 medium	4	0	0	1	1	0	4	0

Description	Serving Size	Cal	Prot (g)	Fat (g)	Carbs (g)	Net Carb(g)	Fiber (g)	Sod (mg)	Chol (mg)
CARROTS (continued)									
Boiled, drained	1/2 cup, sliced	35	1	0	8	6	3	51	0
Canned, no salt added, drained solids	1 cup, mash.	57	1	0	13	9	3	96	0
Canned, regular pack, drained solids	1 cup, mash.	57	1	0	13	9	3	552	0
Frozen, boiled, drained	1 cup, sliced	53	2	0	12	7	5	86	0
Frozen, unprepared	1/2 cup, sliced	25	1	0	6	4	2	38	0
Raw	1 cup, chop.	55	1	0	13	9	4	45	0

Cassava

Description	Serving Size	Cal	Prot (g)	Fat (g)	Carbs (g)	Net Carb(g)	Fiber (g)	Sod (mg)	Chol (mg)
Raw	1 cup	330	3	0	78	75	4	29	0

Catsup

Description	Serving Size	Cal	Prot (g)	Fat (g)	Carbs (g)	Net Carb(g)	Fiber (g)	Sod (mg)	Chol (mg)
Low sodium	1 tbsp	16	0	0	4	4	0	3	0
Regular	1 tbsp	16	0	0	4	4	0	178	0

Cauliflower

Description	Serving Size	Cal	Prot (g)	Fat (g)	Carbs (g)	Net Carb(g)	Fiber (g)	Sod (mg)	Chol (mg)
Boiled, drained	1/2 cup	14	1	0	3	1	2	9	0
Boiled, drained	3 flowerets	12	1	0	2	1	1	8	0
Boiled, drained	3 flowerets	12	1	0	2	1	1	8	0
Green, cooked	1/10 head	29	3	0	6	3	3	21	0
Frozen, boiled, drained	1 cup	34	3	0	7	2	5	32	0
Frozen, unprepared	1/2 cup	16	1	0	3	2	2	16	0
Frozen, unprepared	1 package	68	6	1	13	7	7	68	0
Raw	1 cup	25	2	0	5	3	3	30	0
Raw	1 floweret	3	0	0	1	0	0	4	0

Celeriac

Description	Serving Size	Cal	Prot (g)	Fat (g)	Carbs (g)	Net Carb(g)	Fiber (g)	Sod (mg)	Chol (mg)
Celeriac, boiled, drained	1 cup, pieces	42	1	0	9	7	2	95	0
Raw	1 cup	66	2	0	14	12	3	156	0

Celery

Description	Serving Size	Cal	Prot (g)	Fat (g)	Carbs (g)	Net Carb(g)	Fiber (g)	Sod (mg)	Chol (mg)
Celery, boiled, drained	1 cup, diced	27	1	0	6	4	2	137	0
Celery, boiled, drained	2 stalks	14	1	0	3	2	1	68	0
Raw	1 cup, diced	19	1	0	4	2	2	104	0
Raw	1 cup, strips	20	1	0	5	2	2	108	0

Celtuce

Description	Serving Size	Cal	Prot (g)	Fat (g)	Carbs (g)	Net Carb(g)	Fiber (g)	Sod (mg)	Chol (mg)
Raw	1 leaf	1	0	0	0	0	0	1	0

Chard

Description	Serving Size	Cal	Prot (g)	Fat (g)	Carbs (g)	Net Carb(g)	Fiber (g)	Sod (mg)	Chol (mg)
Swiss, boiled, drained	1 cup, chop.	35	3	0	7	4	4	313	0

Description	Serving Size	Cal	Prot (g)	Fat (g)	Carbs (g)	Net Carb(g)	Fiber (g)	Sod (mg)	Chol (mg)
Swiss, raw	1 cup	7	1	0	1	1	1	77	0
Swiss, raw	1 leaf	9	1	0	2	1	1	102	0

Chayote

Description	Serving Size	Cal	Prot (g)	Fat (g)	Carbs (g)	Net Carb(g)	Fiber (g)	Sod (mg)	Chol (mg)
Fruit, boiled, drained	1 cup	38	1	0	8	4	4	2	0
Fruit, raw	1 chayote	39	2	0	9	6	3	4	0
Fruit, raw	1 cup	25	1	0	6	4	2	3	0

Chicory

Description	Serving Size	Cal	Prot (g)	Fat (g)	Carbs (g)	Net Carb(g)	Fiber (g)	Sod (mg)	Chol (mg)
Greens, raw	1 cup, chop.	41	3	0	8	1	7	81	0
Roots, raw	1/2 cup	33	1	0	8	NA	NA	23	0
Roots, raw	1 root	44	1	0	11	NA	NA	30	0
Witloof, raw	1/2 cup	8	0	0	2	0	1	1	0
Witloof, raw	1 head	9	0	0	2	0	2	1	0

Chives

Description	Serving Size	Cal	Prot (g)	Fat (g)	Carbs (g)	Net Carb(g)	Fiber (g)	Sod (mg)	Chol (mg)
Freeze-dried	1/4 cup	2	0	0	1	0	0	1	0
Freeze-dried	1 tbsp	1	0	0	0	0	0	0	0
Raw	1 tbsp, chop.	1	0	0	0	0	0	0	0

Chrysanthemum

Description	Serving Size	Cal	Prot (g)	Fat (g)	Carbs (g)	Net Carb(g)	Fiber (g)	Sod (mg)	Chol (mg)
Garland, boiled, drained	1 cup	20	2	0	4	2	2	53	0
Garland, raw	1 cup	5	0	0	1	0	1	13	0
Garland, raw	1 stem	3	0	0	1	0	0	7	0
Leaves, raw	1 cup, chop.	12	2	0	2	0	2	60	0
Leaves, raw	1 leaf	4	1	0	1	0	1	21	0

Collards

Description	Serving Size	Cal	Prot (g)	Fat (g)	Carbs (g)	Net Carb(g)	Fiber (g)	Sod (mg)	Chol (mg)
Boiled, drained	1 cup, chop.	49	4	0	9	4	5	17	0
Frozen, chopped, boiled, drained	1 cup, chop.	61	5	0	12	7	5	85	0
Frozen, chopped, unprepared	1 package	94	8	1	18	8	10	136	0
Frozen, chopped, unprepared	1 package	449	37	3	88	39	49	653	0
Raw	1 cup, chop.	11	1	0	2	1	1	7	0

Coriander

Description	Serving Size	Cal	Prot (g)	Fat (g)	Carbs (g)	Net Carb(g)	Fiber (g)	Sod (mg)	Chol (mg)
Coriander (cilantro) leaves, raw	1/4 cup	1	0	0	0	0	0	2	0
Coriander (cilantro) leaves, raw	9 plants	5	0	0	1	0	1	9	0

Corn

Description	Serving Size	Cal	Prot (g)	Fat (g)	Carbs (g)	Net Carb(g)	Fiber (g)	Sod (mg)	Chol (mg)
Corn pudding, home-prepared	2/3 cup	182	7	8	21	NA	NA	92	167
Corn pudding, home-prepared	1 cup	273	11	12	32	NA	NA	138	250

Description	Serving Size	Cal	Prot (g)	Fat (g)	Carbs (g)	Net Carb(g)	Fiber (g)	Sod (mg)	Chol (mg)
CORN (continued)									
Corn salad, raw	1 cup	12	1	0	2	NA	NA	2	0
Corn with red and green peppers, canned, solids and liquids	1 cup	170	5	1	41	NA	NA	788	0
Sweet, white, boiled, drained	1/2 cup, cut	89	3	1	21	18	2	14	0
Sweet, white, boiled, drained	1 ear	83	3	1	19	17	2	13	0
Sweet, white, canned, cream style, no salt added	1/2 cup	92	2	0	23	22	2	4	0
Sweet, white, canned, cream style, regular pack	1 cup	184	4	1	46	43	3	730	0
Sweet, white, canned, vacuum pack, no salt added	1/2 cup	83	3	0	20	18	2	3	0
Sweet, white, canned, vacuum pack, regular pack	1/2 cup	83	3	0	20	18	2	286	0
Sweet, white, canned, whole kernel, drained solids	1 cup	133	4	2	30	27	3	530	0
Sweet, white, canned, whole kernel, no salt added, solids and liquids	1/2 cup	82	2	1	20	19	1	15	0
Sweet, white, canned, whole kernel, regular pack, solids and liquids	1/2 cup	82	2	1	20	18	2	273	0
Sweet, white, frozen, kernels cut off cob, boiled, drained	1/2 cup	66	2	0	16	14	2	4	0
Sweet, white, frozen, kernels cut off cob, boiled, drained	1 package	227	8	1	56	49	7	14	0
Sweet, white, frozen, kernels cut off cob, unprepared	1/2 cup	72	2	1	17	15	2	2	0
Sweet, white, frozen, kernels cut off cob, unprepared	1 package	250	9	2	59	52	7	9	0
Sweet, white, frozen, kernels on cob, boiled, drained	1/2 cup	76	3	1	18	17	2	3	0
Sweet, white, frozen, kernels on cob, boiled, drained	1 ear	59	2	0	14	13	1	3	0
Sweet, white, frozen, kernels on cob, unprepared	1/2 cup	80	3	1	19	17	2	4	0
Sweet, white, frozen, kernels on cob, unprepared	1 ear	123	4	1	29	26	4	6	0
Sweet, white, raw	1 cup	132	5	2	29	25	4	23	0
Sweet, white, raw	1 ear	123	5	2	27	23	4	21	0
Sweet, yellow, boiled, drained	1 baby ear	9	0	0	2	2	0	1	0
Sweet, yellow, boiled, drained	1 cup	177	5	2	41	37	5	28	0
Sweet, yellow, canned, brine pack, regular pack, solids and liquids	1/2 cup	82	2	1	20	18	2	273	0

Description	Serving Size	Cal	Prot (g)	Fat (g)	Carbs (g)	Net Carb(g)	Fiber (g)	Sod (mg)	Chol (mg)
Sweet, yellow, canned, cream style, no salt added	1 cup	184	4	1	46	43	3	8	0
Sweet, yellow, canned, cream style, regular pack	1 cup	184	4	1	46	43	3	730	0
Sweet, yellow, canned, no salt added, solids and liquids	1/2 cup	82	2	1	20	18	2	15	0
Sweet, yellow, canned, vacuum pack, no salt added	1/2 cup	83	3	0	20	18	2	3	0
Sweet, yellow, canned, vacuum pack, regular pack	1/2 cup	83	3	0	20	18	2	286	0
Sweet, yellow, canned, whole kernel, drained solids	1 cup	133	4	2	30	27	3	351	0
Sweet, yellow, frozen, kernels cut off cob, boiled, drained	1/2 cup	66	2	0	16	14	2	4	0
Sweet, yellow, frozen, kernels cut off cob, boiled, drained	1 package	227	8	1	56	49	7	14	0
Sweet, yellow, frozen, kernels cut off cob, unprepared	1/2 cup	72	2	1	17	15	2	2	0
Sweet, yellow, frozen, kernels cut off cob, unprepared	1 package	250	9	2	59	52	7	9	0
Sweet, yellow, frozen, kernels on cob, boiled, drained	1/2 cup	76	3	1	18	16	2	3	0
Sweet, yellow, frozen, kernels on cob, boiled, drained	1 ear	59	2	0	14	12	2	3	0
Sweet, yellow, frozen, kernels on cob, unprepared	1/2 cup	80	3	1	19	17	2	4	0
Sweet, yellow, frozen, kernels on cob, unprepared	1 ear	123	4	1	29	26	4	6	0
Sweet, yellow, raw	1 cup	132	5	2	29	25	4	23	0
Sweet, yellow, raw	1 ear	123	5	2	27	23	4	21	0

Cowpeas

Description	Serving Size	Cal	Prot (g)	Fat (g)	Carbs (g)	Net Carb(g)	Fiber (g)	Sod (mg)	Chol (mg)
Leafy tips, boiled, drained	1 cup, chop.	12	2	0	1	NA	NA	3	0
Leafy tips, raw	1 cup, chop.	10	1	0	2	NA	NA	3	0
Leafy tips, raw	1 leaf	1	0	0	0	NA	NA	0	0
Young pods with seeds, boiled, drained	1 cup	32	2	0	7	NA	NA	3	0
Young pods with seeds, raw	1 cup	41	3	0	9	NA	NA	4	0
Young pods with seeds, raw	1 pod	5	0	0	1	NA	NA	0	0

Cowpeas (Blackeyes)

Description	Serving Size	Cal	Prot (g)	Fat (g)	Carbs (g)	Net Carb(g)	Fiber (g)	Sod (mg)	Chol (mg)
Immature seeds, boiled, drained	1 cup	160	5	0	34	25	8	7	0
Immature seeds, frozen, unprepared	1 cup	222	14	1	40	32	8	10	0
Immature seeds, frozen, unprepared	1 package	395	26	2	71	57	14	17	0

Description	Serving Size	Cal	Prot (g)	Fat (g)	Carbs (g)	Net Carb(g)	Fiber (g)	Sod (mg)	Chol (mg)
COWPEAS (BLACKEYE) (continued)									
Immature seeds, raw	1 cup	131	4	0	27	20	7	6	0

Cress

Description	Serving Size	Cal	Prot (g)	Fat (g)	Carbs (g)	Net Carb(g)	Fiber (g)	Sod (mg)	Chol (mg)
Garden, boiled, drained	1/2 cup	16	1	0	3	2	0	5	0
Garden, boiled, drained	1 cup	31	3	1	5	4	1	11	0
Garden, raw	1 cup	16	1	0	3	2	1	7	0
Garden, raw	1 sprig	0	0	0	0	0	0	0	0

Cucumber

Description	Serving Size	Cal	Prot (g)	Fat (g)	Carbs (g)	Net Carb(g)	Fiber (g)	Sod (mg)	Chol (mg)
Peeled, raw	1 cup, pared	16	1	0	3	2	1	3	0
Peeled, raw	1 cup, sliced	14	1	0	3	2	1	2	0
With peel, raw	1/2 cup, sliced	7	0	0	1	1	0	1	0
With peel, raw	1 cucumber	39	2	0	8	6	2	6	0

Dandelion

Description	Serving Size	Cal	Prot (g)	Fat (g)	Carbs (g)	Net Carb(g)	Fiber (g)	Sod (mg)	Chol (mg)
Greens, boiled, drained	1 cup, chop.	35	2	0	7	4	3	46	0
Greens, raw	1 cup, chop.	25	1	0	5	3	2	42	0

Dock

Description	Serving Size	Cal	Prot (g)	Fat (g)	Carbs (g)	Net Carb(g)	Fiber (g)	Sod (mg)	Chol (mg)
Raw	1 cup, chop.	29	3	0	4	0	4	5	0

Eggplant

Description	Serving Size	Cal	Prot (g)	Fat (g)	Carbs (g)	Net Carb(g)	Fiber (g)	Sod (mg)	Chol (mg)
Boiled, drained	1 cup	28	1	0	7	4	2	3	0
Raw	1 cup, cubes	21	1	0	5	3	2	2	0
Raw	1 eggplant, peeled	119	5	1	28	16	11	14	0

Endive

Description	Serving Size	Cal	Prot (g)	Fat (g)	Carbs (g)	Net Carb(g)	Fiber (g)	Sod (mg)	Chol (mg)
Raw	1/2 cup, chop.	4	0	0	1	0	1	6	0
Raw	1 head	87	6	1	17	1	16	113	0

Epazote

Description	Serving Size	Cal	Prot (g)	Fat (g)	Carbs (g)	Net Carb(g)	Fiber (g)	Sod (mg)	Chol (mg)
Raw	1 sprig	1	0	0	0	0	0	1	0
Raw	1 tbsp	0	0	0	0	0	0	0	0

Eppaw

Description	Serving Size	Cal	Prot (g)	Fat (g)	Carbs (g)	Net Carb(g)	Fiber (g)	Sod (mg)	Chol (mg)
Raw	1 cup	150	5	0	32	NA	NA	12	0

Fennel

Description	Serving Size	Cal	Prot (g)	Fat (g)	Carbs (g)	Net Carb(g)	Fiber (g)	Sod (mg)	Chol (mg)
Bulb, raw	1 bulb	73	3	0	17	10	7	122	0
Bulb, raw	1 cup, sliced	27	1	0	6	4	3	45	0

Description	Serving Size	Cal	Prot (g)	Fat (g)	Carbs (g)	Net Carb(g)	Fiber (g)	Sod (mg)	Chol (mg)
Flour									
Potato flour	1 cup	571	11	0	133	123	9	88	0
Garlic									
Raw	1 cup	203	9	0	45	42	3	23	0
Raw	1 tsp	4	0	0	1	1	0	0	0
Ginger Root									
Raw	1/4 cup, sliced	17	0	0	4	3	0	3	0
Raw	1 tsp	1	0	0	0	0	0	0	0
Gourd									
Dishcloth (towelgourd), boiled, drained	1/2 cup	50	1	0	13	NA	NA	19	0
Dishcloth (towelgourd), boiled, drained	1 cup	100	1	0	26	NA	NA	37	0
Dishcloth (towelgourd), raw	1 cup	19	1	0	4	NA	NA	3	0
Dishcloth (towelgourd), raw	1 gourd	36	2	0	8	NA	NA	5	0
White-flowered (calabash), boiled, drained	1 cup	22	1	0	5	NA	NA	3	0
White-flowered (calabash), raw	1/2 cup	8	0	0	2	NA	NA	1	0
White-flowered (calabash), raw	1 gourd	108	5	0	26	NA	NA	15	0
Grape Leaves									
Canned	1 leaf	3	0	0	0	NA	NA	114	0
Raw	1 cup	13	1	0	2	1	2	1	0
Raw	1 leaf	3	0	0	1	0	0	0	0
Heart of Palm									
Canned	1 cup	41	4	1	7	3	4	622	0
Canned	1 piece	9	1	0	2	1	1	141	0
Horseradish									
Leafy tips, boiled, drained	1 cup, chop.	25	2	0	5	4	1	4	0
Leafy tips, raw	1 cup, chop.	13	2	0	2	1	0	2	0
Pods, boiled, drained	1 cup, sliced	42	2	0	10	5	5	51	0
Pods, raw	1 cup, sliced	37	2	0	9	5	3	42	0
Pods, raw	1 pod	4	0	0	1	1	0	5	0
Hyacinth Beans									
Immature seeds, boiled, drained	1 cup	44	3	0	8	NA	NA	2	0
Immature seeds, raw	1 cup	37	2	0	7	NA	NA	2	0

Description	Serving Size	Cal	Prot (g)	Fat (g)	Carbs (g)	Net Carb(g)	Fiber (g)	Sod (mg)	Chol (mg)
Jute									
Potherb, boiled, drained	1 cup	32	3	0	6	5	2	10	0
Potherb, raw	1 cup	10	1	0	2	NA	NA	2	0
Kale									
Boiled, drained	1 cup, chop.	36	2	0	7	5	3	30	0
Frozen, boiled, drained	1 cup, chop.	39	4	0	7	4	3	20	0
Frozen, unprepared	1/3 package	26	3	0	5	3	2	14	0
Raw	1 cup, chop.	34	2	0	7	5	1	29	0
Scotch, boiled, drained	1 cup, chop.	36	2	0	7	6	2	59	0
Scotch, raw	1 cup, chop.	28	2	0	6	4	1	47	0
Kohlrabi									
Boiled, drained	1 cup, sliced	48	3	0	11	9	2	35	0
Raw	1 cup	36	2	0	8	4	5	27	0
Raw	1 slice	4	0	0	1	0	1	3	0
Lambsquarters									
Boiled, drained	1 cup, chop.	58	6	1	9	5	4	52	0
Leeks									
Bulb and lower leaf-portion, boiled, drained	1/4 cup, chop. or diced	8	0	0	2	2	0	3	0
Bulb and lower leaf-portion, boiled, drained	1 leek	38	1	0	9	8	1	12	0
Bulb and lower leaf-portion, raw	1 cup	54	1	0	13	11	2	18	0
Bulb and lower leaf-portion, raw	1 leek	54	1	0	13	11	2	18	0
Bulb and lower-leaf portion, freeze-dried	1/4 cup	3	0	0	1	1	0	0	0
Bulb and lower-leaf portion, freeze-dried	1 tbsp	1	0	0	0	0	0	0	0
Lentils									
Sprouted, raw	1 cup	82	7	0	17	NA	NA	8	0
Lettuce									
Butterhead (includes Boston and Bibb types), raw	1 cup, shred. or chopped	7	1	0	1	1	1	3	0
Butterhead (includes Boston and Bibb types), raw	1 head	21	2	0	4	2	2	8	0
Cos or Romaine, raw	1/2 cup, shred.	4	0	0	1	0	0	2	0
Cos or Romaine, raw	1 inner leaf	1	0	0	0	0	0	1	0

Description	Serving Size	Cal	Prot (g)	Fat (g)	Carbs (g)	Net Carb(g)	Fiber (g)	Sod (mg)	Chol (mg)
Green leaf, raw	1/2 cup, shred.	5	0	0	1	0	1	3	0
Green leaf, raw	1 leaf	2	0	0	0	0	0	1	0
Iceberg (includes crisphead types), raw	1 cup, shred. or chop.	7	1	0	1	0	1	5	0
Iceberg (includes crisphead types), raw	1 head	91	8	1	16	5	11	68	0

Lima Beans

Description	Serving Size	Cal	Prot (g)	Fat (g)	Carbs (g)	Net Carb(g)	Fiber (g)	Sod (mg)	Chol (mg)
Boiled, drained	1 cup	209	12	0	40	31	9	29	0
Canned, no salt added, solids and liquids	1/2 cup	88	5	0	17	12	4	5	0
Canned, no salt added, solids and liquids	1 can	322	18	1	61	44	16	18	0
Frozen, baby, boiled, drained	1/2 cup	95	6	0	18	12	5	26	0
Frozen, baby, boiled, drained	1 package	327	21	1	60	42	19	90	0
Frozen, baby, unprepared	1/2 cup	108	6	0	21	16	5	43	0
Frozen, baby, unprepared	1 package	375	22	1	71	54	17	148	0
Frozen, ford hook, boiled, drained	1/2 cup	85	5	0	16	11	5	45	0
Frozen, ford hook, boiled, drained	1 package	311	19	1	58	40	18	165	0
Frozen, ford hook, unprepared	1/2 cup	85	5	0	16	11	4	46	0
Frozen, ford hook, unprepared	1 package	301	18	1	56	41	16	165	0
Raw	1 cup	176	11	1	31	24	8	12	0

Lotus Root

Description	Serving Size	Cal	Prot (g)	Fat (g)	Carbs (g)	Net Carb(g)	Fiber (g)	Sod (mg)	Chol (mg)
Boiled, drained	1/2 cup	40	1	0	10	8	2	27	0
Boiled, drained	10 slices	59	1	0	14	12	3	40	0
Raw	1 root	85	3	0	20	14	6	46	0
Raw	10 slices	60	2	0	14	10	4	32	0

Malabar Spinach

Description	Serving Size	Cal	Prot (g)	Fat (g)	Carbs (g)	Net Carb(g)	Fiber (g)	Sod (mg)	Chol (mg)
Cooked	1 bunch	4	1	0	0	0	0	9	0
Cooked	1 cup	10	1	0	1	0	1	24	0

Mixed Vegetables

Description	Serving Size	Cal	Prot (g)	Fat (g)	Carbs (g)	Net Carb(g)	Fiber (g)	Sod (mg)	Chol (mg)
Canned, drained solids	1 cup	77	4	0	15	10	5	243	0
Canned, solids and liquids	1 cup	88	3	0	17	8	9	549	0
Frozen, boiled, drained	1/2 cup	54	3	0	12	8	4	32	0
Frozen, boiled, drained	1 package	162	8	0	36	24	12	96	0
Frozen, unprepared	1 pack	726	38	4	153	107	45	533	0
Frozen, unprepared	1 package	182	9	1	38	27	11	133	0

Description	Serving Size	Cal	Prot (g)	Fat (g)	Carbs (g)	Net Carb(g)	Fiber (g)	Sod (mg)	Chol (mg)
Mountain Yam									
Hawaii, raw	1/2 cup, cubes	46	1	0	11	NA	NA	9	0
Hawaii, raw	1 yam	281	6	0	69	NA	NA	55	0
Hawaii, steamed	1 cup, cubes	119	3	0	29	NA	NA	17	0
Mung Beans									
Mature seeds, sprouted, boiled, drained	1 cup	26	3	0	5	4	1	12	0
Mature seeds, sprouted, raw	1 cup	31	3	0	6	4	2	6	0
Mature seeds, sprouted, raw	1 package	102	10	0	20	14	6	20	0
Mature seeds, sprouted, stir-fried	1 cup	62	5	0	13	11	2	11	0
Mushrooms									
Boiled, drained	1 cup, pieces	42	3	0	8	5	3	3	0
Boiled, drained	1 tbsp	3	0	0	1	0	0	0	0
Brown, Italian, or Crimini, raw	1 piece	3	0	0	1	0	0	1	0
Canned, drained solids	1 can	32	2	0	7	3	3	559	0
Canned, drained solids	1 cup	37	3	0	8	4	4	663	0
Enoki, raw	1 large	2	0	0	0	0	0	0	0
Enoki, raw	1 medium	1	0	0	0	0	0	0	0
Oyster, raw	1 large	55	6	0	9	6	4	46	0
Oyster, raw	1 small	6	1	0	1	1	0	5	0
Raw	1 cup, pieces or slices	18	2	0	3	2	1	3	0
Raw	1 cup, whole	24	3	0	4	3	1	4	0
Shiitake, cooked	1 cup, pieces	80	2	0	21	18	3	6	0
Shiitake, cooked	4 mushrooms	40	1	0	10	9	2	3	0
Shiitake, dried	1 mushroom	11	0	0	3	2	0	0	0
Shiitake, dried	4 mushrooms	44	1	0	11	10	2	2	0
Straw, canned, drained solids	1 cup	58	7	1	8	4	5	699	0
Straw, canned, drained solids	1 piece	2	0	0	0	0	0	21	0
Mustard Greens									
Boiled, drained	1 cup, chop.	21	3	0	3	0	3	22	0
Frozen, boiled, drained	1 cup, chop.	29	3	0	5	0	4	38	0
Frozen, unprepared	1 cup, chop.	29	4	0	5	0	5	42	0
Raw	1 cup, chop.	15	2	0	3	1	2	14	0
Mustard Spinach									
Boiled, drained	1 cup, chop.	29	3	0	5	1	4	25	0
Raw	1 cup, chop.	33	3	0	6	2	4	32	0

Description	Serving Size	Cal	Prot (g)	Fat (g)	Carbs (g)	Net Carb(g)	Fiber (g)	Sod (mg)	Chol (mg)
Nopales									
Cooked	1 cup	22	2	0	5	2	3	30	0
Cooked	1 pad	4	0	0	1	0	1	6	0
Raw	1 cup, sliced	14	1	0	3	1	2	19	0
Okra									
Okra, boiled, drained	1/2 cup, sliced	26	1	0	6	4	2	4	0
Okra, boiled, drained	8 pods	27	2	0	6	4	2	4	0
Okra, frozen, boiled, drained	1/2 cup, sliced	26	2	0	5	3	3	3	0
Okra, frozen, boiled, drained	1 package	71	5	1	15	8	7	8	0
Okra, frozen, unprepared	1 package	85	5	0	19	13	6	9	0
Raw	1 cup	33	2	0	8	4	3	8	0
Raw	8 pods	31	2	0	7	4	3	8	0
Onions									
Boiled, drained	1 cup	92	3	0	21	18	3	6	0
Boiled, drained	1 tbsp, chop.	7	0	0	2	1	0	0	0
Canned, solids and liquids	1/2 cup, chop. or diced	21	1	0	4	3	1	416	0
Canned, solids and liquids	1 onion	12	1	0	3	2	1	234	0
Dehydrated flakes	1/4 cup	49	1	0	12	10	1	3	0
Dehydrated flakes	1 tbsp	17	0	0	4	4	0	1	0
Frozen, chopped, boiled, drained	1/2 cup, chop. or diced	29	1	0	7	5	2	13	0
Frozen, chopped, boiled, drained	1 tbsp, chop.	4	0	0	1	1	0	2	0
Frozen, chopped, unprepared	1 package	82	2	0	19	14	5	34	0
Onion rings, breaded, par fried, frozen, prepared, heated in oven	1 cup	195	3	12	18	18	1	180	0
Onion rings, breaded, par fried, frozen, prepared, heated in oven	10 rings	289	4	17	27	26	1	266	0
Onion rings, breaded, par fried, frozen, unprepared	1 package	1171	14	59	139	130	8	1117	0
Onion rings, breaded, par fried, frozen, unprepared	1 package	658	8	33	78	73	5	627	0
Raw	1 cup, chop.	61	2	0	14	11	3	5	0
Raw	1 cup, sliced	44	1	0	10	8	2	3	0
Spring or scallions (includes tops and bulb), raw	1 cup, chop.	32	2	0	7	5	3	16	0
Spring or scallions (includes tops and bulb), raw	1 tbsp, chop.	2	0	0	0	0	0	1	0

Description	Serving Size	Cal	Prot (g)	Fat (g)	Carbs (g)	Net Carb(g)	Fiber (g)	Sod (mg)	Chol (mg)
Parsley									
Freeze-dried	1/4 cup	4	0	0	1	0	0	5	0
Freeze-dried	1 tbsp	1	0	0	0	0	0	2	0
Raw	1 cup	22	2	0	4	2	2	34	0
Raw	1 tbsp	1	0	0	0	0	0	2	0
Parsnips									
Boiled, drained	1/2 cup, sliced	63	1	0	15	12	3	8	0
Boiled, drained	1 parsnip	130	2	0	31	25	6	16	0
Raw	1 cup, sliced	100	2	0	24	17	7	13	0
Peas									
Boiled, drained	1 cup	67	5	0	11	7	4	6	0
Boiled, drained	1 cup	170	9	2	30	20	9	8	0
Frozen, boiled, drained	1 cup	83	6	0	14	9	5	8	0
Frozen, unprepared	1/2 cup	30	2	0	5	3	2	3	0
Green, boiled, drained	1 cup	134	9	0	25	16	9	5	0
Green, canned, no salt added, drained solids	1/2 cup	59	4	0	11	7	3	2	0
Green, canned, no salt added, solids and liquids	1/2 cup	66	4	0	12	8	4	11	0
Green, canned, regular pack, drained solids	1 cup	117	8	0	21	14	7	428	0
Green, canned, regular pack, solids and liquids	1/2 cup	66	4	0	12	8	4	310	0
Green, canned, seasoned, solids and liquids	1/2 cup	57	4	0	11	8	2	290	0
Green, canned, seasoned, solids and liquids	1 cup	114	7	0	21	16	5	577	0
Green, frozen, boiled, drained	1/2 cup	62	4	0	11	7	4	70	0
Green, frozen, boiled, drained	1 package	197	13	1	36	22	14	220	0
Green, frozen, unprepared	1/2 cup	55	4	0	10	6	3	81	0
Green, frozen, unprepared	1 package	219	15	1	39	26	13	318	0
Green, raw	1 cup	117	8	0	21	14	7	7	0
Raw	1 cup	209	11	2	37	29	8	8	0
Raw	1 cup, chop.	41	3	0	7	5	3	4	0
Raw	1 cup, whole	26	2	0	5	3	2	3	0
Raw	10 seeds	5	0	0	1	1	0	0	0
Sprouted, raw	1 cup	154	11	1	34	NA	NA	24	0

Description	Serving Size	Cal	Prot (g)	Fat (g)	Carbs (g)	Net Carb(g)	Fiber (g)	Sod (mg)	Chol (mg)
Peppers									
Ancho, dried	1 pepper	48	2	1	9	5	4	7	0
Banana, raw	1 cup	33	2	0	7	2	4	16	0
Banana, raw	1 small	9	1	0	2	1	1	4	0
Chili, green, canned	1 cup	29	1	0	6	4	2	552	0
Hot chile, sun-dried	1 cup	120	4	2	26	15	11	34	0
Hot chile, sun-dried	1 pepper	2	0	0	0	0	0	0	0
Hot chili, green, canned, pods, excluding seeds, solids and liquids	1/2 cup, chop. or diced	14	1	0	3	3	1	798	0
Hot chili, green, canned, pods, excluding seeds, solids and liquids	1 pepper	15	1	0	4	3	1	856	0
Hot chili, green, raw	1/2 cup, chop. or diced	30	2	0	7	6	1	5	0
Hot chili, green, raw	1 pepper	18	1	0	4	4	1	3	0
Hot chili, red, canned, excluding seeds, solids and liquids	1/2 cup, chop. or diced	14	1	0	3	3	1	798	0
Hot chili, red, canned, excluding seeds, solids and liquids	1 pepper	15	1	0	4	3	1	856	0
Hot chili, red, raw	1/2 cup, chop. or diced	30	2	0	7	6	1	5	0
Hot chili, red, raw	1 pepper	18	1	0	4	4	1	3	0
Hungarian, raw	1 pepper	8	0	0	2	NA	NA	0	0
Jalapeno, canned, solids and liquids	1 cup, chop.	37	1	1	6	3	4	2273	0
Jalapeno, canned, solids and liquids	1 cup, sliced	28	1	1	5	2	3	1738	0
Jalapeno, raw	1 cup, sliced	27	1	0	5	3	3	1	0
Jalapeno, raw	1 pepper	4	0	0	1	0	0	0	0
Pasilla, dried	1 pepper	24	1	0	4	2	2	6	0
Pimento, canned	1 cup	44	2	0	10	6	4	27	0
Pimento, canned	1 tbsp	3	0	0	1	0	0	2	0
Serrano, raw	1 cup, chop.	34	2	0	7	3	4	11	0
Serrano, raw	1 pepper	2	0	0	0	0	0	1	0
Sweet, green, boiled, drained	1 cup, strips	38	1	0	9	7	2	3	0
Sweet, green, boiled, drained	1 tbsp	3	0	0	1	1	0	0	0
Sweet, green, canned, solids and liquids	1 cup	25	1	0	5	4	2	1917	0
Sweet, green, freeze-dried	1/4 cup	5	0	0	1	1	0	3	0
Sweet, green, freeze-dried	1 tbsp	1	0	0	0	0	0	1	0

Description	Serving Size	Cal	Prot (g)	Fat (g)	Carbs (g)	Net Carb(g)	Fiber (g)	Sod (mg)	Chol (mg)
PEPPERS (continued)									
Sweet, green, frozen, chopped, unprepared	1 package	57	3	0	13	8	5	14	0
Sweet, green, raw	1 cup, chop.	40	1	0	10	7	3	3	0
Sweet, green, raw	1 cup, sliced	25	1	0	6	4	2	2	0
Sweet, red, boiled, drained	1 cup, strips	38	1	0	9	7	2	3	0
Sweet, red, boiled, drained	1 tbsp	3	0	0	1	1	0	0	0
Sweet, red, canned, solids and liquids	1/2 cup, halves	13	1	0	3	2	1	958	0
Sweet, red, canned, solids and liquids	1 cup	25	1	0	5	4	2	1917	0
Sweet, red, freeze-dried	1/4 cup	5	0	0	1	1	0	3	0
Sweet, red, freeze-dried	1 tbsp	1	0	0	0	0	0	1	0
Sweet, red, raw	1 cup, chop.	40	1	0	10	7	3	3	0
Sweet, red, raw	1 cup, sliced	25	1	0	6	4	2	2	0
Sweet, yellow, raw	1 pepper	50	2	0	12	10	2	4	0
Sweet, yellow, raw	10 strips	14	1	0	3	3	0	1	0

Pickles

Description	Serving Size	Cal	Prot (g)	Fat (g)	Carbs (g)	Net Carb(g)	Fiber (g)	Sod (mg)	Chol (mg)
Cucumber, dill	1 cup	28	1	0	6	5	2	1987	0
Cucumber, dill	1 cup, chop. or diced	26	1	0	6	4	2	1833	0
Cucumber, dill, low sodium	1 medium	12	0	0	3	2	1	12	0
Cucumber, dill, low sodium	1 slice	1	0	0	0	0	0	1	0
Cucumber, sour	1 cup	17	1	0	3	2	2	1872	0
Cucumber, sour	1 large	15	0	0	3	1	2	1631	0
Cucumber, sour, low sodium	1 cup	17	1	0	3	2	2	28	0
Cucumber, sour, low sodium	1 cup, chop. or diced	16	0	0	3	2	2	26	0
Cucumber, sweet	1 cup, chop.	187	1	0	51	49	2	1502	0
Cucumber, sweet	1 cup, sliced	199	1	0	54	52	2	1596	0
Cucumber, sweet, low sodium	1 cup, chop. or diced	187	1	0	51	49	2	29	0
Cucumber, sweet, low sodium	1 cup, sliced	199	1	0	54	52	2	31	0
Pickle relish, hamburger	1/2 cup	157	1	1	42	38	4	1337	0
Pickle relish, hamburger	1 tbsp	19	0	0	5	5	0	164	0
Pickle relish, hot dog	1/2 cup	111	2	0	28	27	2	1331	0
Pickle relish, hot dog	1 tbsp	14	0	0	4	3	0	164	0
Pickle relish, sweet	1 cup	319	1	1	86	83	3	1987	0
Pickle relish, sweet	1 tbsp	20	0	0	5	5	0	122	0

Description	Serving Size	Cal	Prot (g)	Fat (g)	Carbs (g)	Net Carb(g)	Fiber (g)	Sod (mg)	Chol (mg)
Poi									
Raw	1 cup	269	1	0	65	64	1	29	0
Pokeberry Shoots									
Boiled, drained	1 cup	33	4	0	5	3	2	30	0
Raw	1 cup	37	4	0	6	3	3	37	0
Potatoes									
Au gratin, dry mix, prepared with water, whole milk and butter	1/6 package	127	3	5	18	16	1	601	21
Au gratin, home-prepared from recipe using butter	1 cup	323	12	18	28	23	4	1061	56
Au gratin, home-prepared from recipe using margarine	1 cup	323	12	18	28	23	4	1061	37
Baked, flesh	1/2 cup	57	1	0	13	12	1	3	0
Baked, flesh	1 potato	145	3	0	34	31	2	8	0
Baked, flesh and skin	1 large	326	7	0	75	68	7	24	0
Baked, flesh and skin	1 medium	188	4	0	44	39	4	14	0
Baked, skin	1 skin	115	2	0	27	22	5	12	0
Boiled, cooked in skin, flesh	1/2 cup	68	1	0	16	14	1	3	0
Boiled, cooked in skin, flesh	1 potato	118	3	0	27	25	2	5	0
Boiled, cooked in skin, skin	1 skin	27	1	0	6	5	1	5	0
Boiled, cooked without skin, flesh	1 large	258	5	0	60	55	5	15	0
Boiled, cooked without skin, flesh	1 medium	143	3	0	33	30	3	8	0
Canned, drained solids	1 cup	108	3	0	24	20	4	394	0
Canned, drained solids	1 potato	21	0	0	5	4	1	77	0
Canned, solids and liquids	1 cup, whole	132	4	0	30	25	4	651	0
Flesh and skin, raw	1 large	96	7	0	19	10	9	26	0
Flesh and skin, raw	1 medium	55	4	0	11	6	5	15	0
French fried, frozen, home-prepared, heated in oven	10 strips	100	2	3	16	14	2	15	0
French fried, frozen, unprepared	10 strips	101	2	3	16	14	2	15	0
Frozen, French fried, par fried, cottage-cut, prepared, heated in oven	10 strips	109	2	4	17	15	2	23	0
Frozen, French fried, par fried, cottage-cut, unprepared	10 strips	99	2	4	16	14	2	21	0
Frozen, French fried, par fried, extruded, prepared, heated in oven	10 strips	167	2	9	20	18	2	307	0
Frozen, French fried, par fried, extruded, unprepared	10 strips	169	2	9	20	17	3	319	0
Frozen, whole, unprepared	1 cup	142	4	0	32	30	2	46	0

Description	Serving Size	Cal	Prot (g)	Fat (g)	Carbs (g)	Net Carb(g)	Fiber (g)	Sod (mg)	Chol (mg)
POTATOES (continued)									
Hashed brown, frozen, plain, prepared	1/2 cup	170	2	9	22	20	2	27	0
Hashed brown, frozen, plain, prepared	1 patty, oval	63	1	3	8	8	1	10	0
Hashed brown, frozen, plain, unprepared	1/2 cup	86	2	0	19	17	1	23	0
Hashed brown, frozen, with butter sauce, unprepared	1 package	230	3	11	31	26	5	131	0
Hashed brown, home-prepared	1 cup	326	4	21	33	30	3	37	0
Mashed, dehydrated, flakes without milk, dry form	1 cup	170	4	0	39	36	3	51	0
Mashed, dehydrated, granules with milk, dry form	1 cup	716	22	2	155	NA	NA	164	4
Mashed, dehydrated, granules without milk, dry form	1 cup	744	16	1	171	157	14	134	0
Mashed, dehydrated, prepared from flakes without milk, whole milk and butter added	1 cup	237	4	11	32	27	5	697	29
Mashed, dehydrated, prepared from granules with milk, water and margarine added	1 cup	166	4	4	28	24	4	491	4
Mashed, dehydrated, prepared from granules without milk, whole milk and butter added	1 cup	227	4	10	30	26	5	540	29
Mashed, home-prepared, whole milk added	1 cup	162	4	1	37	33	4	636	4
Mashed, home-prepared, whole milk and butter added	1 cup	223	4	9	35	31	4	620	25
Mashed, home-prepared, whole milk and margarine added	1 cup	223	4	8	35	31	4	620	4
Mashed, prepared from flakes, without milk, whole milk and margarine	1 cup	237	4	11	32	27	5	697	8
Mashed, prepared from granules, without milk, whole milk and margarine	1 cup	227	4	10	30	26	5	552	6
Microwaved, cooked in skin, flesh	1/2 cup	78	2	0	18	17	1	5	0
Microwaved, cooked in skin, flesh	1 potato	156	3	0	36	34	2	11	0
Microwaved, cooked in skin, flesh and skin	1 potato	212	5	0	49	44	5	16	0
Microwaved, cooked in skin, skin	1 skin	77	3	0	17	14	3	9	0
O'Brien, home-prepared	1 cup	157	5	2	30	NA	NA	421	8
O'Brien, home-prepared	1 recipe	941	27	14	180	NA	NA	2522	46
Potato pancakes, home-prepared	1 pancake	207	5	11	22	20	2	386	73
Potato puffs, frozen, prepared	1 cup	284	4	13	39	35	4	955	0

Description	Serving Size	Cal	Prot (g)	Fat (g)	Carbs (g)	Net Carb(g)	Fiber (g)	Sod (mg)	Chol (mg)
Potato puffs, frozen, prepared	1 puff	16	0	1	2	2	0	52	0
Potato puffs, frozen, unprepared	1 cup	227	3	10	31	28	3	762	0
Potato salad, home-prepared	1 cup	358	7	19	28	25	3	1323	170
Raw, skin	1 skin	22	1	0	5	4	1	4	0
Scalloped, dry mix, prepared with water, whole milk and butter	1/6 package	127	3	6	17	16	2	467	15
Scalloped, dry mix, prepared with water, whole milk and butter	1 cup	228	5	10	31	29	3	835	27
Scalloped, dry mix, unprepared	1/6 package	93	2	1	19	17	2	410	1
Scalloped, dry mix, unprepared	1 package	558	12	5	115	102	13	2462	8
Scalloped, home-prepared with butter	1 cup	211	7	8	26	22	5	821	29
Scalloped, home-prepared with margarine	1 cup	211	7	9	26	22	5	821	15
Sweet potato, baked in skin	1 cup	206	3	0	49	43	6	20	0
Sweet potato, baked in skin	1 large	185	3	0	44	38	5	18	0
Sweet potato, boiled, without skin	1 cup, mashed	344	5	1	80	74	6	43	0
Sweet potato, boiled, without skin	1 medium	159	2	0	37	34	3	20	0
Sweet potato, candied, home-prepared	1 piece	144	1	2	29	27	3	74	8
Sweet potato, canned, mashed	1 cup	258	5	0	59	55	4	191	0
Sweet potato, canned, syrup pack, drained solids	1 cup	212	3	0	50	44	6	76	0
Sweet potato, canned, syrup pack, solids and liquids	1 cup	203	2	0	48	42	6	100	0
Sweet potato, canned, vacuum pack	1 cup, mashed	232	4	0	54	49	5	135	0
Sweet potato, canned, vacuum pack	1 cup, pieces	182	3	0	42	39	4	106	0
Sweet potato, frozen, baked	1 cup, cubes	176	3	0	41	38	3	14	0
Sweet potato, frozen, unprepared	1 cup, cubes	169	3	0	39	36	3	11	0
Sweet potato, raw, unprepared	1 cup, cubes	140	2	0	32	28	4	17	0
Sweet potato, raw, unprepared	1 potato	137	2	0	32	28	4	17	0

Pumpkin

Description	Serving Size	Cal	Prot (g)	Fat (g)	Carbs (g)	Net Carb(g)	Fiber (g)	Sod (mg)	Chol (mg)
Boiled, drained	1 cup, mashed	49	2	0	12	9	3	2	0
Canned, with salt	1 cup	83	3	0	20	13	7	590	0
Canned, without salt	1 cup	83	3	0	20	13	7	12	0
Pumpkin pie mix, canned	1 cup	281	3	0	71	49	22	562	0
Raw	1 cup	30	1	0	8	7	1	1	0

Purslane

Description	Serving Size	Cal	Prot (g)	Fat (g)	Carbs (g)	Net Carb(g)	Fiber (g)	Sod (mg)	Chol (mg)
Boiled, drained	1 cup	21	2	0	4	NA	NA	51	0
Boiled, drained	1 squash	78	6	0	15	NA	NA	190	0

Description	Serving Size	Cal	Prot (g)	Fat (g)	Carbs (g)	Net Carb(g)	Fiber (g)	Sod (mg)	Chol (mg)
PURSLANE (continued)									
Raw	1 cup	7	1	0	1	NA	NA	19	0
Raw	1 plant	0	0	0	0	NA	NA	1	0

Radicchio

Raw	1 cup, shred.	9	1	0	2	1	0	9	0
Raw	1 leaf	2	0	0	0	0	0	2	0

Radishes

Oriental, boiled, drained	1 cup, sliced	25	1	0	5	3	2	19	0
Oriental, dried	1 cup	314	9	1	74	NA	NA	322	0
Oriental, raw	1 radish	61	2	0	14	8	5	71	0
Radish seeds, sprouted, raw	1 cup	16	1	1	1	NA	NA	2	0
Raw	1 cup, sliced	23	1	0	4	2	2	28	0
Raw	1 large	2	0	0	0	0	0	2	0
White icicle, raw	1/2 cup, sliced	7	1	0	1	1	1	8	0
White icicle, raw	1 radish	2	0	0	0	0	0	3	0

Rutabagas

Boiled, drained	1 cup, cubes	66	2	0	15	12	3	34	0
Boiled, drained	1 cup, mashed	94	3	0	21	17	4	48	0
Raw	1 cup, cubes	50	2	0	11	8	4	28	0
Raw	1 large	278	9	1	63	43	19	154	0

Salsify

Boiled, drained	1 cup, sliced	92	4	0	21	17	4	22	0
Raw	1 cup, sliced	109	4	0	25	20	4	27	0

Seaweed

Agar, raw	2 tbsp	3	0	0	1	1	0	1	0
Irishmoss, raw	2 tbsp	5	0	0	1	1	0	7	0
Kelp, raw	2 tbsp	4	0	0	1	1	0	23	0
Laver, raw	10 sheets	9	2	0	1	1	0	12	0
Laver, raw	2 tbsp	4	1	0	1	0	0	5	0
Spirulina, dried	1 cup	44	9	1	4	3	1	157	0
Wakame, raw	2 tbsp	5	0	0	1	1	0	87	0

Sesbania Flower

Raw	1 cup	5	0	0	1	NA	NA	3	0
Raw	1 flower	1	0	0	0	NA	NA	0	0
Steamed	1 cup	23	1	0	5	NA	NA	11	0

Description	Serving Size	Cal	Prot (g)	Fat (g)	Carbs (g)	Net Carb(g)	Fiber (g)	Sod (mg)	Chol (mg)
Shallots									
Freeze-dried	1/4 cup	13	0	0	3	NA	NA	2	0
Freeze-dried	1 tbsp	3	0	0	1	NA	NA	1	0
Raw	1 tbsp, chop.	7	0	0	2	NA	NA	1	0
Soybeans									
Green, boiled, drained	1 cup	254	22	9	20	12	8	25	0
Green, raw	1 cup	376	33	13	28	18	11	38	0
Mature seeds, sprouted, raw	1/2 cup	43	5	2	3	3	0	5	0
Mature seeds, sprouted, raw	10 sprouts	12	1	1	1	1	0	1	0
Mature seeds, sprouted, steamed	1 cup	76	8	4	6	5	1	9	0
Spinach									
Boiled, drained	1 cup	41	5	0	7	2	4	126	0
Canned, drained solids	1 cup	49	6	1	7	2	5	58	0
Canned, no salt added, solids and liquids	1 cup	44	5	1	7	2	5	176	0
Canned, regular pack, solids and liquids	1 cup	44	5	1	7	3	4	746	0
Frozen, chopped or leaf, boiled, drained	1/2 cup	27	3	0	5	2	3	82	0
Frozen, chopped or leaf, boiled, drained	1 package	62	7	0	12	5	7	189	0
Frozen, chopped or leaf, unprepared	1 cup	37	5	0	6	2	5	115	0
New Zealand spinach, boiled, drained	1 cup, chop.	22	2	0	4	NA	NA	193	0
New Zealand spinach, raw	1 cup, chop.	8	1	0	1	NA	NA	73	0
Raw	1 bunch	75	10	1	12	3	9	269	0
Raw	1 cup	7	1	0	1	0	1	24	0
Spinach soufflé, home-prepared	1 cup	219	11	17	3	NA	NA	763	184
Squash									
Summer, all varieties, boiled, drained	1 cup, sliced	36	2	0	8	5	3	2	0
Summer, all varieties, raw	1 cup, sliced	23	1	0	5	3	2	2	0
Summer, all varieties, raw	1 large	65	4	0	14	8	6	6	0
Summer, crookneck and straightneck, boiled, drained	1/2 cup, sliced	18	1	0	4	3	1	1	0
Summer, crookneck and straightneck, boiled, drained	1 cup, sliced	36	2	0	8	5	3	2	0
Summer, crookneck and straightneck, canned, drained, solid	1 cup, diced	27	1	0	6	3	3	11	0
Summer, crookneck and straightneck, canned, drained, solid	1 cup, mashed	31	1	0	7	4	3	12	0
Summer, crookneck and straightneck, frozen, boiled, drained	1 cup, sliced	48	2	0	11	8	3	12	0

Description	Serving Size	Cal	Prot (g)	Fat (g)	Carbs (g)	Net Carb(g)	Fiber (g)	Sod (mg)	Chol (mg)
SQUASH (continued)									
Summer, crookneck and straightneck, frozen, unprepared	1 cup, sliced	26	1	0	6	5	2	7	0
Summer, crookneck and straightneck, raw	1 cup, sliced	25	1	0	5	3	2	3	0
Summer, scallop, boiled, drained	1 cup, mashed	38	2	0	8	3	5	2	0
Summer, scallop, boiled, drained	1 cup, sliced	29	2	0	6	3	3	2	0
Summer, scallop, raw	1 cup, sliced	23	2	0	5	NA	NA	1	0
Summer, zucchini, includes skin, boiled, drained, mashed	1/2 cup	19	1	0	5	3	2	4	0
Summer, zucchini, includes skin, boiled, drained	1 cup, sliced	29	1	0	7	5	3	5	0
Summer, zucchini, includes skin, frozen, boiled, drained	1 cup	38	3	0	8	5	3	4	0
Summer, zucchini, includes skin, frozen, unprepared	1 package	48	3	0	10	7	4	6	0
Summer, zucchini, includes skin, raw	1 cup, chop.	17	1	0	4	2	1	4	0
Summer, zucchini, includes skin, raw	1 cup, sliced	16	1	0	3	2	1	3	0
Summer, zucchini, Italian style, canned	1 cup	66	2	0	16	NA	NA	849	0
Winter, acorn, baked	1 cup, cubes	115	2	0	30	21	9	8	0
Winter, acorn, boiled, mashed	1 cup, mashed	83	2	0	22	15	6	7	0
Winter, acorn, raw	1 cup, cubes	56	1	0	15	12	2	4	0
Winter, acorn, raw	1 squash	172	3	0	45	38	6	13	0
Winter, all varieties, baked	1 cup, cubes	80	2	1	18	12	6	2	0
Winter, all varieties, raw	1 cup, cubes	43	2	0	10	8	2	5	0
Winter, butternut, baked	1 cup, cubes	82	2	0	22	NA	NA	8	0
Winter, butternut, frozen, boiled	1 cup, mashed	94	3	0	24	NA	NA	5	0
Winter, butternut, frozen, unprepared	1 package	194	6	0	49	45	4	7	0
Winter, butternut, raw	1 cup, cubes	63	1	0	16	NA	NA	6	0
Winter, Hubbard, baked	1 cup, cubes	103	5	1	22	NA	NA	16	0
Winter, Hubbard, boiled, mashed	1 cup, mashed	71	3	1	15	8	7	12	0
Winter, Hubbard, raw	1 cup, cubes	46	2	0	10	NA	NA	8	0
Winter, spaghetti, boiled, drained, or baked	1 cup	42	1	0	10	8	2	28	0
Winter, spaghetti, raw	1 cup, cubes	31	1	0	7	NA	NA	17	0
Zucchini, baby, raw	1 large	3	0	0	0	0	0	0	0
Zucchini, baby, raw	1 medium	2	0	0	0	0	0	0	0

Succotash

Description	Serving Size	Cal	Prot (g)	Fat (g)	Carbs (g)	Net Carb(g)	Fiber (g)	Sod (mg)	Chol (mg)
Boiled, drained	1 cup	221	10	1	47	38	9	33	0

Description	Serving Size	Cal	Prot (g)	Fat (g)	Carbs (g)	Net Carb(g)	Fiber (g)	Sod (mg)	Chol (mg)
Canned, with cream style corn	1 cup	205	7	1	47	39	8	652	0
Canned, with whole kernel corn, solids and liquids	1 cup	161	7	1	36	29	7	564	0
Frozen, boiled, drained	1 cup	158	7	1	34	27	7	77	0
Frozen, unprepared	1 cup	145	7	1	31	25	6	70	0

Taro

Description	Serving Size	Cal	Prot (g)	Fat (g)	Carbs (g)	Net Carb(g)	Fiber (g)	Sod (mg)	Chol (mg)
Cooked	1 cup, sliced	187	1	0	46	39	7	20	0
Leaves, raw	1 cup	12	1	0	2	1	1	1	0
Leaves, raw	1 leaf	4	0	0	1	0	0	0	0
Leaves, steamed	1 cup	35	4	0	6	3	3	3	0
Raw	1 cup, sliced	116	2	0	28	23	4	11	0
Shoots, cooked	1 cup, sliced	20	1	0	4	NA	NA	3	0
Shoots, raw	1/2 cup, sliced	5	0	0	1	NA	NA	0	0
Shoots, raw	1 shoot	9	1	0	2	NA	NA	1	0
Tahitian, cooked	1 cup, sliced	60	6	1	9	NA	NA	74	0
Tahitian, raw	1 cup, sliced	55	3	1	9	NA	NA	63	0

Tomatillos

Description	Serving Size	Cal	Prot (g)	Fat (g)	Carbs (g)	Net Carb(g)	Fiber (g)	Sod (mg)	Chol (mg)
Raw	1/2 cup, chop. or diced	21	1	0	4	3	1	1	0
Raw	1 medium	11	0	0	2	1	1	0	0

Tomato Products

Description	Serving Size	Cal	Prot (g)	Fat (g)	Carbs (g)	Net Carb(g)	Fiber (g)	Sod (mg)	Chol (mg)
Canned, paste, with salt added	1/2 cup	107	5	1	25	20	5	1035	0
Canned, paste, with salt added	1 can	139	6	1	33	26	7	1343	0
Canned, paste, without salt added	1 cup	215	10	1	51	40	11	231	0
Canned, paste, without salt added	1 tbsp	13	1	0	3	2	1	14	0
Canned, puree, with salt added	1 can	329	14	1	79	62	16	3280	0
Canned, puree, with salt added	1 cup	100	4	0	24	19	5	998	0
Canned, puree, without salt added	1 can	329	14	1	79	62	16	279	0
Canned, puree, without salt added	1 cup	100	4	0	24	19	5	85	0
Canned, sauce	1 cup	74	3	0	18	14	3	1482	0
Canned, sauce, Spanish style	1 can	140	6	1	31	25	6	2006	0
Canned, sauce, Spanish style	1 cup	81	4	0	18	14	3	1152	0
Canned, sauce, with herbs and cheese	1/2 cup	72	3	2	12	10	3	662	4
Canned, sauce, with herbs and cheese	1 can	251	9	8	44	34	9	2308	13
Canned, sauce, with mushrooms	1 cup	86	4	0	21	17	4	1107	0
Canned, sauce, with onions	1 cup	103	4	0	24	20	4	1350	0

Description	Serving Size	Cal	Prot (g)	Fat (g)	Carbs (g)	Net Carb(g)	Fiber (g)	Sod (mg)	Chol (mg)
TOMATO PRODUCTS (continued)									
Canned, sauce, with onions, green peppers, and celery	1 can	169	4	2	36	30	6	2244	0
Canned, sauce, with onions, green peppers, and celery	1 cup	103	2	1	22	18	4	1365	0
Canned, sauce, with tomato tidbits	1 can	136	6	1	30	24	6	64	0
Canned, sauce, with tomato tidbits	1 cup	78	3	1	17	14	3	37	0

Tomatoes

Description	Serving Size	Cal	Prot (g)	Fat (g)	Carbs (g)	Net Carb(g)	Fiber (g)	Sod (mg)	Chol (mg)
Green, raw	1 cup	43	2	0	9	7	2	23	0
Green, raw	1 large	44	2	0	9	7	2	24	0
Orange, raw	1 cup, chop.	25	2	0	5	4	1	66	0
Orange, raw	1 tomato	18	1	0	4	3	1	47	0
Red, ripe, canned, stewed	1 cup	71	2	0	17	15	3	564	0
Red, ripe, canned, wedges in tomato juice	1 cup	68	2	0	16	14	3	566	0
Red, ripe, canned, whole, no salt added	1 cup	46	2	0	10	8	2	24	0
Red, ripe, canned, whole, no salt added	1 tbsp	3	0	0	1	1	0	2	0
Red, ripe, canned, whole, regular pack	1 cup	46	2	0	10	8	2	355	0
Red, ripe, canned, whole, regular pack	1 tbsp	3	0	0	1	1	0	22	0
Red, ripe, canned, with green chilies	1 cup	36	2	0	9	6	2	966	0
Red, ripe, cooked	1 cup	65	3	1	14	12	2	26	0
Red, ripe, cooked	2 medium	66	3	1	14	12	2	27	0
Red, ripe, raw	1 cup	31	1	0	7	5	2	13	0
Red, ripe, raw	1 cup, chop.	38	2	0	8	6	2	16	0
Red, ripe, stewed	1 cup	80	2	2	13	11	2	460	0
Red, ripe, stewed	1 recipe	477	12	15	79	69	10	2748	0
Sun-dried	1 cup	139	8	1	30	23	7	1131	0
Sun-dried	1 piece	5	0	0	1	1	0	42	0
Sun-dried, packed in oil, drained	1 cup	234	6	14	26	19	6	293	0
Sun-dried, packed in oil, drained	1 piece	6	0	0	1	1	0	8	0
Yellow, raw	1 cup, chop.	21	1	0	4	3	1	32	0
Yellow, raw	1 tomato	32	2	0	6	5	1	49	0

Tree Fern

Description	Serving Size	Cal	Prot (g)	Fat (g)	Carbs (g)	Net Carb(g)	Fiber (g)	Sod (mg)	Chol (mg)
Cooked	1/2 cup, chop.	28	0	0	8	5	3	4	0

Turnips & Turnip Greens

Description	Serving Size	Cal	Prot (g)	Fat (g)	Carbs (g)	Net Carb(g)	Fiber (g)	Sod (mg)	Chol (mg)
Greens and turnips, frozen, boiled, drained	1 cup	28	3	0	5	2	3	24	0

Description	Serving Size	Cal	Prot (g)	Fat (g)	Carbs (g)	Net Carb(g)	Fiber (g)	Sod (mg)	Chol (mg)
Greens and turnips, frozen, unprepared	1 package	60	7	0	10	3	7	51	0
Greens, boiled, drained	1 cup, chop.	29	2	0	6	1	5	42	0
Greens, canned, solids and liquids	1/2 cup	16	2	0	3	1	2	324	0
Greens, frozen, boiled, drained	1 cup	49	5	0	8	3	6	25	0
Greens, frozen, unprepared	1/2 cup, chop. or diced	18	2	0	3	1	2	10	0
Greens, raw	1 cup, chop.	15	1	0	3	1	2	22	0
Turnips, boiled, drained	1 cup, cubes	33	1	0	8	5	3	78	0
Turnips, boiled, drained	1 cup, mashed	48	2	0	11	7	5	115	0
Turnips, frozen, boiled, drained	1 cup	36	2	0	7	4	3	56	0
Turnips, frozen, unprepared	1/3 package	15	1	0	3	1	2	24	0
Turnips, raw	1 cup, cubes	35	1	0	8	6	2	87	0
Turnips, raw	1 large	49	2	0	11	8	3	123	0

Wasabi

Description	Serving Size	Cal	Prot (g)	Fat (g)	Carbs (g)	Net Carb(g)	Fiber (g)	Sod (mg)	Chol (mg)
Root, raw	1 cup, sliced	142	6	0	31	21	10	22	0
Root, raw	1 root	184	8	0	40	27	13	29	0

Water Chestnuts

Description	Serving Size	Cal	Prot (g)	Fat (g)	Carbs (g)	Net Carb(g)	Fiber (g)	Sod (mg)	Chol (mg)
Chinese, (matai), raw	1/2 cup, sliced	60	1	0	15	13	2	9	0
Chinese, canned, solids and liquids	1/2 cup, sliced	35	1	0	9	7	2	6	0

Watercress

Description	Serving Size	Cal	Prot (g)	Fat (g)	Carbs (g)	Net Carb(g)	Fiber (g)	Sod (mg)	Chol (mg)
Raw	1 cup, chop.	4	1	0	0	0	1	14	0

Waxgourd

Description	Serving Size	Cal	Prot (g)	Fat (g)	Carbs (g)	Net Carb(g)	Fiber (g)	Sod (mg)	Chol (mg)
Boiled, drained	1 cup, cubes	23	1	0	5	4	2	187	0
Raw	1 cup, cubes	17	1	0	4	0	4	147	0

Winged Beans

Description	Serving Size	Cal	Prot (g)	Fat (g)	Carbs (g)	Net Carb(g)	Fiber (g)	Sod (mg)	Chol (mg)
Immature seeds, boiled, drained	1 cup	24	3	0	2	NA	NA	2	0
Immature seeds, raw	1 cup, sliced	22	3	0	2	NA	NA	2	0

Yambean (Jicama)

Description	Serving Size	Cal	Prot (g)	Fat (g)	Carbs (g)	Net Carb(g)	Fiber (g)	Sod (mg)	Chol (mg)
Raw	1 cup, sliced	46	1	0	11	5	6	5	0

Yams

Description	Serving Size	Cal	Prot (g)	Fat (g)	Carbs (g)	Net Carb(g)	Fiber (g)	Sod (mg)	Chol (mg)
Boiled, drained, or baked	1 cup, cubes	158	2	0	38	32	5	11	0
Raw	1 cup, cubes	177	2	0	42	36	6	14	0

Yardlong Beans

Description	Serving Size	Cal	Prot (g)	Fat (g)	Carbs (g)	Net Carb(g)	Fiber (g)	Sod (mg)	Chol (mg)
Boiled, drained	1 cup, sliced	49	3	0	10	NA	NA	4	0

Description	Serving Size	Cal	Prot (g)	Fat (g)	Carbs (g)	Net Carb(g)	Fiber (g)	Sod (mg)	Chol (mg)
YARDLONG BEANS (continued)									
Raw	1 cup, sliced	43	3	0	8	NA	NA	4	0

Yautia

Raw	1 cup, sliced	132	2	0	32	30	2	28	0

Description	Serving Size	Cal	Prot (g)	Fat (g)	Carbs (g)	Net Carb(g)	Fiber (g)	Sod (mg)	Chol (mg)
Arby's®									
ROAST BEEF SANDWICHES									
Arby-Q®	1 sandwich	360	18	11	51	49	2	1210	35
Big Montana®1	1 sandwich	590	47	29	41	38	3	2080	115
Giant Roast Beef	1 sandwich	450	32	19	41	39	2	1440	75
Regular Roast Beef	1 sandwich	320	21	13	34	32	2	950	45
Beef 'n Cheddar	1 sandwich	440	22	21	44	42	2	1270	50
Super Roast Beef	1 sandwich	440	22	19	48	45	3	1130	45
Junior Roast Beef	1 sandwich	270	16	9	34	32	2	740	30
French Dip 'n Swiss	1 sandwich	320	35	25	56	53	3	2040	75
Philly Beef Supreme	1 sandwich	450	36	37	59	56	3	1660	95
OTHER SANDWICHES									
Chicken Breast Fillet	1 sandwich	490	25	24	46	44	2	1220	55
Chicken Bacon 'n Swiss	1 sandwich	550	31	27	49	47	2	1640	70
Chicken Cordon Bleu	1 sandwich	570	34	29	46	44	2	1880	85
Chicken Fingers 4 Pack	1 sandwich	640	31	38	42	39	3	1590	70
Grilled Chicken Deluxe	1 sandwich	380	29	12	40	38	2	920	50
Roast Chicken Club	1 sandwich	470	27	25	39	37	2	1320	65
Hot Ham 'n Cheese	1 sandwich	300	23	9	35	34	1	1450	50
MARKET FRESH® SANDWICHES									
Market Fresh® Roast Turkey	1 sandwich	830	49	38	75	70	5	2260	110
Market Fresh® Ultimate BLT	1 sandwich	780	23	46	75	69	6	1570	50
Market Fresh® Roast Beef & Swiss	1 sandwich	780	37	39	74	68	6	1740	90
Market Fresh® Roast Ham & Swiss	1 sandwich	700	36	31	74	69	5	2140	85
Market Fresh® Roast Turkey & Swiss	1 sandwich	720	45	27	74	69	5	1790	90
Market Fresh® Chicken Salad	1 sandwich	860	26	44	92	86	6	1270	60
MARKET FRESH® LOW CARBYS™ WRAPS									
Ultimate BLT Wrap	1 wrap	650	25	47	48	17	31	1730	50
Roast Turkey Ranch & Bacon Wrap	1 wrap	710	51	39	48	18	30	2420	110
Southwest Chicken Wrap	1 wrap	550	35	30	45	15	30	1690	75
Chicken Caesar Wrap	1 wrap	520	33	27	46	16	30	1530	65
MARKET FRESH® SALADS									
Martha's Vineyard™	1 salad	250	26	8	23	19	4	490	60
Raspberry Vinaigrette	1 salad	172	0	12	16	16	0	344	0
Santa Fe™	1 salad	520	27	29	40	35	5	1120	60

Description	Serving Size	Cal	Prot (g)	Fat (g)	Carbs (g)	Net Carb(g)	Fiber (g)	Sod (mg)	Chol (mg)
ARBY'S® (continued)									
Seasoned Tortilla Strips	1 salad	61	1	3	10	10	1	25	0
Santa Fe Ranch Dressing	1 salad	264	1	28	3	3	0	615	19
Asian Sesame™	1 salad	140	NA	1	15	12	3	360	40
Asian Sesame Dressing	1 salad	190	NA	14	15	15	0	463	0
Garden Side Salad	1 salad	35	NA	0	7	2	5	25	0
LIGHT DRESSING CHOICES									
Light Buttermilk Ranch Dressing	1 Packet	100	1	6	12	11	1	486	0
Light Balsamic Vinaigrette	1 Packet	110	NA	6	13	13	0	220	0
Fat Free Italian Dressing	1 Packet	30	NA	0	7	7	0	520	0
PREMIUM POTATOES									
Curly Fries	1 small order	340	4	18	39	35	4	790	0
Homestyle Fries	1 small order	300	3	13	44	41	3	550	0
Potato Cakes	2 cakes	250	2	15	26	24	2	390	0
Baked Potato	1 potato	200	4	0	46	42	4	15	0
Broccoli 'n Cheddar Potato	1 potato	460	11	23	56	50	6	780	50
Deluxe Potato	1 potato	570	18	34	50	45	5	750	90
SIDEKICKERS®									
Jalapeno Bites	Regular (5)	310	5	19	29	27	2	530	30
Mozzarella Sticks	Regular (4)	430	18	23	38	36	2	1370	45
Onion Petals	Regular	330	4	19	35	33	2	330	0
BREAKFAST									
Biscuit– Plain	1 biscuit	230	5	12	26	25	1	710	0
Bacon Biscuit	1 biscuit	300	9	17	27	26	1	950	15
Ham Biscuit	1 biscuit	270	12	27	26	25	1	1080	30
Sausage Biscuit	1 biscuit	390	10	27	26	25	1	1080	30
Bacon 'n Egg Croissant	1 croissant	410	13	26	31	30	1	670	190
Ham 'n Cheese Croissant	1 croissant	350	15	19	30	29	1	870	65
Sausage 'n Egg Croissant	1 croissant	510	14	36	31	30	1	800	210
Sourdough Ham, Egg 'n Swiss	1 sandwich	450	27	23	33	32	1	1750	330
Sourdough Bacon, Egg & Swiss	1 sandwich	500	25	29	33	32	1	1600	325
Sourdough Egg 'n Cheese	1 sandwich	330	15	16	31	30	1	1060	165
DESSERTS & SHAKES									
Apple Turnover (no icing)	1 turnover	250	4	10	35	33	2	200	0
Cherry Turnover (no icing)	1 turnover	250	4	10	35	33	2	200	0
Gourmet Chocolate Cookie	1 cookie	200	2	10	26	25	1	210	15

Description	Serving Size	Cal	Prot (g)	Fat (g)	Carbs (g)	Net Carb(g)	Fiber (g)	Sod (mg)	Chol (mg)
Chocolate Shake	Regular	510	13	13	83	83	0	360	35
Jamocha Shake	Regular	500	13	13	81	81	0	390	35
Strawberry Shake	Regular	500	13	13	81	81	0	360	35
Vanilla Shake	Regular	500	13	13	82	82	0	370	35
SAUCES / CONDIMENTS									
Arby's Sauce® Packet	1 packet	15	0	0	4	4	0	180	0
BBQ Dipping Sauce	1 packet	40	0	0	10	10	0	350	0
Bronco Berry Sauce®	1 packet	120	0	0	30	30	0	35	0
Buffalo Dipping Sauce	1 packet	20	0	1	3	3	0	1600	0
Buttermilk Ranch Dressing	1 packet	290	1	30	3	3	0	580	25
Honey Mustard Dipping Sauce	1 packet	130	0	12	5	5	0	170	10
Horsey Sauce® Packet	1 packet	60	0	5	3	3	0	170	5
Ketchup Packet	1 packet	20	0	0	4	4	0	170	0
Marinara Sauce	1 packet	15	0	0	4	3	1	220	0
Mayonnaise Packet	1 packet	100	0	11	0	0	0	75	10
Red Ranch Sauce	1 packet	70	0	6	5	5	0	105	0
Tangy Southwest Sauce®	1 packet	330	1	35	5	5	0	370	30
Three Pepper Sauce Packet	1 packet	20	0	1	3	3	0	140	0

Auntie Anne's Pretzels® —

Description	Serving Size	Cal	Prot (g)	Fat (g)	Carbs (g)	Net Carb(g)	Fiber (g)	Sod (mg)	Chol (mg)
PRETZELS & MORE									
Almond Pretzel	1 pretzel	400	9	8	72	70	2	400	20
Almond Pretzel without Butter	1 pretzel	350	9	2	72	70	2	390	0
Cinnamon Sugar Pretzel	1 pretzel	450	8	9	83	80	3	430	25
Cinnamon Sugar Pretzel without Butter	1 pretzel	350	9	2	74	72	2	410	0
Garlic Pretzel	1 pretzel	350	9	5	68	66	2	850	10
Garlic Pretzel without Butter	1 pretzel	320	9	1	66	64	2	830	0
Glazin' Raisin® Pretzel	1 pretzel	510	11	4	107	103	4	480	10
Glazin' Raisin® Pretzel without Butter	1 pretzel	470	11	1	104	101	3	460	0
Jalapeño Pretzel	1 pretzel	310	8	5	59	57	2	940	10
Jalapeño Pretzel without Butter	1 pretzel	270	8	1	58	56	2	780	0
Maple Crumb Pretzel	1 pretzel	550	10	6	112	109	3	550	10
Maple Crumb Pretzel without Butter	1 pretzel	520	10	3	100	97	3	550	0
Original Pretzel	1 pretzel	370	10	4	72	69	3	930	10
Original Pretzel without Butter	1 pretzel	340	10	1	72	69	3	900	0
Parmesan Herb Pretzel	1 pretzel	440	10	13	72	63	9	660	30

Description	Serving Size	Cal	Prot (g)	Fat (g)	Carbs (g)	Net Carb(g)	Fiber (g)	Sod (mg)	Chol (mg)
AUNTIE ANNE'S PRETZELS® (continued)									
Parmesan Herb Pretzel without Butter	1 pretzel	390	11	5	74	70	4	780	10
Pretzel Dog	1 pretzel	290	10	16	25	24	1	600	40
Sesame Pretzel	1 pretzel	410	12	12	64	57	7	860	15
Sesame Pretzel without Butter	1 pretzel	350	11	6	63	60	3	840	0
Smart Bites	1 bite	10	1	1	2	1	1	30	0
Sour Cream & Onion Pretzel	1 pretzel	340	9	5	66	64	2	930	10
Sour Cream & Onion Pretzel without Butter	1 pretzel	310	9	1	66	64	2	920	0
Stix - Cinnamon Sugar	Regular	300	5	6	55	53	2	287	17
Stix - Cinnamon Sugar without Butter	Regular	233	6	1	49	48	1	273	0
Stix - Original	Regular	247	7	3	48	46	2	620	7
Stix - Original without Butter	Regular	227	7		48	46	2	600	0
Whole Wheat Pretzel	1 pretzel	370	11	5	72	65	7	1120	10
Whole Wheat Pretzel without Butter	1 pretzel	350	11	2	72	65	7	1100	0
DUTCH ICE®									
Grape Dutch Ice®	20 fl oz	260	0	0	62	62	0	30	0
Kiwi-Banana Dutch Ice®	20 fl oz	270	0	0	70	70	0	40	0
Lemonade Dutch Ice®	20 fl oz	450	0	15	110	110	0	0	0
Mocha Dutch Ice®	20 fl oz	570	0	0	105	105	0	150	0
Orange Crème Dutch Ice®.	20 fl oz	400	0	0	92	92	0	50	0
Piña Colada Dutch Ice®	20 fl oz	360	0	0	82	82	0	30	0
Blue Raspberry Dutch Ice®	20 fl oz	250	0	0	57	55	2	40	0
Strawberry Dutch Ice®	20 fl oz	315	0	0	72	72	0	60	0
Wild Cherry Dutch Ice®	20 fl oz	330	0	0	75	75	0	35	0
DUTCH SHAKE									
Chocolate Dutch Shake	20 fl oz	860	14	41	113	113	0	576	155
Coffee Dutch Shake	20 fl oz	890	14	41	115	115	0	456	155
Strawberry Dutch Shake	20 fl oz	910	14	41	118	118	0	456	155
Vanilla Dutch Shake	20 fl oz	770	15	63	87	87	0	460	155
DUTCH SMOOTHIE									
Grape Dutch Smoothie	20 fl oz	400	5	14	65	65	0	180	55
Kiwi-Banana Dutch Smoothie	20 fl oz	430	5	14	68	68	0	150	55
Lemonade Dutch Smoothie	20 fl oz	540	5	23	95	95	0	150	55
Mocha Dutch Smoothie	20 fl oz	590	5	14	90	90	0	240	55
Orange Creme Dutch Smoothie	20 fl oz	500	5	14	83	83	0	180	55
Pina Colada Dutch Smoothie	20 fl oz	470	5	14	79	79	0	170	55

Description	Serving Size	Cal	Prot (g)	Fat (g)	Carbs (g)	Net Carb(g)	Fiber (g)	Sod (mg)	Chol (mg)
Blue Raspberry Dutch Smoothie.	20 fl oz	400	5	14	61	61	0	180	55
Strawberry Dutch Smoothie	20 fl oz	450	5	14	72	72	0	180	55
Wild Cherry Dutch Smoothie	20 fl oz	450	5	22	74	74	0	170	55
DIPPING SAUCES									
Light Cream Cheese	1 container	70	3	10	1	1	0	140	25
Strawberry Cream Cheese	1 container	110	2	3	4	4	0	105	35
Caramel Dip	1 container	135	1	8	27	27	0	110	5
Cheese Sauce	1 container	100	3	4	4	4	0	510	10
Chocolate Flavored Dip	1 container	130	1	0	24	23	1	65	2
Marinara Sauce	1 container	10	0	2	4	4	0	180	0
Sweet Mustard	1 container	60	1	8	8	8	0	120	40

Blimpie®

SANDWICHES

Description	Serving Size	Cal	Prot (g)	Fat (g)	Carbs (g)	Net Carb(g)	Fiber (g)	Sod (mg)	Chol (mg)
Best Sub on Wheat Cold	1 6-inch sub	410	39	13	47	43	4	1480	50
Best Sub on White Cold	1 6-inch sub	410	39	13	47	43	4	1480	50
Cheese Trio Sub on Wheat Cold	1 6-inch sub	490	26	23	48	43	5	1110	55
Cheese Trio Sub on White Cold	1 6-inch sub	490	25	23	48	45	3	1130	55
Chicken Caesar Wrap	1 wrap	610	26	31	56	53	3	1770	35
Chik Max on Wheat Hot Sub	1 6-inch sub	495	26	13	69	65	4	1370	0
Chik Max on White Hot Sub	1 6-inch sub	483	34	12	70	66	4	1293	0
Club Sub on Wheat Cold	1 6-inch sub	370	23	11	48	43	5	1180	30
Club Sub on White Cold	1 6-inch sub	370	23	10	48	45	3	1200	30
Grille Max on Wheat Hot Sub	1 6-inch sub	425	19	7	71	66	5	900	5
Grille Max on White Hot Sub	1 6-inch sub	413	18	6	72	67	5	823	5
Grilled Chicken Hot Sub	1 6-inch sub	400	28	9	52	50	2	950	30
Ham & Swiss Sub on Wheat Cold	1 6-inch sub	400	26	14	46	41	5	1040	50
Ham & Swiss Sub on White Cold	1 6-inch sub	410	25	14	48	45	3	1050	50
Ham, Salami, & Provolone Sub on Wheat Cold	1 6-inch sub	450	24	20	47	42	5	1350	55
Ham, Salami, & Provolone Sub on White Cold	1 6-inch sub	480	24	20	49	46	3	1370	55
Italian Meatball Hot Sub	1 6-inch sub	500	23	22	52	50	2	970	25
Mexi Max on Wheat Hot Sub	1 6-inch sub	405	25	6	65	60	5	1080	0
Mexi Max on White Hot Sub	1 6-inch sub	393	25	5	66	61	5	1003	0
Roast Beef Sub on Wheat Cold	1 6-inch sub	390	37	8	45	40	5	1380	65
Roast Beef Sub on White Cold	1 6-inch sub	390	37	7	47	44	3	1370	65

Description	Serving Size	Cal	Prot (g)	Fat (g)	Carbs (g)	Net Carb(g)	Fiber (g)	Sod (mg)	Chol (mg)
BLIMPIE® (continued)									
Roast Turkey Cordon Bleu Hot Sub	1 6-inch sub	430	29	14	43	42	1	1180	60
Smokey Cheddar Beef Hot Sub	1 6-inch sub	380	23	12	42	41	1	1200	50
South Western Wrap	1 wrap	590	28	28	56	53	3	1990	75
Steak & Cheese Hot Sub	1 6-inch sub	550	27	26	51	49	2	1080	70
Turkey Sub on Wheat Cold	1 6-inch sub	330	19	7	48	43	5	1190	10
Turkey Sub on White Cold	1 6-inch sub	330	19	6	48	45	3	1200	10
Vegi Max on Wheat Hot Sub	1 6-inch sub	415	24	8	60	55	5	1050	0
Vegi Max on White Hot Sub	1 6-inch sub	403	24	7	61	56	5	980	0
Zesty Italian Wrap	1 wrap	530	24	22	59	56	3	1850	45
BLIMPIE Special Sub Dressing	1 serving	70	0	7	0	0	0	0	0
SALADS									
Chef Salad	1 salad	150	17	6	8	5	3	600	40
Chili Ole Salad	1 salad	480	21	27	42	39	3	1240	45
Club Salad	1 salad	130	14	6	7	4	3	450	30
Cole Slaw	1 serving	180	1	13	13	12	1	230	5
Italian Pasta Supreme Salad	1 salad	180	3	7	20	19	1	840	0
Tossed Green Salad	1 salad	35	2	1	7	4	3	20	0
Turkey Salad	1 salad	90	15	1	8	5	3	580	25
Antipasto Salad	1 salad	200	19	11	9	6	3	950	50
Fat Free Italian Dressing	1 packet	20	0	0	5	5	0	670	0
Potato Salad	1 serving	270	2	19	19	18	1	560	10
Zesty Pesto Turkey Salad	1 salad	370	20	19	31	31	0	1410	40
Guacamole	1 serving	194	2	18	7	6	1	468	1
Roast Beef 'n Bleu Salad	1 salad	390	31	16	29	29	0	1550	70
Mayonnaise	1 packet	100	0	11	1	1	0	60	10
Ham & Swiss Cheese Salad	1 salad	170	16	8	7	4	3	500	40
Roast Beef Salad	1 salad	120	19	3	8	5	3	480	25
BLIMPIE Dressing	1 packet	120	1	8	16	15	1	570	0
Light Italian Dressing	1 packet	20	0	1	3	3	0	810	0
Light Buttermilk Ranch Dressing	1 packet	90	1	5	10	10	0	350	0
Blue Cheese Dressing	1 packet	220	2	24	2	2	0	440	40
Buttermilk Ranch Dressing	1 packet	270	0	29	1	1	0	360	5
Honey French Dressing	1 packet	240	0	20	16	16	0	350	0
Thousand Island Dressing	1 packet	210	0	21	7	7	0	360	25
Mustard Potato Salad	1 serving	160	2	5	21	20	1	660	5
Macaroni Salad	1 serving	360	4	25	25	24	1	660	10

Description	Serving Size	Cal	Prot (g)	Fat (g)	Carbs (g)	Net Carb(g)	Fiber (g)	Sod (mg)	Chol (mg)
SOUPS									
Chicken Noodle Soup	1 bowl	140	8	3	20	18	2	1190	30
Chicken Soup with White & Wild Rice	1 bowl	230	10	12	21	19	2	1210	30
Classic Chili with Beans & Beef	1 bowl	240	14	8	27	17	10	1060	40
Cream of Potato Soup		190	5	9	24	21	3	860	5
CHIPS									
Blimpie Regular Flavored Potato Chips	1 bag	210	3	11	25	23	2	190	0
Blimpie Cheddar & Sour Cream Potato Chips	1 bag	210	3	11	25	24	1	220	5
Blimpie Sour Cream & Onion Potato Chips	1 bag	210	2	11	25	24	1	250	5
Blimpie Zesty Potato Chips	1 bag	210	3	11	25	23	2	220	5
Blimpie Jalapeno Potato Chips	1 bag	210	2	11	25	23	2	250	0
Blimpie Lea & Perrin's Barbecue Potato Chips	1 bag	210	3	10	25	23	2	270	0
DESSERTS									
Peanut Butter Cookie	1 cookie	221	4	12	27	26	1	201	15
Sugar Cookie	1 cookie	330	3	17	24	24	0	290	30
Macadamia White Chunk Cookie	1 cookie	210	2	10	26	25	1	140	20
Chocolate Chunk Cookie	1 cookie	201	2	10	26	25	1	201	15
Oatmeal Raisin Cookie	1 cookie	191	3	8	27	26	1	201	15

Burger King®

Description	Serving Size	Cal	Prot (g)	Fat (g)	Carbs (g)	Net Carb(g)	Fiber (g)	Sod (mg)	Chol (mg)
BURGERS/ SANDWICHES									
Cheeseburger	1 sandwich	360	19	17	31	29	2	790	50
Bacon Cheeseburger	1 sandwich	400	22	20	32	30	2	1010	60
Bacon Double Cheeseburger	1 sandwich	580	35	34	32	30	2	1240	110
Hamburger	1 sandwich	310	17	14	31	29	2	580	40
Whopper Jr.®	1 sandwich	390	17	22	32	30	2	570	45
Whopper Jr.® (w/o Mayo)	1 sandwich	310	17	13	31	29	2	510	40
Whopper Jr.® With Cheese	1 sandwich	440	19	26	32	30	2	790	55
Whopper Jr.® With Cheese (w/o Mayo)	1 sandwich	360	19	17	32	30	2	730	50
WHOPPER®	1 sandwich	710	31	43	52	48	4	980	85
Whopper® With Cheese	1 sandwich	800	36	50	53	49	4	1420	110
Whopper® With Cheese (w/o Mayo)	1 sandwich	640	35	33	53	49	4	1290	95
Whopper® (w/o Mayo)	1 sandwich	550	31	25	52	48	4	860	75
Double Whopper®	1 sandwich	980	52	62	52	48	4	1070	160

Description	Serving Size	Cal	Prot (g)	Fat (g)	Carbs (g)	Net Carb(g)	Fiber (g)	Sod (mg)	Chol (mg)
BURGER KING® (continued)									
Double Whopper® (w/o Mayo)	1 sandwich	820	52	45	52	48	4	950	150
Double Whopper® With Cheese	1 sandwich	1070	57	70	53	49	4	1500	185
Double Whopper® With Cheese (w/o Mayo)	1 sandwich	910	57	52	53	49	4	1380	170
Double Cheeseburger	1 sandwich	540	32	31	32	30	2	1050	100
BK VEGGIE Burger	1 sandwich	340	14	10	47	43	4	950	0
BK FISH FILET Sandwich	1 sandwich	520	18	30	44	42	2	840	55
Flame-Roasted Peppers & Onions	1 sandwich	18	1	1	3	1	2	81	0
Grilled Chicken Caesar Club Sandwich	1 sandwich	540	34	27	40	37	3	1510	65
Smoky BBQ Fire Grilled Chicken Baguette	1 sandwich	350	29	5	48	44	4	1450	45
Santa Fe Fire Grilled Chicken Baguette	1 sandwich	350	29	5	47	43	4	1220	45
Savory Mustard Fire Grilled Chicken Baguette	1 sandwich	350	28	5	47	44	3	1110	45
Chicken WHOPPER®	1 sandwich	580	39	26	48	44	4	1370	75
Chicken WHOPPER® (w/o Mayo)	1 sandwich	420	38	8	47	43	4	1250	60
Original Chicken Sandwich	1 sandwich	560	25	28	52	49	3	1270	60
SALADS									
Side Garden Salad (w/o dressing)	1 salad	25	1	0	5	3	2	15	0
Side Garden Salad (w/o dressing)	1 salad	25	1	0	5	3	2	15	0
Chicken Caesar Salad (w/o dressing)	1 salad	230	36	7	5	2	3	1040	60
SIDES									
French Fries - Medium (salted)	Medium	360	4	18	46	42	4	640	0
Onion Rings - Medium	Medium	320	4	16	40	37	3	460	0
CHICKEN TENDERS®	5 pieces	210	14	12	13	12	1	530	30
CHICKEN TENDERS®	8 pieces	340	22	19	20	19	1	840	50
Chili	1 bowl/cup	190	13	8	17	12	5	1040	25
CONDIMENTS/ DRESSINGS									
Baja BBQ Sauce	1 packet	14	1	1	3	2	1	351	0
Barbecue Dipping Sauce	1 packet	35	0	0	9	9	0	390	0
Breakfast Syrup	1 packet	80	0	0	21	21	0	20	0
Fire Roasted Sauce	1 packet	9	1	1	2	1	1	129	0
Grape Jam	1 packet	30	0	0	7	7	0	0	0
Honey Flavored Dipping Sauce	1 packet	90	0	0	23	23	0	0	0
Honey Mustard Dipping Sauce	1 packet	90	0	6	9	9	0	150	10
Kraft® Catalina Dressing	1 packet	180	0	16	10	10	0	530	0
Kraft® Fat Free Ranch Dressing	1 packet	60	0	0	6	6	0	430	0

CHAINS

Description	Serving Size	Cal	Prot (g)	Fat (g)	Carbs (g)	Net Carb(g)	Fiber (g)	Sod (mg)	Chol (mg)
Kraft® Ranch Dressing	1 packet	220	0	23	2	2	0	410	10
Lite Done Right® Light Italian Dressing	1 packet	50	0	5	4	4	0	360	0
Ranch Dipping Sauce	1 packet	140	1	15	1	1	0	95	5
Savory Mustard Sauce	1 packet	21	1	1	4	3	1	92	2
Signature® Creamy Caesar Dressing	1 packet	140	1	13	4	4	0	340	10
Strawberry Jam	1 packet	30	0	0	7	7	0	0	0
Sweet and Sour Dipping Sauce	1 packet	40	0	0	10	10	0	65	0
Zesty Onion Ring Dipping Sauce	1 packet	150	0	15	3	3	0	210	15
DESSERTS/ SHAKES/ BEVERAGES									
Chocolate Shake (Syrup added)	Medium	790	15	42	89	87	2	380	125
Strawberry Shake (Syrup added)	Medium	780	15	41	88	87	1	300	125
Vanilla Shake	Medium	720	15	41	73	72	1	280	125
Frozen Coca Cola® Classic	Medium	455	0	0	113	113	0	0	0
Frozen Minute Maid® Cherry	Medium	450	0	0	113	113	0	0	0
Nestle® Freshly Baked Choc.Chip Cookies	2 cookies	440	5	16	68	68	0	360	20
Dutch Apple Pie	1 slice	340	2	14	52	51	1	470	0
Hershey's® Sundae Pie	1 slice	300	3	18	31	30	1	190	10
BREAKFAST ITEMS									
Croissan'wich® with Sausage & Cheese	1 sandwich	420	14	31	23	22	1	840	45
Croissan'wich® with Sausage, Egg & Cheese	1 sandwich	520	19	39	24	23	1	1090	210
Croissan'wich® with Egg & Cheese	1 sandwich	320	12	19	24	23	1	730	185
Croissan'wich® with Bacon, Egg & Cheese	1 sandwich	360	15	22	25	24	1	950	195
Croissan'wich® with Ham, Egg & Cheese	1 sandwich	360	18	20	25	24	1	1500	200
Sourdough Sandwich w/ Ham, Egg & Cheese	1 sandwich	380	19	20	30	28	2	1560	195
Sourdough Sandwich w/ Bacon, Egg & Cheese	1 sandwich	380	16	20	30	28	2	990	190
Sourdough Sandwich w/ Sausage, Egg & Cheese	1 sandwich	540	20	39	30	28	2	1140	210
French Toast Sticks	5 sticks	390	7	20	46	44	2	440	0
Hash Brown Rounds	Large	390	3	25	38	34	4	760	0
Hash Brown Rounds	Small	230	2	15	23	21	2	450	0

Description	Serving Size	Cal	Prot (g)	Fat (g)	Carbs (g)	Net Carb(g)	Fiber (g)	Sod (mg)	Chol (mg)
Chick-Fil-A®									
CLASSICS									
Chicken Strips	6 pieces	430	NA	20	21	20	1	1090	100
Chicken Strips	4 pieces	290	29	13	14	13	1	730	65
Chicken Sandwich	1 sandwich	410	28	16	38	37	1	1300	60
Chicken Sandwich(no butter)	1 sandwich	380	28	13	37	36	1	1290	60
Chargrilled Sandwich	1 sandwich	270	28	4	33	30	3	940	65
Chargrilled Chicken Club	1 sandwich	380	35	11	33	30	3	1240	90
Chicken Salad Sandwich	1 sandwich	350	20	15	32	27	5	880	65
Chick-fil-a Nuggets	4-pc kid meal	130	NA	6	6	6	0	550	35
Chick-fil-a Nuggets	6-pc kid meal	200	NA	9	9	8	1	820	50
Chick-fil-a Nuggets	8 pack	260	26	12	12	11	1	1090	70
Chick-fil-a Nuggets 12 pack	12 pack	390	NA	18	18	17	1	1640	100
Chicken (no bun)	1 filet	230	23	11	10	10	0	990	60
Chargrilled Chicken (no bun)	1 filet	100	21	2	1	1	0	610	65
BREAKFAST									
Plain Biscuit	1 biscuit	260	4	11	38	37	1	670	0
Hot Buttered Biscuit	1 biscuit	270	4	12	38	38		680	0
Chicken Biscuit	1 biscuit	400	16	18	43	41	2	1200	30
Chicken Biscuit w/Cheese	1 biscuit	450	19	23	43	41	2	1430	45
Biscuit w/Bacon	1 biscuit	300	6	14	38	37	1	780	5
Biscuit w/ Bacon & Egg	1 biscuit	390	13	20	38	37	1	860	250
Biscuit w/ Bacon Egg & Cheese	1 biscuit	430	16	24	38	37	1	1070	265
Biscuit w/ Egg	1 biscuit	340	11	16	38	37	1	740	245
Biscuit w/Egg & Cheese	1 biscuit	390	13	21	38	37	1	960	260
Biscuit w/Sausage	1 biscuit	410	9	23	42	41	1	740	20
Biscuit w/ Sausage & Egg	1 biscuit	500	15	29	43	42	1	810	265
Biscuit w/Sausage, Egg & Cheese	1 biscuit	540	18	33	43	42	1	1030	280
Biscuit & Gravy	1 biscuit	310	5	13	44	43	1	930	5
Chick-fil-A Chicken Platter	1 platter	589	NA	29	53	51	2	1703	391
Chick-fil-A Bacon Platter	1 platter	525	NA	28	47	46	2	1409	375
Chick-fil-A Sausage Platter	1 platter	603	NA	35	52	50	2	1244	382
Hashbrowns	1 packet	170	2	9	20	18	2	350	10
Danish	1 danish	430	6	17	63	61	2	160	25
COOLWRAPS									
Spicy Chicken Cool Wrap	1 wrap	380	30	6	52	49	3	1090	60
Chargrilled Chicken Cool Wraps	1 wrap	390	29	7	54	51	3	1020	65

Description	Serving Size	Cal	Prot (g)	Fat (g)	Carbs (g)	Net Carb(g)	Fiber (g)	Sod (mg)	Chol (mg)
Chicken Caesar Cool Wraps	1 wrap	460	36	10	52	49	3	1350	80
SALADS									
Chargrilled Chicken Garden Salad	1 salad	180	22	6	9	6	3	620	65
Chicken Strips Salad	1 salad	390	34	18	22	18	4	860	80
Southwest Chargrilled Salad	1 salad	240	25	8	17	12	5	770	60
Garlic & Butter Croutons	1 packet	50	NA	3	6	6	0	90	0
Honey Roasted Sunflower Kernels	1 packet	80	NA	7	3	2	1	38	0
Tortilla Strips	1 packet	70	NA	4	9	8	1	53	0
SIDES									
Chick-Fil-A Waffle Potato Fries	Small	270	3	13	34	30	4	115	0
Fresh Fruit Cup	1 cup	60	1	0	16	14	2	0	0
Carrot & Raisin Salad	1 salad	170	1	6	28	26	2	110	10
Cole Slaw	1 salad	260	2	21	17	15	2	220	25
Side Salad	1 salad	60	3	3	4	2	2	75	10
Hearty Breast of Chicken Soup	Regular	140	8	4	18	17	1	900	25
Hearty Breast of Chicken Soup	Large	250	NA	7	32	29	3	1650	50
Chicken Salad Cup	1 cup	270	NA	18	8	4	4	790	85
DRESSING & SAUCES									
Caesar Dressing	1 packet	160	1	17	1	1	0	240	30
Red. Fat Raspberry Vinaigrette	1 packet	80	0	2	15	15	0	190	0
Buttermilk Ranch Dressing	1 packet	160	0	16	1	1	0	270	5
Blue Cheese Dressing	1 packet	150	1	16	1	1	0	300	20
Spicy Dressing	1 packet	140	0	14	2	2	0	130	5
Thousand Island Dressing	1 packet	150	0	14	5	5	0	250	10
Light Italian Dressing	1 packet	15	0	1	2	2	0	570	0
Fat Free Honey Mustard	1 packet	60	0	0	14	14	0	200	0
Polynesian Sauce	1 packet	110	0	6	13	13	0	210	0
Barbecue Sauce	1 packet	45	0	0	11	11	0	180	0
Honey Mustard	1 packet	45	0	0	10	10	0	150	0
Buttermilk Ranch	1 packet	110	0	12	1	1	0	200	5
Chick-fil-A Buffalo Sauce	1 packet	15	0	2	1	1	0	410	0
Honey Roasted BBQ Sauce	1 packet	60	0	6	2	2	0	90	5
DRINKS									
Chick-fil-A Lemonade	Small	170	0	1	41	41	0	10	0
DESSERTS									
Icedream Cup	1 cup	230	5	6	38	38	0	100	25

Description	Serving Size	Cal	Prot (g)	Fat (g)	Carbs (g)	Net Carb(g)	Fiber (g)	Sod (mg)	Chol (mg)
CHICK-FIL-A® (continued)									
Icedream Cone	1 cone	160	4	4	28	28	0	80	15
Chick-fil-A Cheesecake	1 slice	340	6	21	30	28	2	270	90
Chick-fil-A Lemon Pie	1 slice	320	7	10	51	48	3	220	110
Fudge Nut Brownie	1 brownie	330	4	15	45	43	2	210	20

Church's Chicken™

FRIED CHICKEN

Description	Serving Size	Cal	Prot (g)	Fat (g)	Carbs (g)	Net Carb(g)	Fiber (g)	Sod (mg)	Chol (mg)
Wing	1 piece	250	19	16	8	8	0	540	60
Leg	1 piece	140	13	9	2	2	0	160	45
Thigh	1 piece	230	16	16	5	5	0	520	80
Breast	1 piece	200	19	12	4	4	0	510	65
Krispy Tender Strips™	1 piece	137	11	5	11	11	0	431	25
Tender Crunchers™	1 piece	411	34	15	32	31	1	1294	74

SIDES

Description	Serving Size	Cal	Prot (g)	Fat (g)	Carbs (g)	Net Carb(g)	Fiber (g)	Sod (mg)	Chol (mg)
Honey Butter Biscuits	1 biscuit	250	2	16	26	25	1	640	<5
Mashed Potatoes & Gravy	1 serving	90	1	3	14	13	1	520	
Okra	1 serving	210	3	16	19	15	4	520	
Corn on the Cob	1 serving	139	4	3	24	15	9	15	
Whole Jalapeno Poppers	1 serving	10	0	0	2	1	1	390	
Cole Slaw	1 serving	92	4	6	8	6	2	230	
French Fries	1 serving	210	3	11	29	27	2	60	
Collard Greens	1 serving	25	2	0	5	3	2	170	0
Macaroni & Cheese	1 serving	210	8	11	23	22	1	690	15
C. Fried Steak w/White Gravy	1 serving	470	21	28	36	35	1	1615	65
Sweet Corn Nuggets	1 serving	250	3	12	30	28	2	530	0
Jalapeno Cheese Bombers ®	1 serving	240	8	10	29	26	3	968	28
Cajun Rice	1 serving	130	1	7	16	15	1	260	5

DESSERT

Description	Serving Size	Cal	Prot (g)	Fat (g)	Carbs (g)	Net Carb(g)	Fiber (g)	Sod (mg)	Chol (mg)
Apple Pie	1 slice	280	2	12	41	40	1	340	<5
Edwards Double Lemon Pie	1 slice	300	5	14	39	39	0	15	25
Edward's Strawberry Cream Cheese Pie	1 slice	280	4	15	32	30	2	130	160

Description	Serving Size	Cal	Prot (g)	Fat (g)	Carbs (g)	Net Carb(g)	Fiber (g)	Sod (mg)	Chol (mg)
Denny's®									
BREAKFAST MENU									
Meat Lover's Skillet	1 order	1031	39	74	27	17	10	2374	528
Meat Lover's Breakfast	1 order	1027	44	60	72	69	3	3462	497
Chicken Fajita Skillet	1 order	855	26	49	30	19	11	1863	515
Original Grand Slam	1 order	665	26	49	33	31	2	1106	515
All American Slam	1 order	816	46	67	3	2	1	1826	828
French Slam	1 order	1119	46	77	71	68	3	2265	705
Farmer's Slam	1 order	1200	51	80	82	79	3	3204	704
Grand Slam Slugger	1 order	927	34	55	74	71	3	2399	476
Country Scramble	1 order	1038	42	62	79	75	4	3935	481
Denver Scramble	1 order	940	48	51	75	71	4	3331	551
Fiesta Scramble	1 order	910	40	52	74	70	4	2945	493
Lumberjack Slam w/ hash browns	1 order	1035	51	58	73	70	3	4462	589
Corned Beef Hash Slam	1 order	668	32	55	11	10	1	816	535
Ultimate Omelet	1 order	619	36	50	8	7	1	1214	770
Veggie-Cheese Omelet	1 order	494	30	39	2	0	6	11	747
Veggie-Cheese Omelet w/eggbeaters	1 order	346	25	22	11	8	3	849	23
Ham & Cheddar Omelet	1 order	595	41	47	5	5	0	1200	783
Ham & Cheddar Omelet w/eggbeaters	1 order	468	37	32	5	5	0	1351	58
Oatmeal Deluxe	1 order	460	13	6	95	88	7	87	11
Country Fried Steak & Eggs	1 order	464	29	34	13	7	6	828	527
T-bone Steak & Eggs	1 order	991	73	77	1	0	1	1003	657
Sirloin Steak & Eggs	1 order	675	62	45	1	0	1	368	643
Breakfast Dagwood	1 order	1446	82	90	81	80	1	4003	765
Moons Over My Hammy	1 order	841	54	51	42	40	2	2699	580
Belgian Waffle Platter	1 order	619	22	45	28	28	0	1683	274
Fabulous French Toast Platter	1 order	1146	26	71	104	101	3	2241	297
Buttermilk Pancake Platter	1 order	466	20	23	47	45	2	2077	47
Buttermilk Pancake	1 order	223	6	4	47	45	2	901	0
Country Fried Potatoes	1 order	394	3	20	23	13	10	938	9
Hashed Browns	1 order	197	2	12	20	18	2	446	0
Covered	1 order	280	7	19	2	1	1	21	583
Covered & Smothered	1 order	493	14	25	54	51	3	3524	29
Fresh Fruit Bowl w/ Bagel	1 order	407	13	4	86	81	5	659	0
Grits	1 order	80	2	0	18	18	0	520	0

Description	Serving Size	Cal	Prot (g)	Fat (g)	Carbs (g)	Net Carb(g)	Fiber (g)	Sod (mg)	Chol (mg)
DENNY'S® (continued)									
APPETIZERS									
Sampler ™		1405	47	80	124	120	4	5305	75
Buffalo Wings	9 wings	974	67	72	11	9	2	4049	267
Mozzarella Sticks	8 sticks	710	36	41	49	43	6	5220	48
Smothered Cheese Fries	1 order	767	27	48	69	69	0	875	78
Buffalo Chicken Strips	1 order	734	48	42	43	43	0	1673	96
Chicken Strips	1 order	720	47	33	56	56	0	1666	95
Nacho	1 order	1278	54	64	117	106	11	1654	181
ENTREES									
Mini Burgers (6) w/Onion Rings	1 order	2044	61	122	179	169	10	3834	145
T-bone Steak Dinner	1 order	860	65	65	0	0	0	867	196
Sirloin Steak Dinner	1 order	337	18	28	1	0	1	344	687
Pot Roast Dinner	1 order	292	42	11	5	5	0	927	87
Country Fried Steak	1 order	644	28	46	30	19	11	2149	89
Fried Shrimp & Shrimp Scampi	1 order	346	27	20	15	14	1	1104	241
Steak and Shrimp Dinner	1 order	645	36	42	31	29	2	1143	150
Fried Shrimp Dinner	1 order	219	17	10	18	17	1	774	133
Roast Turkey & Stuffing (incl. gravy)	1 order	435	42	10	62	60	2	4620	100
Shrimp Scampi Skillet Dinner	1 order	289	25	19	3	3	0	766	192
Grilled Chicken Dinner	1 order	200	25	5	15	14	1	824	67
Fish & Chips	1 order	958	34	54	83	77	6	1390	88
Chicken Strips	1 order	635	47	25	55	55	0	1510	95
Fisherman's Platter	1 order	1027	24	62	89	79	10	1103	121
SIDES									
Carrots in sauce	1 order	50	0	1	8	6	2	121	0
Green Beans in sauce	1 order	40	1	1	5	3	2	115	2
Baked Potato, plain w/skin	1 order	220	5	0	51	46	5	16	0
Mashed Potatoes, plain	1 order	168	3	7	23	21	2	498	8
Bread Stuffing, plain	1 order	100	3	1	19	18	1	405	0
Cottage Cheese	1 order	72	9	3	2	2	0	281	10
Applesauce, Musselman's	1 order	60	0	0	15	14	1	13	0
French Fries, unsalted	1 order	423	6	20	57	52	5	221	0
Seasoned Fries	1 order	261	5	12	35	35	0	556	0
Onion Rings	1 order	381	5	23	38	37	1	1003	6
Coleslaw	1 order	274	2	24	14	12	2	588	37

Description	Serving Size	Cal	Prot (g)	Fat (g)	Carbs (g)	Net Carb(g)	Fiber (g)	Sod (mg)	Chol (mg)
SANDWICHES									
Club Sandwich	1 sandwich	602	31	38	45	43	2	2450	41
The Super Bird® Sandwich	1 sandwich	479	24	29	32	30	2	1764	47
Grilled Chicken Sandwich w/o dressing	1 sandwich	476	36	14	56	52	4	1494	77
Bacon, Lettuce & Tomato	1 sandwich	610	15	38	50	48	2	862	35
BBQ Chicken Sandwich	1 sandwich	1089	48	62	86	81	5	1872	103
Classic Burger	1 sandwich	694	40	35	56	52	4	785	100
Classic Burger w/Cheese	1 sandwich	852	49	48	57	53	4	1385	140
Hickory Cheeseburger	1 sandwich	1221	49	71	84	79	5	1133	114
Bacon Cheddar Burger	1 sandwich	875	53	52	58	53	5	1672	163
Patty Melt	1 sandwich	798	45	51	37	33	4	1285	127
Chicken Ranch Melt	1 sandwich	758	44	45	44	41	3	2195	105
Hoagie Chicken Melt	1 sandwich	751	46	44	43	41	2	1834	93
Hoagie Philly Melt	1 sandwich	874	47	50	58	53	5	2444	114
Italian Chicken Melt	1 sandwich	1134	51	62	68	61	7	3735	115
Boca Burger	1 sandwich	601	32	27	64	55	9	1446	14
Mushroom Swiss Burger	1 sandwich	880	51	49	63	58	5	1619	137
Buffalo Chicken Sandwich	1 sandwich	708	37	28	80	75	5	1733	74
Turkey Breast on Multigrain w/o mayo	1 sandwich	277	23	4	41	36	5	1607	15
Ham & Swiss on Rye w/o mayo	1 sandwich	417	32	16	39	34	5	1763	57
Albacore Tuna Melt	1 sandwich	640	30	39	42	39	3	1438	109
Fish Sandwich	1 sandwich	589	22	30	30	27	3	1557	30
SOUPS									
Chicken Noodle	1 order	118	1	5	14	13	1	1130	30
Cream of Broccoli	1 order	574	6	43	41	39	2	1174	0
Clam Chowder	1 order	624	7	42	4	0	7	55	1474
Vegetable Beef	1 order	79	6	1	11	9	2	820	5
SALADS									
Chef's Salad	1 salad	365	41	16	14	10	4	1376	289
Grilled Chicken Breast Salad	1 salad	264	32	11	10	6	4	714	89
Turkey Breast Salad w/o dressing	1 salad	248	31	8	12	8	4	798	86
Fried Chicken Strip Salad	1 salad	438	33	26	26	22	4	1030	78
Side Caesar (w/ dressing)	1 salad	362	11	26	20	17	3	913	23
Side Garden Salad (w/o dressing)	1 salad	113	7	7	6	4	2	144	0
DESSERTS									
Apple Pie	1 slice	7	3	470	47	46	1	0	6
Coconut Cream Pie	1 slice	582	5	33	63	60	3	482	0

Description	Serving Size	Cal	Prot (g)	Fat (g)	Carbs (g)	Net Carb(g)	Fiber (g)	Sod (mg)	Chol (mg)
DENNY'S (continued)									
French Silk Pie	1 slice	690	7	49	54	50	4	225	80
Apple Crisp a la mode	1 slice	723	6	21	133	127	6	394	32
Chocolate Peanut Butter Pie	1 slice	653	15	39	64	61	3	319	27
Cheesecake	1 slice	580	8	38	51	51	0	380	174
Carrot Cake	1 slice	799	9	45	99	97	2	630	125
Hot Fudge Brownie a la mode	1 order	997	12	42	147	141	6	82	14
Banana Split	1 order	894	4	43	121	115	6	177	78
Double Scoop/Sundae	1 sundae	375	6	27	29	29	0	86	74
Single Scoop/Sundae	1 sundae	188	3	14	14	14	0	43	37
Milkshake (van/choc)	1 shake	560	11	26	76	75	1	272	100
Malted Milkshake (van/choc)	1 shake	583	12	26	82	81	1	278	100
Floats (Root beer or Cola)	1 float	280	3	10	47	47	0	109	39
Oreo Blender Blaster	1 order	895	16	46	112	110	2	280	135

Domino's®

CLASSIC HAND TOSSED — 12" MEDIUM

Description	Serving Size	Cal	Prot (g)	Fat (g)	Carbs (g)	Net Carb(g)	Fiber (g)	Sod (mg)	Chol (mg)
Classic Hand Tossed ExtravaganZZa Feast	1 slice	289	13	14	30	28	2	764	28
Classic Hand Tossed MeatZZa Feast	1 slice	281	13	14	29	27	2	740	28
Classic Hand Tossed Bacon Cheeseburger Feast	1 slice	273	12	13	28	26	2	634	27
Classic Hand Tossed w/ Pepperoni & Sausage	1 slice	255	10	12	28	26	2	626	22
Classic Hand Tossed Pepperoni Feast	1 slice	265	11	13	28	26	2	670	24
Classic Hand Tossed America's Favorite Feast	1 slice	257	10	12	29	27	2	626	22
Classic Hand Tossed Barbeque Feast	1 slice	252	11	10	31	30	1	600	20
Classic Hand Tossed w/ Sausage	1 slice	231	9	10	28	26	2	530	17
Classic Hand Tossed Deluxe Feast	1 slice	234	9	10	29	27	2	542	17
Classic Hand Tossed Beef	1 slice	225	9	9	28	26	2	493	16
Classic Hand Tossed w/ Pepperoni	1 slice	223	9	9	28	26	2	522	16
Classic Hand Tossed Veggie Feast	1 slice	218	9	8	29	27	2	489	13
Classic Hand Tossed Hawaiian Feast	1 slice	223	10	8	30	28	2	547	16
Classic Hand Tossed w/ Ham & Pineapple	1 slice	200	9	6	29	27	2	467	12
Classic Hand Tossed w/ Ham	1 slice	198	9	6	28	27	1	492	13

Description	Serving Size	Cal	Prot (g)	Fat (g)	Carbs (g)	Net Carb(g)	Fiber (g)	Sod (mg)	Chol (mg)
Classic Hand Tossed Gr. Pepper, Onion, & Mushroom	1 slice	191	8	6	29	27	2	386	9
Classic Hand Tossed w/ Cheese	1 slice	186	7	6	28	27	1	385	9

CRUNCH THIN CRUST — 12" MEDIUM

Description	Serving Size	Cal	Prot (g)	Fat (g)	Carbs (g)	Net Carb(g)	Fiber (g)	Sod (mg)	Chol (mg)
Crunchy Thin Crust ExtravaganZZa Feast	1 slice	240	11	16	16	15	1	672	29
Crunchy Thin Crust Pepperoni Feast	1 slice	216	9	14	14	13	1	577	26
Crunchy Thin Crust America's Favorite Feast	1 slice	208	8	14	15	14	1	533	23
Crunchy Thin Crust Bacon Cheeseburger Feast	1 slice	224	10	15	14	13	1	542	29
Crunchy Thin Crust w/ Pepperoni & Sausage	1 slice	206	8	14	14	13	1	533	23
Crunchy Thin Crust w/ Sausage	1 slice	181	7	11	14	13	1	438	18
Crunchy Thin Crust Barbeque Feast	1 slice	203	8	12	17	16	1	508	22
Crunchy Thin Crust Deluxe Feast	1 slice	185	7	12	15	14	1	449	19
Crunchy Thin Crust MeatZZa Feast	1 slice	232	11	15	15	14	1	647	29
Crunchy Thin Crust Beef	1 slice	175	7	11	14	13	1	400	17
Crunchy Thin Crust w/ Pepperoni	1 slice	174	7	11	14	13	1	429	17
Crunchy Thin Crust Gr. Pepper, Onion, & Mushroom	1 slice	142	6	8	15	14	1	293	10
Crunchy Thin Crust w/ Ham & Pineapple	1 slice	150	7	8	15	14	1	374	13
Crunchy Thin Crust w/ Ham	1 slice	148	7	8	14	13	1	400	14
Crunchy Thin Crust w/ Cheese	1 slice	137	5	7	14	13	1	293	10
Crunchy Thin Crust Veggie Feast	1 slice	168	7	10	15	14	1	397	14
Crunchy Thin Crust Hawaiian Feast	1 slice	174	8	10	16	15	1	454	17

ULTIMATE DEEP DISH — 12" MEDIUM

Description	Serving Size	Cal	Prot (g)	Fat (g)	Carbs (g)	Net Carb(g)	Fiber (g)	Sod (mg)	Chol (mg)
Ultimate Deep Dish ExtravaganZZa Feast	1 slice	341	14	20	30	28	2	935	31
Ultimate Deep Dish MeatZZa Feast	1 slice	333	14	19	29	27	2	911	31
Ultimate Deep Dish Bacon Cheeseburger Feast	1 slice	325	14	19	28	26	2	805	30
Ultimate Deep Dish Pepperoni Feast	1 slice	317	13	18	29	27	2	841	27
Ultimate Deep Dish America's Favorite Feast	1 slice	309	12	17	29	27	2	797	25
Ultimate Deep Dish w/ Pepperoni & Sausage	1 slice	307	12	17	29	27	2	796	25
Ultimate Deep Dish Barbeque Feast	1 slice	304	12	15	32	30	2	771	23

Description	Serving Size	Cal	Prot (g)	Fat (g)	Carbs (g)	Net Carb(g)	Fiber (g)	Sod (mg)	Chol (mg)
DOMINO'S® (continued)									
Ultimate Deep Dish w/ Sausage	1 slice	283	11	15	29	27	2	701	19
Ultimate Deep Dish Beef	1 slice	277	11	15	28	26	2	664	19
Ultimate Deep Dish w/ Pepperoni	1 slice	275	11	14	28	26	2	692	19
Ultimate Deep Dish Veggie Feast	1 slice	270	11	14	30	28	2	660	15
Ultimate Deep Dish Hawaiian Feast	1 slice	275	12	13	30	28	2	717	19
Ultimate Deep Dish w/ Ham	1 slice	250	11	12	28	26	2	663	16
Ultimate Deep Dish w/ Ham & Pineapple	1 slice	252	10	12	30	28	2	637	15
Ultimate Deep Dish Gr. Pepper, Onion, & Mushroom	1 slice	244	9	11	30	28	2	556	11
Ultimate Deep Dish w/ Cheese	1 slice	238	9	11	28	26	2	556	11

DQ®

BURGERS

Description	Serving Size	Cal	Prot (g)	Fat (g)	Carbs (g)	Net Carb(g)	Fiber (g)	Sod (mg)	Chol (mg)
DQ Homestyle® Hamburger	1 sandwich	290	17	12	29	27	2	1130	45
DQ Homestyle® Cheeseburger	1 sandwich	340	20	17	29	27	2	31	55
DQ Homestyle® Double Cheeseburger	1 sandwich	540	35	31	30	28	2	1130	115
DQ Homestyle® Bacon Double Cheeseburger	1 sandwich	610	41	36	31	29	2	1380	130
DQ Ultimate® Burger	1 sandwich	680	40	43	29	27	2	1210	135

SANDWICHES/BASKETS

Description	Serving Size	Cal	Prot (g)	Fat (g)	Carbs (g)	Net Carb(g)	Fiber (g)	Sod (mg)	Chol (mg)
Grilled Chicken Sandwich	1 sandwich	340	22	16	26	24	2	1000	55
Chicken Strip Basket™, 4-piece	1 basket	920	32	49	92	85	7	2090	40
Chicken Strip Basket™, 6-piece	1 basket	1120	45	60	102	93	9	2450	60

SALADS

Description	Serving Size	Cal	Prot (g)	Fat (g)	Carbs (g)	Net Carb(g)	Fiber (g)	Sod (mg)	Chol (mg)
Crispy Chicken Salad - no dressing	1 salad	350	21	20	21	15	6	620	40
Grilled Chicken Salad - no dressing	1 salad	240	26	10	12	8	4	950	65
Side Salad	1 salad	60	3	25	6	4	2	60	5

FRIES/ONION RINGS

Description	Serving Size	Cal	Prot (g)	Fat (g)	Carbs (g)	Net Carb(g)	Fiber (g)	Sod (mg)	Chol (mg)
French Fries	Medium	380	4	15	56	52	4	880	0
Onion Rings	Medium	470	6	30	45	42	3	740	0

CONES

Description	Serving Size	Cal	Prot (g)	Fat (g)	Carbs (g)	Net Carb(g)	Fiber (g)	Sod (mg)	Chol (mg)
DQ® Vanilla Soft Serve	1/2 cup	140	3	5	22	22	0	70	15
DQ® Chocolate Soft Serve	1/2 cup	150	4	5	22	22	0	75	15
Medium Vanilla Cone	1 cone	330	8	9	53	53	0	160	30

Description	Serving Size	Cal	Prot (g)	Fat (g)	Carbs (g)	Net Carb(g)	Fiber (g)	Sod (mg)	Chol (mg)
Medium Chocolate Cone	1 cone	340	8	11	53	53	0	160	30
Medium Dipped Cone	1 cone	490	8	24	59	58	1	190	30
MALTS, SHAKES AND MISTY®									
Medium Chocolate Malt	1 malt	870	20	22	153	151	2	450	70
Medium Chocolate Shake	1 shake	760	17	20	129	127	2	370	70
Medium Misty® Slush	1 slush	290	0	0	74	74	0	30	0
SUNDAES									
Medium Strawberry Sundae	1 sundae	340	7	9	58	59	<1	160	30
Medium Chocolate Sundae	1 sundae	400	8	10	71	71	0	210	30
ROYAL TREATS®									
Banana Split	1 treat	510	8	12	96	93	3	180	30
Peanut Buster® Parfait	1 treat	730	16	31	99	97	2	400	35
Pecan Praline™ Parfait	1 treat	430	NA	14	70	69	1	360	60
Triple Chocolate Utopia™	1 treat	770	12	39	96	91	5	390	55
Strawberry Shortcake	1 treat	430	7	14	70	69	1	360	60
Brownie Earthquake™	1 treat	740	10	27	112	112	0	350	50
NOVELTIES									
DQ® Sandwich	1 sandwich	200	4	6	31	30	1	140	10
Chocolate Dilly® Bar	1 bar	220	3	13	25	25	0	85	15
Buster Bar®	1 bar	500	11	28	45	43	2	230	15
Starkiss®	1 serving	80	0	0	21	21	0	10	0
DQ® Fudge Bar - No Sugar Added	1 serving	50	4	0	13	13	0	70	0
DQ® Vanilla Orange Bar - No Sugar Added	1 bar	60	2	0	17	17	0	40	0
Lemon DQ Freez'r®	1/2 cup	80	0	0	20	20	0	10	0
BLIZZARD® TREATS									
Medium Oreo® Cookies Blizzard®	Medium	700	13	26	103	102	1	560	45
Medium Chocolate Chip Cookie Dough Blizzard®	Medium	1030	17	40	150	150	0	520	70
Medium Banana Split Blizzard®	Medium	580	12	17	97	96	1	260	50

Hardee's®

BURGERS/ SANDWICHES

Description	Serving Size	Cal	Prot (g)	Fat (g)	Carbs (g)	Net Carb(g)	Fiber (g)	Sod (mg)	Chol (mg)
Hot Ham n Cheese	1 sandwich	420	30	18	39	37	2	1600	55
Big Hot Ham n Cheese	1 sandwich	570	37	23	59	56	3	2020	70
2/3 LB Bacon Cheese Thickburger	1 sandwich	1340	56	96	60	55	5	2110	205

Description	Serving Size	Cal	Prot (g)	Fat (g)	Carbs (g)	Net Carb(g)	Fiber (g)	Sod (mg)	Chol (mg)
HARDEE'S® (continued)									
2/3 LB Double Bacon Cheese Thickburger	1 sandwich	1300	55	96	51	48	3	2110	205
2/3 LB Double Thickburger	1 sandwich	1230	52	90	53	50	3	2090	195
1/2 LB Grilled Sourdough Thickburger	1 sandwich	1100	47	74	61	56	5	1430	155
1/2 LB Six Dollar Burger	1 sandwich	1120	42	73	72	67	5	1870	150
1/3 LB Bacon Cheese Thickburger	1 sandwich	910	33	63	50	47	3	1490	115
1/3 LB Thickburger	1 sandwich	850	30	57	54	51	3	1470	105
1/3 LB Chili Cheese Thickburger	1 sandwich	870	41	54	55	51	4	1840	135
1/3 LB Mushroom and Swiss Thickburger	1 sandwich	720	35	42	48	46	2	1570	100
1/3 LB Cheeseburger	1 sandwich	680	30	39	51	48	3	1320	90
1/3 LB Low Carb Thickburger	1 sandwich	420	30	32	5	3	2	1010	115
Hot Dog	1 sandwich	420	16	30	22	21	1	1200	55
Charbroiled Chicken Sandwich	1 sandwich	590	36	26	53	49	4	1180	80
Regular Roast Beef	1 sandwich	330	19	16	29	27	2	860	40
Big Roast Beef	1 sandwich	470	29	23	38	36	2	1290	60
CHICKEN									
Big Chicken Sandwich	1 sandwich	770	39	36	73	69	4	2000	95
Chicken Strips	3 pieces	380	22	21	27	26	1	1360	55
Chicken Strips	5 pieces	630	37	34	45	43	2	2260	90
Fried Chicken Thigh	1 piece	330	19	15	30	30	0	1000	60
Fried Chicken Breast	1 piece	370	29	15	29	29	0	1190	75
Fried Chicken Wing	1 piece	200	10	8	23	23	0	740	30
Fried Chicken Leg	1 piece	170	13	7	15	15	0	570	45
BBQ Sauce	1 packet	45	1	0	10	10	0	250	0
Honey Mustard Sauce	1 packet	110	0	9	6	6	0	220	10
Kids Meal - Chicken Strips (no sauce)	1 meal	500	19	25	50	47	3	1050	35
Spicey Chicken Sandwich	1 sandwich	430	14	22	46	44	2	1190	40
Sweet N Sour Sauce	1 packet	45	0	0	11	11	0	85	0
Chicken Fillet	1 sandwich	230	19	11	15	14	1	790	55
SIDES									
Cole Slaw	Small	170	1	10	20	18	2	140	10
Chili Cheese Fries	Medium	700	22	39	67	60	7	780	50
Crispy Curls	Medium	410	5	20	52	48	4	1020	0
French Fries	Medium	520	8	24	67	62	5	320	0
French Fries Kids	Small	250	4	12	32	29	3	150	0
Mashed Potatoes	Small	90	1	2	17	17	0	410	0

Description	Serving Size	Cal	Prot (g)	Fat (g)	Carbs (g)	Net Carb(g)	Fiber (g)	Sod (mg)	Chol (mg)
Chicken Gravy	1 serving	20	0	1	3	3	0	220	0
Au Jus Sauce	1 serving	10	0	0	2	2	0	320	0
BREAKFAST ITEMS									
Pancakes	3 Pancakes	300	8	5	55	53	2	830	25
Pancake Syrup	1 packet	90	0	0	21	21	0	0	0
Breakfast Ham	1 order	60	10	3	1	1	0	660	30
Country Ham	1 order	60	9	3	1	1	0	810	35
Grits	1 order	110	2	5	16	16	0	480	0
Hash Rounds	Small	260	3	16	25	23	2	360	0
Scrambled Egg	1 order	160	12	12	1	1	0	100	405
Big Country Breakfast Platter - Bacon	1 platter	980	28	56	90	87	3	2080	435
Big Country Breakfast Platter - Sausage	1 platter	1060	30	64	91	87	4	2140	455
Big Country Breakfast Platter - Chicken	1 platter	1140	44	61	105	101	4	2580	480
Big Country Breakfast Platter - Country Ham	1 platter	970	33	53	90	87	3	2600	460
Big Country Breakfast Platter - Breakfast Ham	1 platter	970	34	52	90	87	3	2450	455
Big Country Breakfast Platter - Country Steak	1 platter	1150	36	68	98	94	4	2260	455
Chicken Filet Biscuit	1 biscuit	600	24	34	50	49	1	1680	55
Country Steak Biscuit	1 biscuit	620	16	41	44	44	0	1360	35
Smoked Sausage Biscuit	1 biscuit	620	15	46	37	37	0	1680	40
Smoked Egg Biscuit	1 biscuit	610	17	44	36	36	0	1290	235
Bacon, Egg and Cheese Biscuit	1 biscuit	560	16	38	37	37	0	1360	225
Bacon Biscuit	1 biscuit	560	16	38	37	37	0	1360	225
Ham, Egg and Cheese Biscuit	1 biscuit	560	23	35	37	37	0	1800	245
Biscuit N Gravy	1 biscuit	530	8	34	47	47	0	1550	10
Loaded Omelet Biscuit	1 biscuit	500	14	33	36	36	0	1140	215
Made from Scratch Biscuit	1 biscuit	370	5	23	35	35	0	890	0
Country Ham Biscuit	1 biscuit	440	14	26	36	36	0	1710	35
Frisco Breakfast Sandwich	1 biscuit	360	24	13	38	36	2	670	230
Sunrise Croissant with Sausage Patty	1 croissant	550	22	38	29	29	0	1030	265
Sunrise Croissant with Bacon	1 croissant	450	19	29	28	28	0	900	240
Sunrise Croissant with Ham	1 croissant	430	23	26	28	28	0	1050	250
DESSERTS/ SHAKES									
Apple Turnover	1 turnover	290	2	15	36	35	1	350	5
Cinnamon Roll	1 roll	390	8	20	96	94	2	780	20
Chocolate Shake (regular)	Regular	710	27	7	137	125	12	550	20

Description	Serving Size	Cal	Prot (g)	Fat (g)	Carbs (g)	Net Carb(g)	Fiber (g)	Sod (mg)	Chol (mg)
HARDEE'S® (continued)									
Strawberry Shake (regular)	Regular	720	25	6	139	129	10	450	20
Vanilla Shake (regular)	Regular	580	28	8	99	89	10	480	30
Chocolate Chip Cookie	1 cookie	290	4	11	44	44	0	270	20

Jack's

SANDWICHES

Description	Serving Size	Cal	Prot (g)	Fat (g)	Carbs (g)	Net Carb(g)	Fiber (g)	Sod (mg)	Chol (mg)
Hamburger	1 sandwich	270	15	8	35	35	NA	570	20
Cheeseburger	1 sandwich	380	22	17	35	35	NA	770	50
Double Cheeseburger	1 sandwich	590	38	33	37	37	NA	1150	60
Big Jack	1 sandwich	500	25	27	40	40	NA	880	35
Double Big Jack Cheese	1 sandwich	930	56	60	43	43	NA	1640	115
Big Bacon	1 sandwich	700	36	42	45	45	NA	1140	70
Chicken Fillet	1 sandwich	640	20	31	69	69	NA	1040	30
Grilled Chicken	1 sandwich	410	25	15	44	44	NA	920	15

FRIES

Description	Serving Size	Cal	Prot (g)	Fat (g)	Carbs (g)	Net Carb(g)	Fiber (g)	Sod (mg)	Chol (mg)
Regular Fries	Regular	250	4	9	38	38	NA	340	0
Medium Fries	Medium	360	5	13	55	55	NA	490	0
Mega Fries	Mega	450	7	17	69	69	NA	600	0

BREAKFAST

Description	Serving Size	Cal	Prot (g)	Fat (g)	Carbs (g)	Net Carb(g)	Fiber (g)	Sod (mg)	Chol (mg)
Biscuit	1 biscuit	250	5	11	31	31	NA	520	0
Biscuit w/butter	1 biscuit	350	5	23	31	31	NA	660	35
Egg & Cheese Biscuit	1 biscuit	550	26	34	35	35	NA	880	340
Eggs	1 order	190	14	13	3	3	NA	160	310
Bacon Biscuit	1 biscuit	290	8	15	31	31	NA	660	5
Sausage Biscuit	1 biscuit	400	13	25	31	31	NA	810	25
Sausage, Egg & Cheese Biscuit	1 biscuit	700	34	48	35	35	NA	1170	360
Bologna Biscuit	1 biscuit	380	10	24	32	32	NA	850	25
Steak Biscuit	1 biscuit	430	14	22	44	44	NA	1150	15
Ham Biscuit	1 biscuit	290	12	13	31	31	NA	1040	10
Grits	1 order	100	1	8	8	8	NA	120	0
Flapjacks	1 order	360	9	11	57	57	NA	600	0
Gravy	1 order	150	2	11	11	11	NA	690	0

CHICKEN

Description	Serving Size	Cal	Prot (g)	Fat (g)	Carbs (g)	Net Carb(g)	Fiber (g)	Sod (mg)	Chol (mg)
Chicken Breast	1 piece	320	28	19	9	9	NA	620	45
Chicken Leg	1 piece	150	11	10	5	5	NA	240	25
Chicken Thigh	1 piece	260	13	19	9	9	NA	370	25

Description	Serving Size	Cal	Prot (g)	Fat (g)	Carbs (g)	Net Carb(g)	Fiber (g)	Sod (mg)	Chol (mg)
Chicken Wings	1 piece	170	9	12	6	6	NA	270	25
Chicken Fingers	3 pieces	470	30	24	33	33	NA	1400	25
SIDE ITEMS									
Mashed Potatoes	4 oz	70	0	1	15	15	NA	260	0
Brown Gravy	1 oz	10	0	0	2	2	NA	135	0
Green Beans	4 oz	25	0	0	5	5	NA	270	0
Coleslaw	4 oz	210	1	16	17	17	NA	200	0
Biscuit	1 biscuit	250	5	11	31	31	NA	520	0
DESSERTS									
Apple Pie	1 pie	250	3	10	37	37	NA	300	0
Lemon Pie	1 pie	230	3	8	39	39	NA	260	0

KFC®

Description	Serving Size	Cal	Prot (g)	Fat (g)	Carbs (g)	Net Carb(g)	Fiber (g)	Sod (mg)	Chol (mg)
EXTRA CRISPY									
Extra Crispy Chicken - Breast	1 piece	470	34	28	19	19	0	1230	135
Extra Crispy Chicken - Thigh	1 piece	370	21	26	12	12	0	710	120
Extra Crispy Chicken - Whole Wing	1 piece	190	10	12	10	10	0	390	55
Extra Crispy Chicken - Drumstick	1 piece	160	12	10	5	5	0	415	70
ORIGINAL RECIPE									
Original Recipe Sandwich w/ sauce	1 sandwich	450	29	22	33	31	2	940	70
Original Recipe Chicken - Breast	1 piece	370	40	19	11	11	0	1145	145
Original Recipe Sandwich w/o sauce	1 sandwich	360	29	13	21	20	1	890	60
Original Recipe Chicken - Thigh	1 piece	360	22	25	12	12	0	1060	165
Original Recipe Chicken - Whole Wing	1 piece	145	11	9	5	5	0	370	60
Original Recipe Chicken - Drumstick	1 piece	140	14	8	4	4	0	440	75
CRISPY STRIPS									
Blazin Strips	3 strips	315	26	16	21	20	1	1541	56
Honey BBQ Strips	3 strips	377	27	15	33	29	4	1709	45
Colonel's Crispy Strips	3 strips	340	28	16	20	20	0	1140	70
Spicy Crispy Strips	3 strips	335	25	15	23	22	1	1140	70
ENTREES									
Chunky Chicken Pot Pie	1 piece	770	29	42	69	64	5	2160	70
Honey BBQ Pieces	6 pieces	607	33	38	33	32	1	1145	193
Hot Wing Pieces	6 pieces	471	27	33	18	16	2	1230	150
Popcorn Chicken	Small	362	17	23	21	21	0	610	43

Description	Serving Size	Cal	Prot (g)	Fat (g)	Carbs (g)	Net Carb(g)	Fiber (g)	Sod (mg)	Chol (mg)
KFC® (continued)									
Popcorn Chicken	Large	620	30	40	36	36	0	1046	73
HOT & SPICY CHICKEN									
Hot & Spicy Chicken - Breast	1 piece	450	33	27	20	20	0	1450	130
Hot & Spicy Chicken - Drumstick	1 piece	140	13	9	4	4	0	380	65
Hot & Spicy Chicken - Thigh	1 piece	390	20	28	14	14	0	1240	125
Hot & Spicy Chicken - Whole Wing	1 piece	180	11	11	9	9	0	420	60
SANDWICHES									
Crispy Caesar Twister	1 sandwich	744	27	41	66	61	5	1616	55
Blazin Twister	1 sandwich	719	30	43	56	52	4	1986	70
Honey BBQ Crunch Melt	1 sandwich	556	33	26	48	46	2	1010	60
Honey BBQ Flavored Sandwich w/ sauce	1 sandwich	310	28	6	37	35	2	560	125
Tender Roast Sandwich w/o sauce	1 sandwich	270	31	5	23	22	1	690	65
Tender Roast Sandwich w/ sauce	1 sandwich	350	32	15	26	25	1	880	75
Triple Crunch Sandwich w/ sauce	1 sandwich	490	28	29	39	37	2	710	70
Triple Crunch Sandwich w/o sauce	1 sandwich	390	25	15	29	27	2	650	50
Triple Crunch Zinger Sandwich w/ sauce	1 sandwich	550	28	32	39	37	2	830	85
w/o sauce	1 sandwich	390	25	15	36	34	2	650	50
Twister	1 sandwich	600	22	34	52	48	4	1430	50
SIDES									
Biscuit	1 biscuit	180	4	10	20	19	1	560	0
Cole Slaw	1 order	232	2	14	26	23	3	284	8
Potato Salad	1 order	230	4	14	23	20	3	540	15
Macaroni & Cheese	1 order	180	7	8	21	19	2	860	10
Corn on the cob	1 order	150	5	2	35	33	2	20	0
Mashed Potato w/ gravy	1 order	120	1	6	17	15	2	440	1
Mean Beans	1 order	70	4	3	11	6	5	650	10
Green Beans	1 order	45	1	2	7	4	3	730	5
BBQ Baked Beans	1 order	190	6	3	33	27	6	760	5
Potato Wedges	1 order	376	6	15	53	48	5	1323	4
DESSERTS									
Double Choc. Chip Cake	1 slice	320	4	16	41	40	1	230	55
Colonels Pies - Apple	1 slice	310	2	14	44	44	0	280	0
Colonels Pies - Strawberry Creme	1 slice	280	4	15	32	30	2	130	15
Colonels Pies - Pecan Pie Slice	1 slice	490	5	23	66	64	2	510	65

Description	Serving Size	Cal	Prot (g)	Fat (g)	Carbs (g)	Net Carb(g)	Fiber (g)	Sod (mg)	Chol (mg)
Little Bucket Parfait - Chocolate Cream	1 parfait	290	3	15	37	35	2	330	15
Little Bucket Parfait - Fudge Brownie	1 parfait	280	3	10	44	43	1	190	145
Little Bucket Parfait - Strawberry Shortcake	1 parfait	200	1	7	33	32	1	220	10
Little Bucket Parfait - Lemon Crème	1 parfait	410	7	14	62	58	4	290	20

Krystal

BREAKFAST

Description	Serving Size	Cal	Prot (g)	Fat (g)	Carbs (g)	Net Carb(g)	Fiber (g)	Sod (mg)	Chol (mg)
Krystal Sunriser	1 sandwich	240	12	14	14	12	2	460	255
Plain Biscuit	1 biscuit	270	5	13	33	33	0	660	0
Sausage Biscuit	1 biscuit	480	12	33	33	33	0	980	40
Bacon Egg Cheese Biscuit	1 biscuit	390	11	23	33	33	0	1090	40
Biscuit and Gravy	1 biscuit	280	5	14	34	34	0	710	0
Chik Biscuit	1 biscuit	360	13	15	40	40	0	1030	20
Kryspers	1 order	190	1	13	17	15	2	340	10
Country Breakfast	1 order	660	24	42	46	38	8	1450	590
Scrambler	1 order	440	20	26	33	30	3	840	255
4 Carb Scrambler (bacon)	1 order	370	24	29	4	3	1	830	595
4 Carb Scrambler (sausage)	1 order	600	32	51	4	2	2	1040	600

SANDWICHES

Description	Serving Size	Cal	Prot (g)	Fat (g)	Carbs (g)	Net Carb(g)	Fiber (g)	Sod (mg)	Chol (mg)
Cheese Krystal	1 sandwich	180	9	9	17	15	2	430	25
Double Krystal	1 sandwich	260	13	13	24	22	2	550	40
Double Cheese Krystal	1 sandwich	310	16	16	26	25	1	800	65
Bacon Cheese Krystal	1 sandwich	190	10	10	16	14	2	430	25
B.A. Burger	1 sandwich	470	22	27	39	37	2	760	55
B.A. Burger w/Cheese	1 sandwich	530	25	32	40	38	2	1020	55
Double B.A. Burger	1 sandwich	800	44	53	41	39	2	1600	115
Krystal Chik	1 sandwich	240	11	11	24	22	2	640	25
Chik'n Bites	1 sandwich	310	17	19	16	15	1	790	55
Plain Pup	1 pup	170	6	9	15	14	1	500	25
Chili Cheese Pup	1 pup	210	9	12	17	15	2	510	40
Corn Pup	1 pup	260	5	19	19	18	1	480	50

SALADS

Description	Serving Size	Cal	Prot (g)	Fat (g)	Carbs (g)	Net Carb(g)	Fiber (g)	Sod (mg)	Chol (mg)
Chik'n Bites Salad	1 salad	290	20	20	12	8	4	490	65

SIDES

Description	Serving Size	Cal	Prot (g)	Fat (g)	Carbs (g)	Net Carb(g)	Fiber (g)	Sod (mg)	Chol (mg)
Regular Fries	Medium	470	4	20	53	46	7	90	20

Description	Serving Size	Cal	Prot (g)	Fat (g)	Carbs (g)	Net Carb(g)	Fiber (g)	Sod (mg)	Chol (mg)
KRYSTAL (continued)									
Chili Cheese Fries	Medium	540	13	28	59	53	6	800	45
Krystal Chili	Regular	200	13	7	22	15	7	1130	25
DESSERTS									
Fried Apple Turnover	1 turnover	220	3	10	31	29	2	300	<5
Lemon Icebox Pie	1 slice	260	5	9	41	39	2	180	25

McDonald's®

SANDWICHES

Description	Serving Size	Cal	Prot (g)	Fat (g)	Carbs (g)	Net Carb(g)	Fiber (g)	Sod (mg)	Chol (mg)
Hamburger	1 sandwich	280	12	10	36	34	2	550	30
Cheeseburger	1 sandwich	330	15	14	36	34	2	790	45
Double Cheeseburger	1 sandwich	490	25	26	38	36	2	1220	85
Quarter Pounder®	1 sandwich	430	23	21	38	35	3	770	70
Quarter Pounder® with Cheese	1 sandwich	540	29	29	39	36	3	1240	95
Double Quarter Pounder® with Cheese	1 sandwich	770	46	47	39	36	3	1440	165
Big Mac®	1 sandwich	600	25	33	50	46	4	1050	85
Big N' Tasty®	1 sandwich	540	24	32	38	35	3	780	80
Filet-O-Fish®	1 sandwich	410	15	20	41	40	1	660	45
Chicken McGrill®	1 sandwich	400	27	16	37	34	3	1020	70
Crispy Chicken	1 sandwich	510	22	26	47	44	3	1090	50
McChicken®	1 sandwich	430	14	23	41	38	3	830	45
Hot 'n Spicy McChicken®	1 sandwich	450	15	26	40	39	1	820	45

FRENCH FRIES

Description	Serving Size	Cal	Prot (g)	Fat (g)	Carbs (g)	Net Carb(g)	Fiber (g)	Sod (mg)	Chol (mg)
Small French Fries	Small	220	3	11	28	25	3	150	0
Chicken McNuggets®	4 piece	170	10	10	10	10	0	450	25
Chicken McNuggets®	6 piece	250	15	15	15	15	0	670	35
Barbeque Sauce	1 packet	45	0	0	10	10	0	250	0
Honey	1 packet	45	0	0	12	12	0	0	0
Hot Mustard Sauce	1 packet	60	<1	4	7	6	1	240	5
Sweet 'N Sour Sauce	1 packet	50	0	0	11	11	0	140	0
Chicken Selects® Premium Breast Strips	5 piece	630	38	32	47	47	0	1590	85
Spicy Buffalo Sauce	1 packet	60	0	7	2	2	0	430	0
Creamy Ranch Sauce	1 packet	210	0	22	2	2	0	310	10
Tangy Honey Mustard Sauce	1 packet	70	<1	3	12	12	0	170	10

Description	Serving Size	Cal	Prot (g)	Fat (g)	Carbs (g)	Net Carb(g)	Fiber (g)	Sod (mg)	Chol (mg)
SALADS									
Grilled Chicken Bacon Ranch Salad	1 salad	250	31	10	9	6	3	930	85
Crispy Chicken Bacon Ranch Salad	1 salad	350	26	19	20	17	3	1000	65
Bacon Ranch Salad (without chicken)	1 salad	130	10	8	7	4	3	280	25
Grilled Chicken Caesar Salad	1 salad	200	29	6	9	6	3	820	70
Crispy Chicken Caesar Salad	1 salad	310	23	16	20	17	3	890	50
Caesar Salad (without chicken)	1 salad	90	7	4	7	4	3	170	10
Grilled Chicken California Cobb Salad	1 salad	270	33	11	9	6	3	1060	145
Crispy Chicken California Cobb Salad	1 salad	370	27	21	20	17	3	1130	125
California Cobb Salad (without chicken)	1 salad	150	11	9	7	4	3	410	85
Side Salad	1 salad	15	1	0	3	2	1	10	0
Butter Garlic Croutons	1 packet	50	1	2	8	8	0	140	0
Fiesta Salad (without Sour Cream and Salsa)	1 salad	360	21	22	19	15	4	580	80
SALAD DRESSINGS									
Newman's Own® Cobb Dressing	1 packet	120	1	9	9	9	0	440	10
Newman's Own® Creamy Caesar Dressing	1 packet	190	2	18	4	4	0	500	20
Newman's Own® Low Fat Balsamic Vinaigrette	1 packet	40	0	3	4	4	0	730	0
Newman's Own® Ranch Dressing	1 packet	170	1	15	9	9	0	530	20
Newman's Own® Salsa	1 packet	30	1	0	7	6	1	290	0
BREAKFAST									
Egg McMuffin®	1 sandwich	300	18	12	28	26	2	850	235
Sausage McMuffin®	1 sandwich	370	14	23	28	26	2	790	50
English Muffin	1 sandwich	150	5	2	27	25	2	260	0
Bacon, Egg & Cheese Biscuit	1 biscuit	430	18	26	31	30	1	1230	240
Sausage Biscuit	1 biscuit	410	10	28	30	29	1	930	35
Biscuit	1 biscuit	240	4	11	30	29	1	640	0
Bacon, Egg & Cheese McGriddles™	1 sandwich	440	19	21	43	42	1	1270	240
Sausage, Egg & Cheese McGriddles™	1 sandwich	550	20	33	43	42	1	1290	260
Sausage McGriddles™	1 sandwich	420	11	23	42	41	1	970	35
Ham, Egg & Cheese Bagel	1 sandwich	550	26	23	58	56	2	1500	255
Spanish Omelet Bagel	1 sandwich	710	27	40	59	56	3	1520	275
Steak, Egg & Cheese Bagel	1 sandwich	640	31	31	57	55	2	1540	265
Bagel (plain)	1 bagel	260	9	1	54	52	2	520	0
Big Breakfast®	1 order	700	24	47	45	42	3	1430	455
Deluxe Breakfast	1 order	1190	30	61	130	127	3	1990	470

Description	Serving Size	Cal	Prot (g)	Fat (g)	Carbs (g)	Net Carb(g)	Fiber (g)	Sod (mg)	Chol (mg)
McDONALD'S® (continued)									
Sausage Burrito	1 burrito	290	13	16	24	22	2	680	170
Hotcakes and Sausage	1 order	780	15	33	104	104	0	1060	50
Hash Browns	1 order	130	1	8	14	13	1	330	0
Warm Cinnamon Roll	1 roll	440	7	19	60	58	2	330	80
DESSERTS/SHAKES									
Fruit 'n Yogurt Parfait	1 parfait	160	4	2	30	29	1	85	5
Apple Dippers with Low Fat Caramel Dip	1 order	100	0	1	22	22	0	35	5
Apple Dippers	1 order	35	0	0	8	8	0	0	0
Low Fat Caramel Dip	1 order	70	0	1	14	14	0	35	5
Vanilla Reduced Fat Ice Cream Cone	1 cone	150	4	5	23	23	0	75	20
Kiddie Cone	1 cone	45	1	2	7	7	0	20	5
Strawberry Sundae	1 sundae	290	7	7	50	49	1	95	30
Hot Caramel Sundae	1 sundae	360	7	10	61	61	0	180	35
Hot Fudge Sundae	1 sundae	340	8	12	52	51	1	170	30
M&M® McFlurry®	12 oz cup	630	16	23	90	89	1	210	75
Oreo® McFlurry®	12 oz cup	570	15	20	82	81	1	280	70
Baked Apple Pie	1 pie	260	3	13	34	33	1	200	0
McDonaldland® Chocolate Chip Cookies	1 cookie	280	3	14	37	36	1	170	40
McDonaldland® Cookies	1 cookie	230	3	8	38	37	1	250	0
Chocolate Chip Cookie	1 cookie	160	2	8	22	21	1	125	5
Oatmeal Raisin Cookie	1 cookie	150	2	6	23	22	1	100	5
Sugar Cookie	1 cookie	140	2	6	20	20	0	120	10

Milo's®

SANDWICHES

Description	Serving Size	Cal	Prot (g)	Fat (g)	Carbs (g)	Net Carb(g)	Fiber (g)	Sod (mg)	Chol (mg)
Hamburger	1 sandwich	370	1	16	36	30	6	640	45
Cheeseburger	1 sandwich	430	1	21	37	31	6	920	60
Double Hamburger	1 sandwich	530	1	26	39	32	7	830	70
Double Cheeseburger	1 sandwich	580	1	31	40	33	7	1120	90
Toasted Cheese	1 sandwich	270	0	12	30	27	3	840	30
Chicken Sandwich	1 sandwich	460	0	18	54	51	3	1370	35

CHICKEN

Description	Serving Size	Cal	Prot (g)	Fat (g)	Carbs (g)	Net Carb(g)	Fiber (g)	Sod (mg)	Chol (mg)
Chicken Tender	1 tender	150	0	8	13	13	0	550	15
Chicken Tenders	4 tenders	600	0	32	52	52	0	2200	60

Description	Serving Size	Cal	Prot (g)	Fat (g)	Carbs (g)	Net Carb(g)	Fiber (g)	Sod (mg)	Chol (mg)
FRIES									
Regular	Regular	320	0	13	45	45	0	440	20
Mega	Mega	510	0	21	72	72	0	710	30
PIES									
Apple	1 pie	260	50	13	33	26	7	320	0
Peach	1 pie	290	30	14	37	29	8	220	0
Lemon	1 pie	290	0	13	39	31	8	260	0
SAUCE									
"Dine in" Sauce	1 container	15	0	0	4	2	2	220	0
"To-Go" Sauce	1 packet	35	0	0	8	3	5	450	0

O'Charley's®

Description	Serving Size	Cal	Prot (g)	Fat (g)	Carbs (g)	Net Carb(g)	Fiber (g)	Sod (mg)	Chol (mg)
APPETIZERS									
Buffalo Tenders	1 order	715		22	92	87	5	3056	57
Chicken Tenders	1 order	580		15	74	71	3	2644	57
Chipotle BBQ Tenders	1 order	724		11	123	118	5	3231	54
Chips & Salsa	1 order	455		23	60	52	8	784	0
Combo Appetizer	1 order	1030		55	82	77	5	3249	136
Crispy Fried Onion Tanglers	1 order	420		29	36	31	5	450	0
Fried Cheese Wedges	1 order	265		15	21	20	1	581	50
Loaded Potato Skins	1 order	563		40	19	16	3	2218	120
Southwestern Chicken Quesidilla	1 order	1133		81	52	47	5	2017	162
Spinach & Artichoke Dip	1 order	661		41	66	58	8	1222	12
Three Cheese Shrimp Dip	1 order	625		38	59	51	8	1104	100
SIDES									
Bacon Strips	1 order	109		9	0	0	0	303	16
Baked Potato, Plain	1 potato	200		0	46	42	4	15	0
Vegetable medley	1 order	689		17	69	63	6	3052	132
Coleslaw	1 order	215		14	21	19	2	566	5
Dinner Rolls	1 order	162		2	32	31	1	112	0
French Fries	1 order	402		21	51	47	4	449	0
Fresh vegetables, steamed w/dressing	1 order	725		36	90	75	15	2710	0
Fried Eggs	2 eggs	274		23	1	1	0	265	501
Loaded Baked Potato	1 potato	490		25	53	49	4	891	25
Rice Pilaf	1 order	221		6	38	37	1	623	0
Loaded Potato Soup	1 bowl	404		22	38	37	1	2561	24

Description	Serving Size	Cal	Prot (g)	Fat (g)	Carbs (g)	Net Carb(g)	Fiber (g)	Sod (mg)	Chol (mg)
O'CHARLEY'S (continued)									
Smashed Potatoes	1 order	340		14	45	41	4	1098	20
BRUNCH MENU									
Strawberry Waffles	1 order	971		33	158	153	5	1622	29
Ultimate Omelet	1 order	970		66	50	43	7	1498	798
Bavarian Waffles w/syrup	1 order	831		24	143	141	2	1572	0
Brunch Potatoes	1 order	198		10	27	23	4	222	0
Cajun Chicken Omelet	1 order	1142		80	48	41	7	1262	832
Chicken Teriyaki on rice pilaf w/Ham & Cheese Omelet	1 order	949		67	41	36	5	1640	804
Pecan Waffles w/syrup	1 order	1225		63	156	151	5	1621	29
Spanish Omelet	1 order	956		70	47	40	7	1262	791
Steak & Eggs Brunch	1 order	975		54	43	38	5	824	672
Sausage Links	1 order	96		8	0	0	0	336	22
CHICKEN ENTREES									
Cajun Chicken Pasta	1 order	1615		95	96	88	8	2276	183
Chicken Florentine on Linguini w/vegetable medley	1 order	960		38	79	68	11	1483	165
Chicken Tenders Dinner	1 order	1359		34	178	171	7	6320	137
Chicken Potatoes w/vegetable medley	1 order	689		17	69	63	6	3052	132
Chicken Parmesan on linguini w/vegetable medley	1 order	841		27	90	78	12	1894	116
SALADS									
Southern fried BLT Chicken Salad	1 salad	848		21	110	104	6	3646	88
Black and Bleu Caesar Salad	1 salad	1008		66	15	11	4	2065	220
Cajun Chicken Salad	1 salad	979		78	21	17	4	2219	143
Chicken Caesar	1 salad	620		40	11	7	4	678	112
Classic Caesar Salad	1 salad	464		38	11	7	4	584	30
House Salad	1 salad	245		14	14	11	3	1232	39
Island Chicken Salad	1 salad	1464		30	225	212	13	5560	109
Salmon Caesar Salad	1 salad	773		52	11	7	4	680	151
Southern Fried Chicken Salad	1 salad	1803		85	173	163	10	5883	167
SANDWICHES									
Bacon & Cheese Trio Chicken	1 sandwich	760		45	36	34	2	1420	155
Buffalo Chicken Sandwich	1 sandwich	559		14	64	60	4	1763	83
Cajun Chicken Sandwich	1 sandwich	483		21	38	35	3	1542	91
Chicken Sandwich	1 sandwich	470		21	35	33	2	594	91

Description	Serving Size	Cal	Prot (g)	Fat (g)	Carbs (g)	Net Carb(g)	Fiber (g)	Sod (mg)	Chol (mg)
Club w/Honey Mustard	1 sandwich	1194		90	45	42	3	2169	113
Fisherman's TLC w/ Sauce	1 sandwich	672		25	71	66	5	1732	259
Half Pound Cheeseburger	1 sandwich	1129		73	35	33	2	1107	234
Roast Beef Stack	1 sandwich	930		64	33	30	3	639	161
Three Cheese Bacon Burger	1 sandwich	1304		88	36	34	2	1410	268

SEAFOOD

Description	Serving Size	Cal	Prot (g)	Fat (g)	Carbs (g)	Net Carb(g)	Fiber (g)	Sod (mg)	Chol (mg)
Blackened Rainbow Trout	1 order	424		24	2	2	0	664	134
Chipotle BBQ Salomon Filet	1 order	594		32	16	16	0	871	167
Fried Shrimp Platter	1 order	549		28	26	25	1	780	401
Fisherman's Platter	1 order	1892		95	180	169	11	4061	588
Grilled Salmon Filet	6 oz	324		20	1	1	0	569	100
Grilled Shrimp Platter	1 order	387		18	40	39	1	1511	85
Grilled Tuna	1 order	410		16	7	7	0	926	115
Lunch Chipotle BBQ Salmon	1 order	768		34	74	68	6	1945	100
Lunch Salmon	1 order	680		34	52	46	6	1613	100

STEAK & RIBS ENTREES

Description	Serving Size	Cal	Prot (g)	Fat (g)	Carbs (g)	Net Carb(g)	Fiber (g)	Sod (mg)	Chol (mg)
3 Story Chopped Steak	1 order	1427		97	43	39	4	1201	263
Blackened Prime Rib	1 order	1172		100	1	1	0	823	238
Choice Cut Sirloin	1 order	447		18	1	1	0	499	192
Filet Mignon	1 order	756		53	1	1	0	479	219
Petite Sirloin	1 order	317		13	1	1	0	456	134
Prime Rib	8 oz	932		80	0	0	0	147	191
Prime Rib	10 oz	1165		100	0	0	0	184	238
Prime Rib	16 oz	1864		159	0	0	0	295	381
Ribeye	1 order	903		71	1	1	0	547	228
Steak & Fried Shrimp Combo	1 order	620		28	17	16	1	1023	347
Steak & Grilled Shrimp Combo	1 order	570		19	40	39	1	1120	177
Steak & Rib Combo	1 order	1498		91	57	56	1	3257	435
Steak Tips Monterey on Rice	1 order	1143		82	46	44	2	1333	169
Ribs, Full Rack (w/fries & slaw)	1 order	2872		190	160	152	8	5885	607
Ribs, Half Rack (w/fries & slaw)	1 order	1763		113	120	113	7	3687	306

Papa John's®

ORIGINAL CRUST PIZZA

Description	Serving Size	Cal	Prot (g)	Fat (g)	Carbs (g)	Net Carb(g)	Fiber (g)	Sod (mg)	Chol (mg)
Original Crust Pizza - Six Cheese	1 slice	425	23	21	38	36	2	1066	51
Original Crust Pizza w/ All the Meats	1 slice	390	18	19	37	35	2	1096	41

Description	Serving Size	Cal	Prot (g)	Fat (g)	Carbs (g)	Net Carb(g)	Fiber (g)	Sod (mg)	Chol (mg)
PAPA JOHN'S (continued)									
Original Crust Pizza w/ Cheese	1 slice	283	13	10	37	35	2	717	20
Original Crust Pizza - The Works	1 slice	342	16	15	38	36	2	943	32
Original Crust Pizza - Spinach Alfredo	1 slice	333	17	14	35	34	1	677	36
Original Crust Pizza w/ Sausage	1 slice	322	14	14	37	35	2	877	28
Original Crust Pizza - Garden Special	1 slice	280	12	10	38	36	2	713	16
Original Crust Pizza w/ Pepperoni	1 slice	303	13	12	37	35	2	793	23
THIN CRUST PIZZA									
Thin Crust Pizza - Spinach Alfredo	1 slice	293	15	17	20	19	1	476	39
Thin Crust Pizza w/ All the Meats	1 slice	393	19	26	22	21	1	1051	50
Thin Crust Pizza w/ Sausage	1 slice	283	12	17	22	21	1	697	30
Thin Crust Pizza w/ Pepperoni	1 slice	266	11	16	22	21	1	621	26
Thin Crust Pizza - The Works	1 slice	322	15	20	24	22	2	871	37
Thin Crust Pizza w/ Cheese	1 slice	233	11	13	22	21	1	496	20
Thin Crust Pizza - Garden Special	1 slice	226	10	12	24	22	2	496	16
Thin Crust Pizza - Six Cheese	1 slice	375	21	24	23	22	1	848	51
APPETIZERS									
Bread Sticks	1 order	140	4	2	26	25	1	260	0
Cheese Sticks	1 order	180	8	8	20	19	1	380	13
Pizza Sauce	1 order	25	0	2	3	1	2	125	0
Garlic Sauce	1 order	235	0	26	0	0	0	300	0
Papa's Chicken Strips	1 order	83	6	4	5	4	1	178	13
Honey Mustard Sauce	1 order	190	0	19	6	6	0	150	10
Ranch Sauce	1 order	140	1	14	2	2	0	280	15
Cheese Sauce	1 order	60	4	5	0	0	0	300	19
BBQ Sauce	1 order	48	0	0	10	10	0	310	0
Buffalo Sauce	1 order	25	0	1	3	3	0	1470	0

Pizza Hut®

Description	Serving Size	Cal	Prot (g)	Fat (g)	Carbs (g)	Net Carb(g)	Fiber (g)	Sod (mg)	Chol (mg)
APPETIZERS									
Breadsticks	1 order	115	2	6	12	12	0	122	0
Cheesy Bread	1 order	123	4	7	13	13	0	162	6
Barbeque Buffalo Wings	1 order	50	6	3	2	2	0	176	26
Hot Buffalo Wings	1 order	45	5	3	1	1	0	255	26
Garlic Sauce	1 order	441	0	49	0	0	0	380	0
Buffalo Chicken Kickers	1 order	47	4	2	3	3	0	163	9

Description	Serving Size	Cal	Prot (g)	Fat (g)	Carbs (g)	Net Carb(g)	Fiber (g)	Sod (mg)	Chol (mg)
Marinara Dipping Sauce	1 order	25	1	0	5	5	0	263	0
Hot Dipping Sauce	1 order	15	0	0	4	4	0	1820	0
Blue Cheese Dipping Sauce	1 order	223	1	24	2	2	0	417	20
DESSERTS						0			
CinnaStix®	1 order	123	2	6	15	14	1	111	0
Sweet Icing	1 order	250	0	3	57	57	0	0	0
APPETIZERS									
Breadstick	1 order	150	4	6	20	19	1	220	0
Cheese Breadstick	1 order	200	7	10	21	20	1	340	15
Bread Stick Dipping Sauce	3 oz	50	1	0	11	9	2	370	0
Mild Wings	2 pieces	110	11	7	1	1	0	320	70
Hot Wings	2 pieces	110	11	6	1	1	0	450	70
Wing Ranch Dipping Sauce	1 1/2 oz	210	1	22	4	4	0	340	10
Wing Blue Cheese Dipping Sauce	1 1/2 oz	230	2	24	2	2	0	550	25
PERSONAL PAN PIZZAS									
Personal Pan Pizza® w/ Cheese Only	6-inch pizza	160	7	7	18	17	1	310	15
Personal Pan Pizza® w/ Quartered Ham	6-inch pizza	150	7	6	18	17	1	330	15
Personal Pan Pizza® w/ Pepperoni	6-inch pizza	170	7	8	18	17	1	340	15
Sausage Lover's® Personal Pan Pizza®	6-inch pizza	190	8	10	18	17	1	400	20
Chicken Supreme Personal Pan Pizza®	6-inch pizza	160	8	6	19	18	1	320	15
Veggie Lover's® Personal Pan Pizza®	6-inch pizza	150	6	6	19	18	1	280	10
Meat Lover's® Personal Pan Pizza®	6-inch pizza	200	9	10	18	17	1	470	20
Pepperoni Lover's® Personal Pan Pizza®	6-inch pizza	200	9	10	18	17	1	440	25
Super Supreme Personal Pan Pizza®	6-inch pizza	200	9	10	19	18	1	480	20
Supreme Personal Pan Pizza®	6-inch pizza	190	8	9	19	18	1	420	20
PZONE									
PZONE® - Meat Lover's®	1/2 PZONE	680	38	28	70	67	3	1540	65
PZONE® - Pepperoni	1/2 PZONE	610	34	22	69	66	3	1280	55
PZONE® - Classic	1/2 PZONE	610	33	21	71	68	3	1210	50
PZONE® - Marinara Dipping Sauce	1 order	45	2	0	9	7	2	380	0
FIT 'N DELICIOUS – MEDIUM									
Fit 'N Delicious - Ham, Pineapple and Diced Red Tomato	1 slice	160	8	4	24	22	2	470	15
Fit 'N Delicious - Ham, Red Onion and Mushroom (12in)	1 slice	160	8	5	22	20	2	470	15

Description	Serving Size	Cal	Prot (g)	Fat (g)	Carbs (g)	Net Carb(g)	Fiber (g)	Sod (mg)	Chol (mg)
PIZZA HUT® (continued)									
Fit 'N Delicious - Tomato, Mushroom and Jalapeno (12in)	1 slice	150	6	4	22	20	2	590	10
Fit 'N Delicious - Green Pepper, Red Onion and Diced Red Tomato (12in)	1 slice	150	6	4	24	22	2	360	10
Fit 'N Delicious - Diced Chicken, Mushroom and Jalapeno (12in)	1 slice	170	10	5	22	20	2	690	15
Fit 'N Delicious - Diced Chicken, Red Onion and Green Pepper (12in)	1 slice	170	10	5	23	21	2	460	15
THIN 'N CRISPY PIZZA — 12" MEDIUM									
Supreme Thin 'N Crispy Pizza	1 slice	240	11	11	22	20	2	640	25
Thin 'N Crispy Pizza w/ Pepperoni	1 slice	210	10	10	21	20	1	550	25
Thin 'N Crispy Pizza w/ Quartered Ham	1 slice	180	9	6	21	20	1	530	20
Thin 'N Crispy Pizza w/ Cheese	1 slice	200	10	8	21	20	1	490	25
Veggie Lover's Thin 'N Crispy Pizza	1 slice	180	8	7	23	21	2	480	15
Meat Lover's® Thin 'N Crispy Pizza	1 slice	270	13	14	21	19	2	740	35
Chicken Supreme Thin 'N Crispy Pizza	1 slice	200	12	7	22	21	1	520	25
Sausage Lover's Thin 'N Crispy Pizza	1 slice	240	11	13	21	19	2	630	30
Pepperoni Lover's® Thin 'N Crispy Pizza	1 slice	260	13	14	21	19	2	690	40
Super Supreme Thin 'N Crispy Pizza	1 slice	260	13	13	23	21	2	760	35
PAN PIZZA — MEDIUM									
Pan Pizza w/ Pepperoni	1 slice	290	11	15	29	27	2	560	25
Pepperoni Lover's® Pan Pizza	1 slice	340	15	19	29	27	2	700	40
Super Supreme Pan Pizza	1 slice	340	14	18	30	28	2	760	35
Meat Lover's® Pan Pizza	1 slice	340	15	19	29	27	2	750	35
Sausage Lover's Pan Pizza	1 slice	330	13	17	29	27	2	640	30
Supreme Pan Pizza	1 slice	320	13	16	30	28	2	650	25
Chicken Supreme Pan Pizza	1 slice	280	13	12	30	28	2	530	25
Pan Pizza w/ Cheese	1 slice	280	11	13	29	28	1	500	25
Pan Pizza w/ Quartered Ham	1 slice	260	11	11	29	28	1	540	20
Veggie Lover's® Pan Pizza	1 slice	260	10	12	30	28	2	470	15
HAND TOSSED — MEDIUM									
Pepperoni Lover's® Hand Tossed Style Pizza	1 slice	300	15	13	30	28	2	710	40
Super Supreme Hand Tossed Style Pizza	1 slice	300	15	13	31	29	2	780	35

Description	Serving Size	Cal	Prot (g)	Fat (g)	Carbs (g)	Net Carb(g)	Fiber (g)	Sod (mg)	Chol (mg)
Meat Lover's® Hand Tossed Style Pizza	1 slice	300	15	13	29	27	2	760	35
Sausage Lover's® Hand Tossed Style Pizza	1 slice	280	13	12	30	28	2	650	30
Supreme Hand Tossed Style Pizza	1 slice	270	13	11	30	28	2	660	25
Hand Tossed Style Pizza w/ Pepperoni	1 slice	250	12	9	29	27	2	570	25
Hand Tossed Style Pizza w/ Cheese	1 slice	240	12	8	30	28	2	520	25
Chicken Supreme Hand Tossed Style Pizza	1 slice	230	14	6	30	28	2	550	25
Hand Tossed Style Pizza w/ Quartered Ham	1 slice	220	12	6	29	27	2	550	20
Veggie Lover's® Hand Tossed Style Pizza	1 slice	220	10	6	31	29	2	490	15
STUFFED CRUST PIZZA — 14" MEDIUM									
Stuffed Crust Pizza w/Cheese	1 slice	360	18	13	43	41	2	920	40
Stuffed Crust Pizza w/Pepperoni	1 slice	370	18	15	42	39	3	970	45
Stuffed Crust Pizza w/Quartered Ham	1 slice	340	18	11	42	40	2	960	40
Supreme Stuffed Crust Pizza	1 slice	400	20	16	44	41	3	1070	45
Super Supreme Stuffed Crust Pizza	1 slice	440	21	20	45	42	3	1270	50
Meat Lover's® Stuffed Crust Pizza	1 slice	450	21	21	43	40	3	1250	55
Sausage Lover's® Stuffed Crust Pizza	1 slice	430	19	19	43	40	3	1130	50
Pepperoni Lover's® Stuffed Crust Pizza	1 slice	420	21	19	43	40	3	1120	55
Chicken Supreme Stuffed Crust Pizza	1 slice	380	20	13	44	41	3	1020	40
Veggie Lover's® Stuffed Crust Pizza	1 slice	360	16	14	45	42	3	980	35
EXTRA LARGE PIZZAS — 16" PIZZA									
Extra Large Sausage Lover's® Pizza	1 slice	510	23	23	51	48	3	1330	55
Extra Large Meat Lover's® Pizza	1 slice	500	24	22	51	48	3	1400	60
Extra Large Super Supreme Pizza	1 slice	490	23	21	53	49	4	1430	55
Extra Large Supreme Pizza	1 slice	460	22	19	52	48	4	1250	45
Extra Large Pizza w/ Pepperoni	1 slice	430	19	17	50	47	3	1130	45
Extra Large Pizza w/ Cheese	1 slice	420	20	15	51	48	3	1080	45
Extra Large Chicken Supreme Pizza	1 slice	400	22	12	52	49	3	1070	40
Extra Large Veggie Lover's® Pizza	1 slice	390	17	12	53	49	4	1030	30
Extra Large Pizza w/ Quartered Ham	1 slice	380	19	12	50	47	3	1110	40
DESSERTS									
Apple Dessert Pizza	1 slice	260	4	4	53	52	1	250	0
Cherry Dessert Pizza	1 slice	240	4	4	47	46	1	250	0

Description	Serving Size	Cal	Prot (g)	Fat (g)	Carbs (g)	Net Carb(g)	Fiber (g)	Sod (mg)	Chol (mg)
PIZZA HUT® (continued)									
Cinnamon Sticks	2 sticks	170	4	5	27	26	1	170	0
White Icing Dipping Cup	2 oz	190	0	0	46	46	0	0	0

Subway®

SUBS AND WRAPS

Description	Serving Size	Cal	Prot (g)	Fat (g)	Carbs (g)	Net Carb(g)	Fiber (g)	Sod (mg)	Chol (mg)
Barbecue Pulled Pork Sub	6-inch sub	440	31	13	54	50	4	1300	70
BBQ Rib Patty Sub	6-inch sub	420	20	19	47	43	4	820	50
Buffalo Chicken Sub	6-inch sub	400	25	15	45	41	4	1420	50
Cheddar Cheese	for 6-inch sub	60	4	5	0	0	0	95	15
Chicken Bacon Ranch Wrap (Atkins® - Friendly)	1 wrap	480	40	27	19	8	11	1340	90
Chicken Pizziola Sub	6-inch sub	450	31	16	48	43	5	1530	80
Chipotle Southwest Steak & Cheese Sub	6-inch sub	440	24	19	49	44	5	1160	45
Cold Cut Trio Sub	6-inch sub	440	21	21	47	43	4	1680	55
Dijon Horseradish Melt Sub	6-inch sub	470	26	21	48	43	5	1620	55
Double Meat Chicken Sub	6-inch sub	430	38	8	50	45	5	1500	90
Double Meat Cold Cut Trio Sub	6-inch sub	580	31	32	49	45	4	2540	100
Double Meat Ham Sub	6-inch sub	350	28	7	47	43	4	2030	50
Double Meat Italian BMT® Sub	6-inch sub	670	34	38	49	45	4	2980	100
Double Meat Meatball Sub	6-inch sub	780	35	41	61	56	5	1760	85
Double Meat Roast Beef Sub	6-inch sub	360	29	7	46	42	4	1310	40
Double Meat Steak & Cheese Sub	6-inch sub	480	37	17	51	45	6	1580	65
Double Meat Subway Club® Sub	6-inch sub	410	39	8	50	46	4	2010	60
Double Meat Subway Melt® Sub	6-inch sub	520	39	20	50	46	4	2620	80
Double Meat Subway Seafood & Crab® Sub	6-inch sub	520	20	24	60	55	5	1730	35
Double Meat Tuna Sub	6-inch sub	620	29	35	49	44	5	1540	75
Double Meat Turkey Breast & Ham Sub	6-inch sub	360	30	7	48	44	4	1930	45
Extreme Chipotle Southwest Steak & Cheese Sub	6-inch sub	530	37	22	46	40	6	1530	70
Extreme Dijon Horseradish Melt Sub	6-inch sub	540	36	23	50	45	5	2330	80
Extreme Red Wine Vinaigrette Club Sub	6-inch sub	450	39	9	55	51	4	2300	70
Extreme Sweet Onion Chicken Teriyaki Sub	6-inch sub	450	43	7	59	55	4	1400	100
Gardenburger® Sub	6-inch sub	390	19	7	66	57	9	960	5
Ham on Deli Round	1 deli round	210	11	4	35	32	3	770	10
Ham Sub	6-inch sub	290	18	5	46	42	4	1270	25

Description	Serving Size	Cal	Prot (g)	Fat (g)	Carbs (g)	Net Carb(g)	Fiber (g)	Sod (mg)	Chol (mg)
Hoisin Chicken Sub	6-inch sub	340	26	5	52	48	4	1000	50
Honey Mustard Ham Sub	6-inch sub	310	18	5	51	47	4	1260	25
Italian BMT® Sub	6-inch sub	480	23	24	47	43	4	1900	55
Lloyd's BBQ Chicken Sub	6-inch sub	330	16	6	52	47	5	1020	25
Meatball Sub	6-inch sub	540	23	26	53	48	5	1290	45
Mediterranean Chicken Sub	6-inch sub	470	29	19	48	43	5	1550	70
Pastrami Sub	6-inch sub	570	32	29	49	44	5	1890	50
Poblano Cheddar Turkey Sub	6-inch sub	310	22	7	46	42	4	850	30
Processed American Cheese	for 6-inch sub	40	2	4	1	1	0	200	10
Provolone Cheese	for 6-inch sub	50	4	4	0	0	0	125	10
Red Wine Vinaigrette Club Sub	6-inch sub	350	24	6	53	49	4	1520	35
Roast Beef on Deli Round	1 deli round	220	13	5	35	32	3	660	15
Roast Beef Sub	6-inch sub	290	19	5	45	41	4	910	20
Roasted Chicken Breast Sub	6-inch sub	330	24	5	47	43	4	1010	47
Savory Chicken Caesar Sub	6-inch sub	490	28	23	46	42	4	1150	70
Seafood & Crab® Sub	6-inch sub	410	16	17	53	48	5	1280	25
Spicey Italian Sub	6-inch sub	480	21	25	46	42	4	1660	55
Steak & Cheese Sub	6-inch sub	390	24	14	48	43	5	1200	35
Subway Club® Sub	6-inch sub	320	24	6	46	42	4	1300	35
Subway Melt Sub	6-inch sub	410	25	15	47	43	4	1720	45
Sweet Onion Chicken Teriyaki Sub	6-inch sub	370	26	5	59	55	4	1090	50
Swiss Cheese	for 6-inch sub	50	4	5	0	0	0	30	15
Thai Sesame Chicken Sub	6-inch sub	370	26	10	48	44	4	1050	55
Tuna on Deli Round	1 deli round	330	13	16	36	33	3	830	25
Tuna Sub	6-inch sub	460	20	23	47	43	4	1190	45
Turkey Bacon Melt Wrap (Atkins® - Friendly)	1 wrap	430	32	25	22	10	12	1650	65
Turkey Breast & Ham Sub	6-inch sub	290	20	5	46	42	4	1220	25
Turkey Breast on Deli Round	1 deli round	220	13	4	36	33	3	730	15
Turkey Breast Sub	6-inch sub	280	18	5	46	42	4	1010	20
Veggie Delite® Sub	6-inch sub	230	9	3	44	40	4	510	0
Veggi-Max Sub	6-inch sub	390	24	8	56	49	7	1030	10
BREAKFAST ITEMS									
Cheese & Egg (Breakfast Sandwich)	6-inch sub	440	27	19	42	39	3	730	570
Cheese & Egg (Breakfast Sandwich)	1 deli round	320	14	15	34	31	3	550	185
Cheese & Egg Omelet	1 omelet	240	19	17	2	2	0	370	570
French Toast w/ Syrup	1 order	350	14	8	57	55	2	350	280
Ham & Egg (Breakfast Sandwich)	6-inch sub	430	29	17	42	39	3	900	575

Description	Serving Size	Cal	Prot (g)	Fat (g)	Carbs (g)	Net Carb(g)	Fiber (g)	Sod (mg)	Chol (mg)
SUBWAY (continued)									
Ham & Egg (Breakfast Sandwich) on Deli Round	1 deli round	310	16	13	34	31	3	720	190
Ham & Egg Omelet	1 omelet	230	21	14	2	2	0	550	575
Steak & Egg (Breakfast Sandwich)	6-inch sub	460	33	18	43	39	4	750	575
Steak & Egg (Breakfast Sandwich) on Deli Round	1 deli round	330	19	14	35	32	3	570	190
Steak & Egg Omelet	1 omelet	250	24	15	3	2	1	390	580
Vegetable & Egg (Breakfast Sandwich)	6-inch sub	410	25	16	44	40	4	610	560
Vegetable & Egg (Breakfast Sandwich)	1 deli round	290	12	12	36	33	3	430	175
Vegetable & Egg Omelet	1 omelet	210	17	14	4	3	1	250	560
Western & Egg Omelet	1 omelet	220	19	14	4	3	1	360	565
Western Egg (Breakfast Sandwich)	6-inch sub	430	27	17	44	40	4	710	565
Western Egg (Breakfast Sandwich) on Deli Round		300	14	12	36	33	3	530	180
Bacon & Egg (Breakfast Sandwich)	6-inch sub	450	28	19	42	39	3	700	570
Bacon & Egg (Breakfast Sandwich) on Deli Round	1 deli round	320	15	15	34	31	3	520	185
Bacon & Egg Omelet	1 omelet	240	20	17	2	2	0	350	570
SALADS									
Cold Cut Trio Salad	1 salad	230	14	15	12	9	3	1370	55
Ham Salad	1 salad	110	11	3	11	8	3	1070	25
Italian BMT® Salad	1 salad	280	16	19	12	9	3	1590	55
Meatball Salad	1 salad	330	16	20	18	15	3	980	45
Roast Beef Salad	1 salad	120	12	3	10	7	3	720	20
Roasted Chicken Breast Salad	1 salad	150	16	3	12	9	3	810	45
Seafood & Crab® Salad	1 salad	200	9	11	17	13	4	970	25
Steak & Cheese Salad	1 salad	180	17	8	13	9	4	890	35
Subway Club® Salad	1 salad	150	17	4	12	9	3	1110	35
Subway Melt Salad	1 salad	200	18	10	12	9	3	1410	45
Tuna Salad	1 salad	250	13	17	12	9	3	870	45
Turkey Breast & Ham Salad	1 salad	120	13	3	11	8	3	1030	25
Turkey Breast Salad	1 salad	100	11	2	11	8	3	820	20
Veggie Delite® Salad	1 salad	50	2	1	9	6	3	310	0
SOUPS									
Cream of Broccoli Soup	1 serving	130	5	6	15	13	2	860	10
Cream of Potato with Bacon Soup	1 serving	210	5	12	20	16	4	970	20
Cheese with Ham and Bacon Soup	1 serving	230	8	16	13	11	2	1270	20

Description	Serving Size	Cal	Prot (g)	Fat (g)	Carbs (g)	Net Carb(g)	Fiber (g)	Sod (mg)	Chol (mg)
Chili Con Carne Soup	1 serving	310	17	14	28	19	9	900	35
Chicken and Dumpling Soup	1 serving	130	7	5	16	15	1	1030	30
Golden Broccoli Cheese Soup	1 serving	180	6	12	12	3	9	910	10
Minestrone Soup	1 serving	70	3	1	11	9	2	1080	5
New England Style Clam Chowder	1 serving	140	5	5	19	12	7	900	15
Roasted Chicken Noodle Soup	1 serving	90	7	4	7	6	1	1180	20
Vegetable Beef Soup	1 serving	90	5	2	14	12	2	1340	10
Vegetarian Vegetable Soup	1 serving	80	2	1	17	14	3	1130	0

DESSERTS

Description	Serving Size	Cal	Prot (g)	Fat (g)	Carbs (g)	Net Carb(g)	Fiber (g)	Sod (mg)	Chol (mg)
Apple Pie	1 slice	245	0	10	37	36	1	290	0
Chocolate Chip Cookie	1 cookie	210	2	10	30	29	1	160	15
Chocolate Chunk Cookie	1 cookie	220	2	10	30	29	1	105	10
Fruit Roll Up	1 roll up	50	0	1	12	12	0	55	0
Double Chocolate Chip Cookie	1 cookie	210	2	10	30	29	1	170	15
M & M Cookie	1 cookie	210	2	10	30	29	1	105	15
Oatmeal Raisin Cookie	1 cookie	200	3	8	30	28	2	170	15
Peanut Butter Cookie	1 cookie	220	4	12	26	25	1	200	10
Sugar Cookie	1 cookie	230	2	12	28	28	0	135	15
White Macadamia Nut Cookie	1 cookie	220	2	11	28	27	1	160	15

DRESSINGS/ SAUCES

Description	Serving Size	Cal	Prot (g)	Fat (g)	Carbs (g)	Net Carb(g)	Fiber (g)	Sod (mg)	Chol (mg)
Chipotle Southwest Sauce	for 6-inch sub	90	0	9	2	2	0	220	10
Dijon Horseradish Sauce	for 6-inch sub	90	0	10	1	1	0	160	10
Fat Free French Dressing	1 packet	70	0	0	17	17	0	390	0
Fat Free Honey Mustard Sauce	for 6-inch sub	30	0	0	7	7	0	140	0
Fat Free Italian Dressing	1 packet	20	0	0	4	4	0	610	0
Fat Free Ranch Dressing	1 packet	60	0	0	14	14	0	530	0
Fat Free Red Wine Vinaigrette Sauce	for 6-inch sub	30	0	0	6	6	0	340	0
Fat Free Sweet Onion Sauce	for 6-inch sub	40	0	0	9	9	0	100	0

Wendy's®

SALADS

Description	Serving Size	Cal	Prot (g)	Fat (g)	Carbs (g)	Net Carb(g)	Fiber (g)	Sod (mg)	Chol (mg)
Mandarin Chicken Salad	1 salad	190	22	3	17	14	3	740	50
Spring Mix Salad	1 salad	180	11	11	12	7	5	230	30
Chicken BLT Salad	1 salad	360	34	19	10	10		1140	95
Taco Supremo Salad	1 salad	360	27	16	29	21	8	1090	65
Homestyle Chicken Strips Salad	1 salad	450	29	22	34	29	5	1190	70

Description	Serving Size	Cal	Prot (g)	Fat (g)	Carbs (g)	Net Carb(g)	Fiber (g)	Sod (mg)	Chol (mg)
WENDY'S® (continued)									
Side Salad	1 salad	35	2	0	7	4	3	20	0
Caesar Side Salad	1 salad	70	6	5	2	1	1	190	10
SALAD DRESSINGS									
Caesar Dressing	1 packet	150	1	16	1	1	0	240	20
Creamy Ranch Dressing	1 packet	230	1	23	5	5	0	580	15
Fat Free French Style	1 packet	80	0	0	19	19	0	210	0
Honey Mustard Dressing	1 packet	280	1	26	11	11	0	350	25
House Vinaigrette Dressing	1 packet	190	0	18	8	8	0	750	0
Reduced Fat Creamy Ranch	1 packet	100	1	8	6	5	1	550	15
Low Fat Honey Mustard	1 packet	110	0	3	21	21	0	340	0
Oriental Sesame Dressing	1 packet	250	1	19	19	19	0	560	0
FROSTY									
Small	12 oz cup	330	8	8	56	56	0	150	35
HOMESTYLE CHICKEN STRIPS/NUGGETS									
Homestyle Chicken Strips	3 strips	410	28	18	33	33	0	1470	60
Chicken Nuggets (kid's meal)	4 pieces	180	8	11	10	10	0	390	25
Chicken Nuggets	5 pieces	220	10	14	13	13	0	490	35
SIDE SELECTIONS									
Baked Potato - Plain	1 potato	270	7	0	61	54	7	25	0
Sour Cream & Chives Potato	1 potato	340	8	6	62	55	7	40	15
Broccoli & Cheese Potato	1 potato	440	10	15	70	61	9	540	10
Bacon & Cheese Potato	1 potato	560	16	25	67	60	7	910	35
Chili	Small	200	17	5	21	16	5	870	35
Fries	Medium	390	4	17	56	50	6	340	0
Fries	Biggie	440	5	19	63	56	7	380	0
Fries	Great Biggie	530	6	23	75	67	8	450	0
Jr. Hamburger	1 sandwich	270	15	9	34	32	2	610	30
Jr. Cheeseburger	1 sandwich	310	17	12	34	32	2	820	45
Jr. Cheeseburger Deluxe	1 sandwich	350	18	15	36	36		880	45
Jr. Bacon Cheeseburger	1 sandwich	380	20	19	34	32	2	830	55
Hamburger	1 kid's meal	270	15	9	33	32	1	610	30
Cheeseburger	1 kid's meal	310	17	12	33	32	1	820	45
Classic Single® w/ Everything	1 sandwich	410	25	19	37	35	2	910	70
Big Bacon Classic	1 sandwich	580	33	29	45	42	3	1430	95
Ultimate Chicken Grill Sandwich	1 sandwich	360	31	7	44	42	2	1100	75

Description	Serving Size	Cal	Prot (g)	Fat (g)	Carbs (g)	Net Carb(g)	Fiber (g)	Sod (mg)	Chol (mg)
Spicy Chicken Fillet Sandwich	1 sandwich	510	29	19	57	55	2	1480	55
Homestyle Chicken Fillet Sandwich	1 sandwich	540	29	22	57	55	2	1320	55
CONDIMENTS									
Deli Honey Mustard Sauce	1 packet	170	0	16	6	6	0	190	15
Spicy Southwest Chipotle Sauce	1 packet	140	0	13	5	5	0	170	20
Heartland Ranch Sauce	1 packet	200	0	21	1	1	0	280	20
Barbecue Sauce	1 packet	40	1	0	10	10	0	160	0
Sweet & Sour Sauce	1 packet	45	0	0	12	12	0	120	0
Honey Mustard Sauce	1 packet	130	0	12	6	6	0	220	10